U•X•L Encyclopedia of Diseases and Disorders

U•X•L Encyclopedia of Diseases and Disorders

VOLUME 3: H-L

Rebecca J. Frey
Larry I. Lutwick, Editor

U·X·L
A part of Gale, Cengage Learning

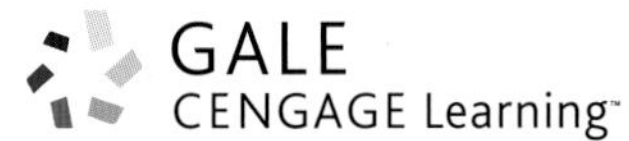

Detroit • New York • San Francisco • New Haven, Conn • Waterville, Maine • London

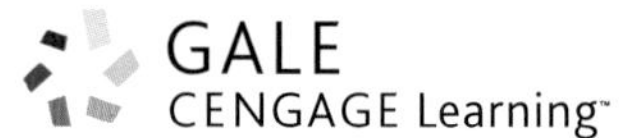

U•X•L Encyclopedia of Diseases and Disorders

Rebecca J. Frey, Author
Larry I. Lutwick, Editor

Project Editor: Kristine Krapp

Editorial: Debra Kirby, Kathleen Edgar, Elizabeth Manar, Kimberley McGrath

Rights Acquisition and Management: Robyn Young

Composition: Evi Abou-El-Seoud, Mary Beth Trimper

Manufacturing: Rita Wimberley

Product Manager: Julia Furtaw

Art Director: Jennifer Wahi

Product Design: CMB Design Partners

For product information and technology assistance, contact us at
Gale Customer Support, 1-800-877-4253.
For permission to use material from this text or product,
submit all requests online at **www.cengage.com/permissions.**
Further permissions questions can be e-mailed to
permissionrequest@cengage.com

Cover photographs: Images courtesy of Dreamstime and Getty.

LIBRARY OF CONGRESS CATALOGING-IN-PUBLICATION DATA

Frey, Rebecca J.
UXL encyclopedia of diseases and disorders / Rebecca J. Frey, author ; Larry I. Lutwick, editor.
p. cm. –
Includes bibliographical references and index.
ISBN 978-1-4144-3065-2 (set : hardcover) – ISBN 978-1-4144-3066-9 (v. 1 : hardcover) – ISBN 978-1-4144-3067-6 (v. 2 : hardcover) – ISBN 978-1-4144-3068-3 (v. 3 : hardcover) – ISBN 978-1-4144-3069-0 (v. 4 : hardcover) – ISBN 978-1-4144-3070-6 (v. 5 : hardcover)
1. Diseases–Encyclopedias. I. Lutwick, Larry I. II. Title. III. Title: Encyclopedia of diseases and disorders.

RB155.5.F74 2009
616.003–dc22 2008047947

Gale
27500 Drake Rd.
Farmington Hills, MI, 48331-3535

ISBN-13: 978-1-4144-3065-2 (set) ISBN-10: 1-4144-3065-5 (set)
ISBN-13: 978-1-4144-3066-9 (vol. 1) ISBN-10: 1-4144-3066-3 (vol. 1)
ISBN-13: 978-1-4144-3067-6 (vol. 2) ISBN-10: 1-4144-3067-1 (vol. 2)
ISBN-13: 978-1-4144-3068-3 (vol. 3) ISBN-10: 1-4144-3068-X (vol. 3)
ISBN-13: 978-1-4144-3069-0 (vol. 4) ISBN-10: 1-4144-3069-8 (vol. 4)
ISBN-13: 978-1-4144-3070-6 (vol. 5) ISBN-10: 1-4144-3070-1 (vol. 5)

This title is also available as an e-book.
ISBN-13: 978-1-4144-3074-4 (set) ISBN-10: 1-4144-3074-4 (set)
Contact your Gale sales representative for ordering information.

Printed in China
1 2 3 4 5 6 7 13 12 11 10 09

Table of Contents

VOLUME 2

VOLUME 3

VOLUME 5

List of Entries by Type of Disease

Please Read—Important Information

The *U•X•L Encyclopedia of Diseases and Disorders* is a medical reference product designed to inform and educate readers about a wide variety of health issues related to diseases and injuries. Cengage Gale believes the product to be comprehensive, but not necessarily definitive. It is intended to supplement, not replace, consultation with a physician or other healthcare professional. While Cengage Gale has made substantial efforts to provide information that is accurate, comprehensive, and up-to-date, Cengage Gale makes no representations or warranties of any kind, including with limitation, warranties of merchantability or fitness for a particular purpose, nor does it guarantee the accuracy, comprehensiveness, or timeliness of the information contained in this product. Readers should be aware that the universe of medical knowledge is constantly growing and changing, and that differences of medical opinion exist among authorities. They are also advised to seek professional diagnosis and treatment for any medical condition, and to discuss information obtained from this book with their healthcare provider.

Preface

"Only the curious will learn and only the resolute overcome the obstacles to learning. The quest quotient has always excited me more than the intelligence quotient." - Eugene S. Wilson (1968)

Eugene "Bill" Wilson (1900–1981) was Dean of Admission at Amherst College. He was known for his sense of humor and his genuine interest in the welfare of each student. This quote attributed to him, published in *Reader's Digest* in April of 1968, summarizes education to me, that is, it is learning itself that is most exciting, not the knowledge per se that one gathers from it. It is truly the lifelong ride of learning, not the final destination, that makes us what we are.

As both a college and medical student and now as a medical educator, I have personally seen numerous, and far too many, individuals whose goal is not learning for learning sake but rather come to me, my brilliant lecturer-wife Suzanne, or any other instructor with the unfortunately all-to-common request of "what do I have to know to pass the exam?"

Would you consult a physician who only knows what he needed to pass the test? Would you hire a tax preparer that could pass the qualifying exam but knew no more? Would you allow your child to drive an automobile with only the knowledge acquired in the Driver's Education manual? The answer to all these questions should be a resounding no.

Whether or not you are using this reference text because you are thinking about, or even planning, a career in a medical field, remember that books such as this one are limited in scope. That is, the information here should be a starting place for anyone who has the true desire to understand the topic. Each entry includes further references for some additional reading, and you are encouraged to follow up on the topic. Additionally, remember that textbooks provide a snapshot of the information available at that time. The half-life of truth can be short because new information appears. Currency, that is, being current, is vital in understanding issues.

As the editor of this text, I wish each of its readers success in your future plans. "Earning a living," so to speak, implies working to live. I hope that you will have the opportunity, as I do, to truly live to work. A career can more than a job, more than just a way of paying the bills. By living to work, the work is not really work in the true sense but rather it is what you do, it is part of your essence. As it is said, "Those who love their jobs do not work a day in their lives."

Remember life is all about the ride, not the destination. Those who feel that "he who dies with the most toys wins" have missed all the scenery. Keep your eyes wide open.

Larry I. Lutwick, editor

Reader's Guide

The *U*X*L Encyclopedia of Diseases and Disorders* is devoted to helping younger students and general readers understand the nature of diseases and disorders of every type, including communicable diseases, genetic disorders, common conditions, and injuries.

This book is a collection of more than 200 entries on diseases, from avian flu, to cystic fibrosis, to warts. The entries start with a definition section and highlight the basic facts of the disease to explain the causes, symptoms, and treatments. Other sections give a more detailed description, talk about demographics, and discuss the future of the disease, for example, if any new treatments are under development or if the disease is becoming more or less prevalent.

The *U*X*L Encyclopedia of Diseases and Disorders* uses everyday language when possible, and explains medical terms as they arise. Terms are also defined in Words to Know sidebars within entries, and a collected Words to Know section is included in the beginning of each book. Entries are designed to instruct, challenge, and excite less-experienced students, while providing a solid foundation and reference for students already captivated by medicine.

Essential features of U*X*L Encyclopedia of Diseases and Disorders

This book contains 192 main entries and 18 overview entries. Overview entries are short descriptions of a group of disorders, like learning disorders. Each overview entry points the reader to specific entries that are part of that group. All articles in the book are meant to be understandable by anyone with a curiosity about diseases.

Entries are arranged alphabetically throughout the volumes. *See also* references at the end of entries alert the readers to related entries across the three-volume set that may provide additional resources or insights each topic.

A *List of Entries by Disease Type* section allows readers to quickly identify diseases by types, such as infectious or genetic. Each entry contains a *Words to Know* section to help students understand important or complex terms. A general compendium of these terms is also included in the book.

A *Where To Learn More* section lists helpful print material and Web sites, while a comprehensive *General Index* guides the reader to topics and terms mentioned in the book.

Photos and color illustrations are included throughout the book where they might stimulate interest or understanding.

Advisors and Contributors

While compiling this volume, the editors relied on the expertise and contributions of Rebecca J. Frey, medical writer. Frey is a freelance writer and editor who has contributed to Gale/Cengage health and medical publications since 1997. A member of the American Medical Writers Association, she completed her B.A. at Mount Holyoke College and her Ph.D. at Yale University. She lives in New Haven, Connecticut.

The editor would like to thank his contacts at Gale, Kristine Krapp and Debra Kirby, for their invaluable assistance in the technical aspects of putting this collection together. Personally, he is indebted to his wife Suzanne for her love and encouragement during this project and to their children Rachel, Zachary, Arielle, and Nina for setting such examples of how to pursue goals in life based on happiness potential, not financial reward. To their grandchildren Talora and Zev, they hope that the information in this collection serves to spark intellectual curiosity so you two will follow your hearts and minds in making this a better world.

Larry I. Lutwick, editor
Brooklyn, New York
December 2008

Larry I. Lutwick MD is an academically trained Infectious Diseases physician who is Director of the Infectious Disease Section at the Brooklyn Campus of the Veterans Affairs New York Harbor Health Care

System. He is also Professor of Medicine at the State University of New York, Downstate Medical School, also in Brooklyn, New York. Dr. Lutwick has authored or coauthored more than 100 scientific papers, 26 book chapters, and is the editor of several books, including (along with his wife Suzanne) *Beyond Anthrax: The Weaponization of Infectious Diseases*. He is also the creator of the medical educational tool, "Bug of the Month," in which the protagonist, a politically incorrect Infectious Disease physician named Dr. Schmeckman, solves medical mysteries.

Words to Know

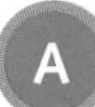

Abscess: A collection of pus that has formed in a body cavity or hollow.

Abstinence: 1.) Complete stopping of alcohol consumption. 2.) Not having sexual intercourse with anyone.

Acclimation: The process of adjusting to seasonal climate changes or to a new climate.

Accommodation: The medical term for the eye's ability to change its focus automatically for viewing objects at different distances.

Acetaldehyde: A colorless liquid chemical that is produced when the body begins to digest alcohol. A chemical that causes hangovers after heavy drinking, it also contributes to fetal alcohol syndrome.

Achilles tendon: The tendon that connects the calf muscle to the back of the heel. Tendinitis in the Achilles tendon is common in sports that involve running and jumping.

Acromegaly: A condition in which a person's body produces too much growth hormone in adult life.

Actinic keratosis: A patch of thickened or scaly skin caused by sun exposure. It is not itself a form of skin cancer but may develop progressively into a skin cancer.

Acupuncture: A form of alternative medicine in which very fine needles are inserted into the skin at specific points on the body for pain relief.

Acute: Referring to a disease or symptom that is severe or quickly worsens.

Addiction: A chronic disease characterized by compulsive drug use and by long-lasting chemical changes in the brain.

Adipose tissue: Fatty tissue.

Adrenaline: A hormone that can be used in medicine to open the breathing passages in patients with severe tissue swelling. It is also called epinephrine.

Affective disorder: A type of mental disorder characterized by disturbed emotions and feelings rather than problems with memory, thinking, or learning.

After drop: A term that doctors use to refer to lowering of the body's core temperature that continues while the person is being rewarmed.

Against-the-rule astigmatism: A type of astigmatism in which the eye sees horizontal lines more clearly than vertical lines.

Agoraphobia: An irrational fear of venturing outside the home or into open spaces, so strong that a large number of activities outside the home are limited or avoided altogether. Agoraphobia is often associated with panic attacks.

Allergen: A substance that causes an allergic reaction in individuals who are sensitive to it.

Alveoli (singular, alveolus): Tiny air sacs in the lungs where carbon dioxide in the blood is exchanged for oxygen from the air.

Amaranth: An herb that produces seeds used as grain in India, Nepal, Mexico, and parts of South America.

Amblyopia: Dimness of sight in one eye without any change in the structure of the eye. It is also known as lazy eye.

Amenorrhea: Stopping of normal menstrual periods.

Amino acids: A group of twenty compounds that are the building blocks of proteins in humans and other animals.

Ammonia: A chemical produced during the breakdown of protein in the body. It is usually converted in the liver to another chemical called urea and then discharged from the body in the urine.

Amputation: Surgical removal of a limb.

Anabolic: Referring to tissue building. Anabolic steroids build up muscle and bone tissue.

Anaerobic: Capable of living in the absence of oxygen.

Anaphylaxis: A severe allergic reaction to a trigger (most commonly a food, medication, insect sting, or latex) that involves most major body systems.

Androgen: The generic term for the group of male sex hormones produced by the body.

Anemia: A condition in which a person's blood does not have enough volume, enough red blood cells, or enough hemoglobin in the cells to keep body tissues supplied with oxygen.

Aneurysm: A weak or thin spot on the wall of an artery.

Angina: Chest pain caused by an inadequate supply of blood to the heart muscle.

Angioedema: The medical term for the swelling of tissues can be part of an allergic reaction.

Antibody: A protein found in blood that is specific to a particular foreign substance, which may be an allergen or a disease organism. The antibody identifies that antigen and neutralizes it.

Anticipation: A condition in which the symptoms of a genetic disorder appear earlier and earlier in each successive generation.

Antidepressant: A type of drug given to treat eating disorders as well as mood disorders like anxiety and depression.

Antiemetic: A type of drug given to control nausea and vomiting.

Anti-psychotics: A group of drugs used to treat schizophrenia. The older anti-psychotic drugs are also called neuroleptics.

Antispasmodic: A type of drug given to relieve the cramping of the intestines or other muscles.

Aorta: The large artery that carries blood away from the heart to be distributed to the rest of the body.

Aortic dissection: A tear in the wall of the aorta that allows blood to seep between the layers of tissue that form the artery and push the layers apart.

Aphthous ulcer: The medical term for canker sore.

Apnea: Temporary stopping of breathing.

Appendectomy: Surgical removal of the appendix.

Arboviruses: A family of viruses spread by blood-sucking insects.

Area postrema: The part of the brain stem that controls vomiting.

Arson: The intentional setting of a fire in a building or other property. Arson is a criminal act in the United States.

Arthroscopy: The use of a small device called an arthroscope to look inside and diagnose or treat an arthritic joint.

Aseptic meningitis: A term that is sometimes used for meningitis that is not caused by bacteria.

Aspie: An informal name for a person with Asperger syndrome.

Aspiration: The entry of food, liquids, or other foreign substances into the lungs during the breathing process.

Astigmatism: A vision problem caused by irregularities in the shape of the cornea or the lens of the eye.

Asymptomatic: Having no symptoms.

Atherosclerosis: Stiffening or hardening of the arteries caused by the formation of plaques within the arteries.

Atopic disease: Any allergic disease that affects parts of the body that are not in direct contact with the allergen. Asthma, eczema, and hay fever are all atopic diseases.

Atopy: The medical term for an allergic hypersensitivity that affects parts of the body that are not in direct contact with an allergen. Hay fever, eczema, and asthma are all atopic diseases.

Atrium (plural, atria): One of the two upper chambers of the heart.

Audiologist: A health care professional who is specially trained to evaluate hearing disorders.

Auditory: Pertaining to the sense of hearing.

Aura: A symptom that precedes migraine headaches in some people. The person may see flashing or zigzag lights, or have other visual disturbances.

Autism: A developmental disorder that appears by three years of age and is characterized by limited communication skills, difficulties in communicating with others, and difficulties forming relationships.

Autoantibody: An antibody formed in reaction against the tissues of the individual producing it.

Autoimmune disease: A disease in which the body's immune system attacks its own cells and tissues.

Autoimmune disorder: A disorder characterized or caused by autoantibodies that attack the cells or organs of the organism producing them.

Automatic behavior: Activity that a person with narcolepsy can carry out while partially awake but is not conscious of at the time and cannot recall afterward.

Autopsy: The examination of a body after death to determine the cause of death.

Avian: Pertaining to birds.

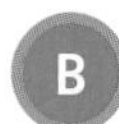

B

B cell: A type of white blood cell produced in the bone marrow that makes antibodies against viruses.

Babesiosis: A malaria-like disease that can be transmitted by ticks.

Baby blues: An informal term for the temporary sad feelings some mothers feel for a week or so after childbirth. It is less serious than postpartum depression and usually goes away by itself.

Bacteremia: The presence of bacteria in the bloodstream.

Bedsore: A type of wet gangrene that develops when a bedridden person cannot turn over to relieve pressure on soft tissue caused by the weight of the body. Bedsores are sometimes called pressure ulcers.

Benign: Not cancerous.

Benign prostatic hypertrophy (BPH): A noncancerous condition in which the swelling of the prostate gland squeezes the urethra and causes difficulty in urination.

Beta blockers: A group of drugs given to treat abnormal heart rhythms and reduce the risk of aortic dilation in MFS patients.

Bile: A yellow-green fluid secreted by the liver that aids in the digestion of fats.

Binge: An episode of eating in which a person consumes a larger amount of food within a limited period of time than most people would eat in similar circumstances.

Binge drinking: A period of heavy drinking that lasts for two days or longer.

Biofeedback: An alternative treatment for headaches (and other conditions) that consists of teaching patients to consciously control their blood pressure, muscle tension, temperature, and other body processes.

Biological therapy: An approach to cancer treatment that is intended to strengthen the patient's own immune system rather than attack the cancer cells directly.

Biomarker: A substance produced by the body that is distinctive to a particular disease and can be used to identify its presence or track its progress.

Bioterrorism: The use of disease agents to frighten or attack civilians.

Biphasic reaction: A recurrence of the symptoms of anaphylaxis about six to eight hours after the first episode.

Blackout: Alcohol-related memory loss.

Bladder: A hollow organ in the lower abdomen that collects urine from the kidneys and stores it prior to urination.

Blunt: A cigar that has been cut open and refilled with marijuana.

Body mass index: BMI. An indirect measurement of the amount of body fat. The BMI of adults is calculated in English measurements by multiplying a person's weight in pounds by 703.1, and dividing that number by the person's height in inches squared.

Bone marrow: The soft spongy tissue inside the long bones of the body where blood cells are formed.

Bong: A water pipe used to smoke marijuana.

Botulism: A rare but potentially fatal paralytic illness caused by a bacterial toxin in contaminated food.

Brain stem: The lowest part of the brain that connects directly to the spinal cord. It controls such basic life functions as breathing, blood pressure, and heart beat.

Bronchiole: A very small thin-walled air passage in the lungs that branches off from a bronchus.

Bronchodilator: A type of drug that opens up the bronchi, increasing airflow and relieving wheezing and other asthma symptoms.

Bronchoscope: A flexible lighted tube that can be inserted into the passages leading to the lungs for examination or treatment.

Bronchus (plural, bronchi): One of the two major divisions of the airway that lead into the right and left lungs.

Bubo: A swollen lymph node in the neck, armpit, or groin area.

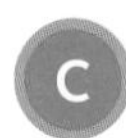

Café-au-lait spots: Brownish-white birthmarks that appear as part of a nervous system disorder that can cause scoliosis in some children. Café au lait is the French expression for "coffee with milk" and describes the color of the spots.

Capsule: The outermost layer of the lens of the eye.

Carcinoma: The medical term for any type of cancer that arises from the skin or from the tissues that line body cavities.

Carcinoma in situ: A cancer that has not spread or is still in one location in the body.

Cardiac arrest: Heart attack; a condition in which the circulation of the blood stops abruptly because the heart stops beating.

Carditis: Inflammation of the heart.

Caries: The medical name for tooth cavities.

Carrier: A person who is infected with a disease and can spread it to others but who has no symptoms of the disease.

Cartilage: A type of dense connective tissue that serves to cushion bones within joints.

Case management: An approach to healthcare based on personalized services to patients.

Cataplexy: Sudden loss of tone in the voluntary muscles.

Catatonia: A condition in which a person sits motionless for long periods of time and does not respond to others.

Catheter: A thin tube inserted into the urethra to drain urine from the bladder.

Cerebellum: The part of the brain at the lower back of the head just above the brain stem.

Cerebral cortex: The part of the brain that controls thinking, memory, paying attention, decision making, and using language.

Cervix: The neck or lowermost part of a woman's uterus that opens into the vagina.

Chancre: A painless ulcer that forms on the skin during the early stage of syphilis.

Chelation therapy: A form of treatment to reduce overly high levels of iron (or other metals) in the body by giving the patient a chemical that allows the body to get rid of the excess metal in urine or stool.

Chiropractic: A form of alternative medicine that treats disorders of the joints and muscles by adjusting the patient's spine or other joints.

Chlamydia: A sexually transmitted disease caused by a bacterium that is a common cause of eye infections.

Cholesterol: A fatty substance produced naturally by the body that is found in the membranes of all body cells and is carried by the blood.

Chorea: A general term for movement disorders marked by loss of coordination and involuntary motions of the head and limbs.

Chorionic villus sampling (CVS): A prenatal test that involves taking a small sample of the placenta, the organ that forms inside the uterus during pregnancy and supplies the baby with oxygen and nutrients carried by the blood.

Chronic: Referring to a disease or symptom that goes on for a long time, tends to recur, and usually gets worse slowly.

Circadian rhythm: The medical name for the daily sleep/wake cycle in humans.

Cirrhosis: Disruption of normal liver function by the formation of scar tissue and nodules in the liver. It is most commonly caused by alcoholism or hepatitis C.

Clap: A slang term for gonorrhea.

Clinically isolated syndrome (CIS): A term applied to patients who have had one episode of illness that suggests they have a disease but do not yet meet the full criteria for diagnosis.

Closed-head injury: An injury to the head in which the skull is not broken or penetrated.

Clubbing: Thickening of the tips of the fingers or toes.

Coagulation cascade: The complex process in which platelets, coagulation factors, and other chemicals in the blood interact to form a clot when a blood vessel is injured.

Coagulation factors: Proteins in blood plasma involved in the chain of chemical reactions leading to the formation of blood clots. They are also called clotting factors.

Cochlea: A snail-shaped fluid-filled chamber in the inner ear.

Cognitive: Related to thinking, memory, and other conscious intellectual activities or processes.

Cognitive-behavioral therapy (CBT): An approach to therapy that aims at changing distorted thinking patterns, beliefs, and behaviors in order to change the patient's feelings.

Colon: The part of the large intestine that extends from the cecum to the rectum.

Colonization: The process by which bacteria form colonies in or on the bodies of humans and other animals.

Comedo (plural, comedones): The medical term for a whitehead or blackhead.

Community-acquired: Referring to a disease that a person gets in the course of ordinary activities rather than in a hospital or clinic.

Compression fracture: A fracture caused by the collapse of a vertebra in the spinal column, usually caused either by trauma or by weakening of the bone in osteoporosis.

Compulsion: A repeated behavior or mental act carried out to control or neutralize obsessions.

Conditioning: The process of becoming physically fit through a program of diet, exercise, and rest.

Congenital: Present at birth.

Congenital rubella syndrome (CRS): A group of birth defects that may affect a baby born to a mother who had rubella during the first three months of pregnancy.

Conjunctiva (plural, conjunctivae): The clear membrane that covers the white part of the eyeball and lines the eyelids.

Contact dermatitis: Inflammation of the skin caused by direct contact with an allergen or irritating substance, such as poison ivy, certain dyes, or certain metals.

Contracture: Shortening or tightening of the muscles surrounding certain joints that limits the movement of the joints.

Cooley's anemia: Another name for the most severe form of beta-thalassemia.

Coprolalia: The medical term for uncontrollable cursing or use of dirty words.

Cornea: The transparent front part of the eye where light enters the eye.

Cortex: The part of the lens underneath the capsule.

Cortisol: A hormone produced by the adrenal glands near the kidneys in response to stress.

Co-sleeping: Allowing a baby to sleep in the same bed as its parents. It is also called bed sharing.

Crabs: A slang term for pubic lice.

Cretinism: A form of hypothyroidism found in some newborns.

Cryotherapy: The use of extreme cold to destroy cancerous tumors or other diseased tissue. It is also called cryosurgery.

Cushing syndrome: A disorder caused by the excess secretion of cortisol by the pituitary gland.

Cutaneous: Pertaining to the skin.

Cyanosis: A blue discoloration of the lips, inside of the mouth, and nail beds caused by lack of oxygen in the blood vessels near the skin surface.

Cycling: Using steroids in periods of several weeks or months (a time cycle) separated by short rest phases of not using the drugs.

Cyclothymia: A mild form of bipolar disorder.

Cyst: A capsule or sac containing a parasite in its resting stage.

Cystitis: The medical term for an infection of the urinary bladder.

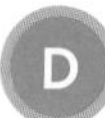

Dander: Tiny skin, feather, or fur particles from household pets that cause allergic reactions in some people.

Debridement: The medical term for the surgical removal of dead or damaged soft tissue.

Decibel (dB): A unit of measurement for expressing the relative intensity of sounds.

Decoding: In education, the ability to associate letters of the alphabet with sounds.

Degenerative disorder: A type of disorder in which a person gradually loses certain abilities that he or she had acquired at an earlier age.

Dehydration: Loss of water from the body. It may be caused by fever, vomiting, diarrhea, or excessive sweating.

Delirium: A suddenly developing mental disturbance characterized by confused thinking, difficulty focusing attention, and disorientation.

Delirium tremens: A severe physical reaction to withdrawal from alcohol in which the person hallucinates and has unstable blood pressure and breathing patterns.

Delusion: In medicine, a false belief that a person holds to despite evidence or proof that it is false.

Dementia: Loss of memory and other mental functions related to thinking or problem-solving.

Dengue: A tropical disease caused by a virus similar to the virus that causes West Nile infection. It is also spread by mosquitoes.

Dentin: A firm tissue that lies between the enamel and the pulp of a tooth.

Dermabrasion: Technique for making acne scars less noticeable by removing the top layer of skin with a rapidly rotating wire brush or a sandy material.

Dermatitis: The medical term for inflammation of the skin.

Dermatographism: A type of hives produced by scratching or stroking the skin.

Dermatologist: A doctor who specializes in diagnosing and treating diseases and disorders of the skin.

Dermatology: The branch of medicine that deals with skin problems and disorders.

Dermis: The lower layer of skin that contains blood vessels, sweat glands, and hair follicles.

Desensitization: A form of treatment for allergies that involves a series of shots containing the allergen to reduce the patient's sensitivity to that particular trigger. Desensitization is also called immunotherapy.

Detoxification: A process or treatment program for clearing an alcoholic's body of alcohol. It usually includes medications to help manage the physical symptoms of withdrawal.

Diagnosis of exclusion: A diagnosis that the doctor arrives at by ruling out other diseases one by one rather than making the diagnosis on the basis of laboratory tests or imaging studies, or other test results.

Dialysis: A process in which the blood of a patient with kidney failure is cleansed of the body's waste products by being pumped through a machine that filters the blood and then returns it to the body.

Diaphragm: A sheet of muscle extending across the bottom of the rib cage that separates the chest from the abdomen.

Diastolic blood pressure: The blood pressure when the heart is resting between beats.

Directly observed therapy (DOT): Treatment in which nurses or health care workers administer medications to patients in a clinic or doctor's office to make sure that the patients take the drugs correctly.

Disseminated gonococcal infection (DGI): A complication of gonorrhea in which the disease organisms get into the bloodstream and cause arthritis, eye disease, skin rashes, or inflammation of the heart valves.

Diuretic: A type of drug that increases the body's production of urine.

Dopamine: A chemical produced in the brain that is needed to produce smooth and controlled voluntary movements.

Dronabinol: A medication that contains synthetic THC, given to relieve nausea and improve appetite in AIDS and cancer patients.

Duodenum: The first part of the small intestine.

Dysthymia: A mood disorder characterized by a long-term low-key depression.

Dystrophin: A protein found in muscle whose absence or defectiveness is one of the causes of muscular dystrophy.

E

Echinacea: A plant native to the eastern United States that is thought by some to be a useful cold remedy. It is also known as purple coneflower.

Ectopic pregnancy: A pregnancy in which the fertilized egg starts growing outside the uterus, usually in the abdomen or in the tubes leading to the uterus.

Effusion: The medical term for an abnormal collection of fluid in a body cavity.

Ehrlichiosis: A tick-borne disease found primarily in dogs that can also be transmitted to humans.

Electroconvulsive therapy (ECT): A form of treatment for severe depression that consists of passing a low dose of electric current through the patient's brain under anesthesia.

Electrolytes: Minerals that are essential for proper body functioning. They include potassium, sodium, calcium, and magnesium.

Embolus: The medical term for a clot that forms in the heart and travels through the circulatory system to another part of the body.

Embryo: The medical term for an unborn baby from the time of conception to the end of its first eight weeks of life.

Emerging infectious disease (EID): A disease that has become more widespread around the world in the last twenty years and is expected to become more common in the future.

Enamel: The hard, smooth, white outer surface of a tooth.

Encephalitis: Inflammation of the brain.

Endemic: A term applied to a disease that maintains itself in a particular area without reinforcement from outside sources of infection.

Endocarditis: An inflammation of the tissues lining the inside of the heart and its valves.

Endocrine system: A system of small organs located throughout the body that regulate metabolism, growth and puberty, tissue function, and mood. The thyroid gland is part of the endocrine system.

Endocrinologist: A doctor who specializes in disorders of the pancreas and other glands.

Endophthalmitis: Inflammation of the tissues inside the eyeball.

Epidemiology: The branch of medicine that deals with the frequency, distribution, and control of disease in a population.

Epidermis: The outermost layer of the skin.

Eradication: The complete elimination of a disease.

Erythema chronicum migrans (EM): The medical name for the distinctive rash that is often seen in early-stage Lyme disease.

Esophagus: The muscular tube that carries food downward from the lower throat to the stomach.

Essential hypertension: High blood pressure that is not caused by medications, pregnancy, or another disease.

Estrogen: A female hormone produced in the ovaries.

Euphoria: An exaggerated feeling of well-being.

Eustachian tube: The passageway that connects the middle ear with the upper throat.

Eustress: A term that is sometimes used to refer to positive stress.

Euthanasia: Sometimes called mercy killing; the act of killing a hopelessly ill human or pet in a painless way.

Eversion injury: An ankle injury caused when the foot is suddenly forced to roll outward.

Exophthalmos: Abnormal protrusion of the eyeballs.

Exotoxin: A toxin secreted by a bacterium or other disease organism into the body tissues of an infected individual.

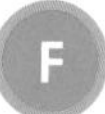

Failure to thrive: A term used to describe children whose present weight or rate of weight gain is markedly lower than that of other children of their age and sex.

Fascia: A sheet of connective tissue that covers and binds together the muscles, glands, blood vessels, and internal organs of the body.

Fasting hypoglycemia: A type of hypoglycemia in people without diabetes that is caused by hormone deficiencies, medication side effects, or tumors rather than by reaction to a sugar-rich meal.

Fatal familial insomnia (FFI): A very rare inherited disease in which the person dies of sleeplessness.

Fatigue: A feeling of weariness or tiredness after work, exercise, or emotional stress.

Female athlete triad: A group of three symptoms that often occur together in female athletes: amenorrhea, osteoporosis, and disordered eating.

Fibro fog: A term that has been coined to describe memory loss and difficulty concentrating in fibromyalgia patients.

Fibroblast: A type of cell that provides structure during the healing of a broken bone or other wound.

Fibrosis: The medical term for the formation of scar tissue.

Filaggrin: A protein in the skin that is defective or lacking in some patients with eczema.

Filovirus: The category of viruses that includes Ebola and Marburg viruses. Filoviruses look like long pieces of thread under a microscope.

Fistula: An abnormal tunnel or passage that forms between one part of the intestine and another or between the intestine and the body surface.

Fixation: The medical term for holding a broken bone in its correct position to speed healing and prevent further injury.

Flare: A return or worsening of symptoms.

Flashback: A temporary reliving of a traumatic event.

Folic acid: A form of vitamin B_9 that helps to prevent spina bifida.

Follicle: Small canal in the skin surrounding the root of a hair.

Forchheimer spots: Tiny reddish spots that appear inside the mouth of a patient with scarlet fever.

Fragility fracture: A fracture that occurs as a result of a fall from standing height or less. A person with healthy bones would not suffer a broken bone falling from a standing position.

Fulminant: Referring to any disease or condition that strikes rapidly and is severe to the point of being life-threatening.

Fundoplication: A surgical procedure in which the upper part of the stomach is wrapped around the lower end of the esophagus to prevent stomach acid from rising into the esophagus.

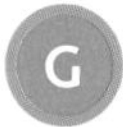

Gait: A person's characteristic pattern of walking.

Gangrene: Decay and death of soft tissue due to loss of blood supply.

Gastric: Related to the stomach.

Gastroenterologist: A doctor who specializes in diagnosing and treating diseases of the digestive system.

Gene therapy: An approach to treating disease by inserting healthy genes into a person's genetic material or by inactivating defective genes.

Genotype: The genetic makeup of a cell or organism.

Germ cell: A cell involved in reproduction. In humans the germ cells are the sperm (male) and egg (female). Unlike other cells in the body, germ cells contain only half the standard number of chromosomes.

Gestational: Pertaining to pregnancy.

Gestational age: An infant's age at birth counting from the date of the mother's last menstrual period.

Gigantism: Excessive production of growth hormone in children who are still growing.

Gingivitis: The medical term for inflammation of the gums.

Glial cells: Cells in brain tissue that hold nerve cells in place, supply them with oxygen and nutrients, and remove dead nerve cells.

Glioma: A type of brain tumor that starts in the glial cells.

Glucagon: A hormone secreted by the pancreas that raises blood sugar levels by signaling the liver to convert glycogen to glucose.

Glucometer: A small blood testing device that can be used to screen for diabetes or used at home to monitor blood sugar levels.

Gluten: A protein found in certain grains, particularly wheat, barley, and rye.

Glycogen: A form of glucose that is stored in the liver as an energy reserve.

Goiter: A swelling in the neck caused by an enlarged thyroid gland.

Gonococcus: The bacterium that causes gonorrhea.

Gout: A disorder of the large toe or other joints caused by deposits of uric acid crystals in the affected joint.

Group A streptococcus: A sphere-shaped bacterium that grows in long chains and causes strep throat as well as scarlet fever and some forms of tonsillitis.

Growth plate: A cartilage plate in the long bones of children where the lengthening of bone takes place.

Guarding: Stiffening of the muscles in response to a doctor's touch.

Gumma: A soft noncancerous growth of tissue found in patients with tertiary syphilis.

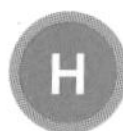

Hair cells: Special cells in the cochlea that convert the movement of the fluid inside the cochlea into electrical signals that travel to the brain via the auditory nerve.

Hallucination: Perceiving something that is not really there. Hallucinations can affect any of the five senses.

Hard palate: A thin bony plate located in the front portion of the roof of the mouth.

Hashish: A concentrated resin prepared from the flowering tops of hemp plants.

Hashitoxicosis: A temporary phase in some patients with Hashimoto disease in which there is too much thyroid hormone in the blood due to leakage from damaged and dying cells in the thyroid gland.

Heat illness: A general term for heat-related disorders, ranging from heat cramps (the mildest) to heat stroke (the most serious).

Heelstick: A method for taking a sample of blood from a newborn by pricking the baby's heel with a needle and collecting a drop or two of blood on special filter paper.

Hematocrit: The proportion of blood volume occupied by red blood cells.

Hematologist: A doctor who specializes in diagnosing and treating disorders of the blood.

Hemoglobin: An iron-containing protein in red blood cells that carries oxygen from the lungs to the rest of the body.

Hepatitis: A general term for inflammation of the liver. It can be caused by toxic substances or alcohol as well as infections.

Herpetiform: Resembling blisters caused by herpes.

Hiatal hernia: A condition in which the upper part of the stomach bulges upward into the chest cavity through a weak spot in the diaphragm.

Highly active antiretroviral therapy (HAART): An individualized combination of three or more antiretroviral drugs used to treat patients with HIV infection. It is sometimes called a drug cocktail.

Histamine: A chemical contained in mast cells that is released during an allergic reaction.

Hit: A single intake of marijuana smoke from a joint or bong.

Holoprosencephaly: A disorder in which a baby's forebrain does not develop normally. The infant's brain fails to divide into two cerebral hemispheres; this failure in turn leads to facial deformities and abnormal brain structure and function.

Hormone: Any chemical produced by living cells that stimulates organs or tissues in parts of the body at some distance from where it is produced.

Hospice: A facility or program for meeting the spiritual as well as the physical needs of people who are terminally ill.

Host: An organism that is infected by a virus, bacterium, or parasite.

Hydrocephalus: Abnormal accumulation of cerebrospinal fluid within the cavities inside the brain.

Hydrops fetalis: The most severe form of alpha thalassemia, leading to death before or shortly after birth.

Hyperammonemia: Overly high levels of ammonia in the blood; it often indicates liver damage.

Hyperarousal: A state of increased emotional tension and anxiety, often including jitteriness and being easily startled.

Hyperbaric oxygen (HBO): Oxygen that is delivered to a patient in a special chamber at two to three times normal atmospheric pressure.

Hyperextension: Stretching or moving a part of the body beyond its normal range of motion.

Hyperopia: The medical term for farsightedness.

Hyperthyroidism: A disease condition in which the thyroid gland produces too much thyroid hormone.

Hypnagogic: Referring to the period of partial alertness on the boundary between sleeping and waking.

Hypocretin: A protein produced by certain brain cells that promotes wakefulness and helps to regulate the sleep/wake cycle. It is also known as orexin.

Hypomania: A less severe form of mania that does not interfere with normal functioning.

Hypothalamus: The part of the brain that controls body temperature, hunger, thirst, and response to stress.

Hypothyroidism: A disease condition in which the thyroid gland does not produce enough thyroid hormone.

Hypotonia: The medical term for poor muscle tone.

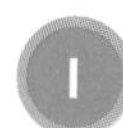

Ideal weight: Weight corresponding to the lowest death rate for individuals of a specific height, gender, and age.

Identical twins: Twins that develop from a single fertilized egg that divides to form two separate embryos.

Idiopathic: The medical term for a disorder whose cause is unknown.

Immunoglobulin E (IgE): An antibody in blood that activates mast cells during an allergic reaction.

Incest: Sexual activity between closely related persons, often within the immediate family.

Indolent: The medical term for a tumor or disease that grows or develops slowly.

Infestation: A condition in which a parasite develops and multiplies on the body of its host rather than inside the body.

Inhalation: The part of the breathing cycle in which a person takes in air from the outside.

Insulin: A hormone secreted by the pancreas that causes the cells in the liver, muscle and fatty tissues of the body to use the glucose carried in the bloodstream after a meal.

Intractable: Referring to a disease or disorder that cannot be easily treated or cured.

Inversion injury: A type of ankle injury caused when the foot is suddenly forced to roll inward.

Involuntary: Not under the control of the will.

Iris: The circular colored structure at the front of the eyeball that controls the amount of light entering the eye by changing the size of the pupil.

Irradiation: A technique for treating raw meat and poultry with gamma rays, x rays, or electron beams to destroy disease organisms.

Ischemia: Loss of blood supply to a tissue or organ resulting from the blockage of a blood vessel.

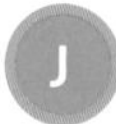

Jaundice: A yellowish discoloration of the skin and whites of the eyes caused by increased levels of bile pigments from the liver in the patient's blood.

Jet lag: A sleep disorder or disturbance in the sleep/wake cycle related to rapid travel across time zones.

Joint: A cigarette made with marijuana instead of tobacco.

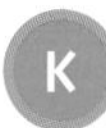

Karyotype: A photomicrograph of the chromosomes in a single human cell. Making a karyotype is one way to test for genetic disorders.

Keratoconus: An eye disorder in which the tissue of the cornea grows thinner over time.

Koplik spots: Small reddish spots with white centers seen on the tissues lining the cheeks in early-stage measles.

Kuru: A fatal brain disease related to CJD that was epidemic in Papua New Guinea in the mid-1950s. Kuru is thought to have been spread by cannibalism.

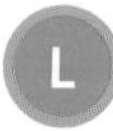

Lactase: An enzyme that breaks down lactose into simpler sugars during the process of digestion.

Lactose: A complex sugar found in milk and other dairy products. It is sometimes called milk sugar.

Lactose intolerance: An inability to digest lactose, the form of sugar found in milk and milk products.

Laparoscope: A fiberoptic instrument resembling a telescope that can be inserted through a small incision to allow a doctor to see the inside of the abdomen during surgery.

Larva: The immature form of an insect.

Larynx: The medical name for the voice box located at the base of the throat.

Latent: Referring to a disease that is inactive.

Lesion: A general term for any skin injury.

Levothyroxine: The chemical name for the synthetic thyroid hormone given to treat Hashimoto disease.

Ligament: A tough fibrous band of tissue that joins bones together.

Lobule: One of the glands in the breast that produce milk.

Lymph nodes: Part of the lymphatic system, the lymph nodes trap foreign particles and are important to defend the body from disease.

Lymphocyte: A type of white blood cell that fights infection. Lymphocytes are divided into two types, T cells (produced in the thymus gland) and B cells (produced in the bone marrow).

Lymphoma: A type of cancer that affects the lymphatic system.

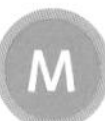

Macule: A spot on the skin or patch that is different in color from normal skin but is usually not raised up above the skin surface.

Mad cow disease: A prion disease that affects cattle and can be transmitted to humans by eating meat from infected cattle.

Malabsorption: Inability to absorb the nutrients in food through the digestive tract.

Malar rash: The medical term for the butterfly-shaped facial rash found in lupus.

Malignant: Cancerous.

Mania: The high-energy phase of bipolar disorder.

Mast cells: Specialized white blood cells that are found in connective tissue and contain histamine.

Mastectomy: Surgical removal of the breast.

Meconium: A dark greenish type of stool passed by a newborn during the first few days of life.

Medulloblastoma: A type of malignant brain tumor that develops in the cerebellum. It is the most common type of brain tumor in children.

Melanin: A brownish or dark reddish pigment that is the primary determinant of skin, hair, and eye color in humans.

Melanocyte: A type of skin cell that produces melanin.

Melanoma: The most serious form of skin cancer. Sunburn increases the risk of melanoma.

Melatonin: A hormone produced in the pineal gland in the brain that regulates the sleep/wake cycle.

Meninges (singular, meninx): The protective membranes that cover the brain and spinal cord.

Meningioma: A type of brain tumor that starts in the meninges.

Meningitis: Inflammation of the membranes that cover the brain and line the brain and spinal cord.

Metabolism: The chemical changes in living cells in which new materials are taken in and energy is provided for vital processes,

Metastasis (plural, metastases): The spread of a cancer from its original location to other organs or parts of the body.

Migraine: A type of primary headache characterized by severe pain, nausea and vomiting, and sensitivity to light. It may occur on only one side of the head.

Milestone: A physical development or accomplishment that most children reach within a specific age range.

Mixed state: A condition in which a person with bipolar disorder has the energy of the manic phase of the disorder combined with the hopeless and sad mood of the depressed phase.

Mohs surgery: A technique for removing skin cancers in very thin layers one at a time in order to minimize damage to healthy skin.

Monosomy: A type of genetic disorder in which a cell contains only one copy of a particular chromosome instead of the normal two.

Mosaicism: A condition in which a person has some body cells containing an abnormal number of chromosomes and other cells containing the normal number. Mosaicism results from random errors during the process of cell division that follows conception.

Motor neuron: A type of cell in the central nervous system that controls the movement of muscles either directly or indirectly.

Mucous membrane: Soft tissues that line the nose, throat, stomach, and intestines.

Multiple chemical sensitivity (MCS): A controversial health condition related to a patient's belief that his or her symptoms are caused by exposure to environmental chemicals.

Mutate: A change in the genetic material of an organism. Viruses can mutate rapidly.

Mutation: A change in the genetic material of an organism.

Mycoplasma: A very small bacterium that causes a mild but long-lasting form of pneumonia.

Myelin: A fatty substance that insulates nerve fibers and allows for speedy and accurate transmission of nerve impulses.

Myeloid: Relating to bone marrow.

Myocardial infarction: The medical term for a heart attack.

Myopia: The medical term for nearsightedness.

Myosin: A protein involved in muscle movement.

Myxedema: A synonym for hypothyroidism. Myxedema coma is a condition in which a person with untreated hypothyroidism loses consciousness. It is potentially fatal.

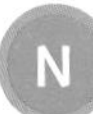

Nebulizer: A device that delivers medication in a fine spray or mist.

Necrotizing: Causing the death of soft tissue.

Neglect: Failing to meet a child's basic needs for food, clothing, shelter, and medical care.

Negri bodies: Round or oval bodies found within the nerve cells of animals infected by the rabies virus. They were first described by Dr. Adolchi Negri in 1903.

Neonatal: The medical term for newborn.

Neural tube: The medical term for the folds of tissue in the human embryo that eventually form the brain and spinal cord.

Neurologic: Pertaining to the nervous system.

Neurologist: A doctor who specializes in diagnosing and treating disorders of the nervous system.

Neurology: The branch of medicine that studies and treats disorders of the nervous system.

Neurotransmitters: Chemicals produced in the brain that transmit nerve impulses to other nerve cells and eventually to muscles.

Nicotine: A chemical found in tobacco that acts as a stimulant in humans.

Nits: The eggs of lice.

Nodule: The medical term for a small rounded lump of tissue.

Nondisjunction: A genetic error in which one or more pairs of chromosomes fail to separate during the formation of germ cells, with the result that both chromosomes are carried to one daughter cell and none to the other.

Non-rapid eye movement (NREM) sleep: The first phase of a sleep cycle, in which there is little or no eye movement.

Norepinephrine: A brain chemical that affects a person's ability to pay attention.

Nosocomial: Referring to a disease that a person gets while hospitalized.

Nucleotide excision repair (NER): A mechanism that allows cells to remove damage caused by ultraviolet light to the cell's DNA.

Nucleotides: The basic structural units of DNA and RNA, a cell's genetic material.

Nucleus: The innermost part of the lens of the eye.

Nymph: The second stage in the life cycle of the deer tick.

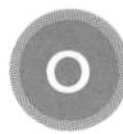

Obsession: A recurrent, distressing, intrusive thought, image, or impulse.

Occult: The medical term for a cancer that is too small to produce a visible tumor.

Oncogene: A gene that has the potential to cause a normal cell to become cancerous.

Ophthalmia neonatorum: The medical name for bacterial conjunctivitis in newborn babies caused by a sexually transmitted infection in the mother.

Ophthalmologist: A doctor who specializes in diagnosing and treating eye disorders and can perform eye surgery.

Opportunistic infection: An infection that occurs only in people with weakened immune systems.

Optician: An eye care professional who fills prescriptions for eyeglasses and corrective lenses.

Optometrist: An eye care professional who diagnoses refractive errors and other eye problems and prescribes corrective lenses.

Orphan drug: A drug defined by the Food and Drug Administration (FDA) as intended to treat a disease or condition that affects less than 200,000 people in the United States, or a disease or condition that affects more than 200,000 people and there is no reasonable expectation that the company can recover the costs of developing the drug.

Orthokeratology: A treatment for astigmatism that consists of wearing hard contact lenses overnight to reshape the cornea during sleep. The lenses are removed during the day.

Orthopaedics (also spelled orthopedics): The branch of medicine that diagnoses and treats disorders of or injuries to the bones, muscles, and joints.

Ossicles: A group of three small bones in the middle ear that transmit sound waves to the cochlea.

Osteopenia: The medical name for low bone mass, a condition that often precedes osteoporosis.

Osteophyte: A bony outgrowth or spur that develops in a joint affected by osteoarthritis. Osteophytes usually cause pain and limit the motion of the joint.

Osteoporosis: A disease in which bones lose their density and are more likely to break or fracture under stress.

Otitis: The medical term for inflammation of the ear.

Otolaryngologist: A doctor who specializes in diagnosing and treating diseases of the ears, nose, and throat.

Otoscope: An instrument with a light and magnifying lens that allows a doctor to examine the eardrum and ear canal.

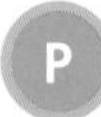

Paget disease: A chronic disorder caused by a slow virus infection that results in deformed or enlarged bones.

Pancolitis: Ulcerative colitis that affects the entire colon.

Pancreas: A small organ that lies between the stomach and the liver and secretes insulin.

PANDAS disorders: A group of disorders with psychiatric symptoms that develop in some children after strep throat or scarlet fever. The acronym stands for Pediatric Autoimmune Neuropsychiatric Disorders Associated with Streptococcal infections.

Pandemic: A disease epidemic that spreads over a wide geographical area and affects a large proportion of the population.

Panic attack: An episode of intense fear that lasts for several minutes and is accompanied by physical symptoms or temporary disturbances of thinking.

Pap test: A screening test for cervical cancer devised by Giorgios Papanikolaou (1883–1962) in the 1940s.

Papule: A small cone-shaped pimple or elevation of the skin.

Paradoxical undressing: A symptom sometimes seen in people with moderate or severe hypothermia, thought to be caused by a malfunction of the hypothalamus. The person becomes confused, disoriented, and begins to remove clothing.

Paraplegia: Paralysis that affects only the lower body.

Parotid glands: Glands that produce saliva, located on each side of the face below and in front of the ear.

Pasteurization: A process in which milk or fruit juice is partially sterilized by heating to a temperature that destroys disease bacteria without causing major changes in appearance and taste.

Pastia's lines: Bright red lines that appear in the body folds of a patient with scarlet fever after the rash develops.

Patent: The medical term for open or unobstructed.

Peak airflow meter: A handheld device that asthma patients can use at home to monitor their lung capacity in order to treat the warning signs of an asthma attack as soon as possible.

Pelvic inflammatory disease (PID): Inflammation of the uterus, fallopian tubes, and ovaries caused by chlamydia or gonorrhea. It can lead to permanent inability to have children if not treated.

Peptic ulcer: The medical term for an ulcer in the digestive tract.

Perinatal: Related to the period around the time of a baby's birth.

Periodontitis: The medical term for gum disease that involves the connective tissue and bone beneath the gums.

Peritonitis: Inflammation of the membrane that lines the abdominal cavity and covers some of the internal organs.

Pertussis: The medical name for whooping cough.

Pervasive developmental disorder (PDD): A diagnostic category for a group of childhood disorders characterized by problems in communication skills and social interactions.

Petechiae: Tiny reddish or purplish spots in the skin caused by the breaking of small blood vessels during intense coughing or vomiting.

Pewter: A metal made mostly of tin and small quantities of copper. Modern pewter is no longer made with lead.

Phacoemulsification: A technique for removing cataracts by breaking up the lens of the eye with ultrasound waves and removing the pieces of the lens by suction.

Pharyngitis: The medical term for sore throat.

Phenylalanine: The amino acid that cannot be used by the bodies of people with phenylketonuria.

Philadelphia chromosome: A genetic abnormality in chromosome 9 associated with CML. Its name comes from the location of the University of Pennsylvania School of Medicine, where it was discovered in 1960.

Phlegm: Thick mucus secreted in the throat and lungs during an upper respiratory infection.

Phobia: An unfounded or morbid dread of a specific object or situation that arouses feelings of panic.

Photophobia: A feeling of discomfort or pain in the eyes during exposure to light.

Photopter: A device positioned in front of a patient's eyes during an eye examination that allows the examiner to place various lenses in front of the eyes to determine the strength of corrective lenses required.

Phototherapy: Method of treating skin disorders by exposing the affected skin to daylight or to specific wavelengths of visible or ultraviolet light.

Pica: An abnormal craving for substances that are not normally considered food, like soil, chalk, paper, or ice cubes.

Pinna: The visible part of the outer ear.

Pitch: The highness or lowness of the voice or a musical note.

Pituitary gland: A pea-sized gland located at the base of the brain behind the nose that secretes growth hormone and other hormones that affect sexual development and the body's response to stress.

Plantar: Located on or referring to the sole of the foot.

Plaque (arterial): A deposit of cholesterol and dead white cells along the inside wall of an artery.

Plaque (dental): A film that forms on the surface of teeth containing bacteria, saliva, and dead cells.

Plasma: The liquid part of blood, about 55 percent of blood by volume.

Platelet: A small flat disk-shaped body in human blood that helps to form blood clots by sticking to other platelets and to damaged tissue at the site of an injury. Platelets are also called thrombocytes.

Plumbism: The medical name for lead poisoning.

Polymyositis: Inflammation of the muscles that causes weakness and difficulty in moving or swallowing.

Polyp: A growth of tissue protruding from a mucous membrane such as the colon.

Polysomnograph: A machine used in a sleep laboratory to monitor chest movement, air flow, brain waves, heart rhythm, and other data relevant to diagnosing sleep disorders.

Popcorn cell: An abnormal cell found in nodular lymphocyte predominant Hodgkin disease (NLPHD).

Post-concussion syndrome (PCS): A condition characterized by several weeks or months of headache following a head injury.

Postexposure prophylaxis (PEP): A treatment given after exposure to the rabies virus. It consists of one dose of rabies immune globulin and five doses of rabies vaccine.

Postmortem: Referring to the period following death.

Postpartum: Referring to the period of time after giving birth.

Postpartum depression: A type of depression that some women experience after the birth of a baby.

Postpartum psychosis: A severe mental disorder in which the mother suffers from delusions or hallucinations.

Prader-Willi syndrome: A rare genetic disorder characterized by mental retardation and an uncontrollable appetite for food.

Premutation: An abnormally large number of repeated triplets in certain genes that does not cause obvious symptoms of a genetic disorder but can expand into a full mutation when transmitted to offspring.

Prenatal: Before birth.

Presbyopia: Age-related farsightedness caused by loss of flexibility in the lens of the eye.

Pressure points: Specific locations on the body where people with fibromyalgia feel pain even with light pressure.

Primary disease: A disease that develops by itself and is not caused by a previous disease or injury.

Prion: An abnormal infectious protein particle.

Proctitis: The medical term for ulcerative colitis limited to the rectum.

Prodrome: A period before the acute phase of a disease when the patient has some characteristic warning symptoms.

Progeria: A disease characterized by abnormally rapid aging. The term can be used to refer specifically to Hutchinson-Gilford syndrome or to a group of diseases characterized by accelerated aging.

Progressive: Referring to a disease or disorder that gets worse over time.

Prophylaxis: The use of a medication or other therapy to maintain health and prevent disease.

Prostate: A walnut-sized gland in males that secretes seminal fluid.

Protozoan (plural, protozoa): A one-celled animal-like organism with a central nucleus enclosed by a membrane. Many protozoa are parasites that can cause disease in humans.

Pseudostrabismus: A condition in which a child may seem to have strabismus because of certain facial features that change as the child's face matures.

Psychosis: Severe mental illness marked by hallucinations and loss of contact with the real world.

Psychostimulant: A type of drug that increases the activity of the parts of the brain that produce dopamine.

Pulp: The soft living material in the center of a tooth that contains blood vessels and nerve endings.

Pupil: The circular opening in the center of the iris.

Pus: A whitish-yellow material produced by the body in response to a bacterial infection. It consists of tissue fluid and dead white blood cells.

Pyelonephritis: The medical term for a urinary tract infection that has spread from the bladder or other parts of the urinary tract upward to the kidneys.

Quadriplegia: Paralysis that affects both arms and both legs. It is also known as tetraplegia.

Quarantine: The practice of isolating people with a contagious disease for a period of time to prevent the spread of the disease.

Quinoa: A plant grown in Peru and Bolivia for its edible seeds. It is high in protein and easy to digest.

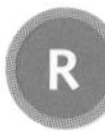

Radiologist: A doctor who specializes in medical imaging techniques to diagnose or treat disease.

Radon: A colorless and odorless gas produced by the breakdown of uranium known to cause lung cancer.

Rapid cycling: Four or more episodes of illness within a 12-month period.

Rapid eye movement (REM) sleep: The phase of a sleep cycle in which dreaming occurs; it is characterized by rapid eye movements.

Raynaud's phenomenon: Discoloration of the fingers and toes caused by blood vessels going into spasm and decreasing the flow of blood to the affected digits.

Reactive hypoglycemia: A condition in which a person develops hypoglycemia between two and five hours after eating foods containing high levels of glucose.

Rebound tenderness: Pain experienced when the doctor releases pressure on the abdomen.

Rectum: The lowermost portion of the large intestine, about 6 inches (15.2 centimeters) long in adults.

Reed-Sternberg cell: An abnormal type of B lymphocyte that is found in classic Hodgkin lymphoma.

Reefer: Another name for a marijuana cigarette.

Reflux: The medical term for the backward flow of stomach acid from the stomach into the esophagus.

Refractive error: A general term for vision problems caused by the eye's inability to focus light correctly.

Regurgitation: Throwing up; effortless flow of undigested stomach contents back up the esophagus into the mouth.

Reiter's syndrome: A type of arthritis than can develop in untreated people with chlamydia. It is characterized by inflammation of the genitals and the eyelids as well as sore and aching joints.

Relapse: Recurrence of an illness after a period of improvement.

Remission: A period in the course of a disease when symptoms disappear for a time.

Reservoir: The term used by biologists for the natural host species of a disease organism. Bats are thought to be the reservoir of viral hemorrhagic fevers.

Resilience: The capacity to recover from trauma and other stressful situations without lasting damage.

Resorption: The removal of old bone from the body.

Retina: The light-sensitive layer of tissue at the back of the eyeball.

Retinal detachment: A disorder in which the retina pulls away from its underlying tissues at the back of the eye.

Rheumatoid factor (RF): An antibody that attacks the body's own tissues that is found in some patients with rheumatoid arthritis and is measured as part of the diagnostic process.

Rheumatologist: A doctor who diagnoses and treats diseases of the muscles, joints, and connective tissue.

Rheumatologist: A doctor who specializes in diagnosing and treating arthritis and other diseases of the muscles and joints.

Rheumatology: The branch of medicine that deals with disorders of the muscles, joints, and connective tissue.

Rhinitis: The medical term for inflammation of the mucous tissues lining the nose. It can be caused by infections or chemical irritants as well as by allergies.

RNA virus: A virus whose genetic material is composed of ribonucleic acid (RNA) and does not need DNA to copy itself and multiply.

Rocker-bottom feet: Abnormally long and slender feet with pointed heels turned outward like the bottom rails of a rocker.

Rotator cuff: A group of four muscles that attach the arm to the shoulder blade.

Scald: A burn caused by steam or a hot liquid.

Scaling: Scraping tartar away from the teeth around the gum line.

Scintigraphy: A technique for detecting the location and extent of soft-tissue injury by injecting a small quantity of a radioactive element and following its distribution in the tissue with a scanner.

Sclera: The opaque white portion of the eyeball.

Scleroderma: A disorder of connective tissue characterized by thickening and tightening of the skin as well as damage to internal organs.

Sclerosis: Hardening or scarring of tissue.

Scoliosis: Abnormal curvature of the spine from side to side.

Scrapie: A prion disease of sheep and goats.

Sebum: An oily lubricant secreted by glands in the skin.

Secondary disease: A disease that is caused by another disease or condition or by an injury.

Selective serotonin reuptake inhibitors (SSRIs): A group of antidepressants that work by increasing the amount of serotonin available to nerve cells in the brain.

Senile cataract: Another term for cataracts caused by the aging process.

Sepsis: The presence of bacteria or their toxic products in the bloodstream or other tissues, leading to inflammation of the entire body.

Septum (plural, septa): A partition that separates two cavities or chambers in the body.

Serotonin: A brain chemical that influences mood, anger, anxiety, body temperature, and appetite.

Shingles: A skin inflammation caused by reactivation of the chickenpox virus remaining in the nervous system.

Shock: A medical emergency in which there is a drop in blood pressure and a reduced volume of blood circulating in the body.

Shunt: A flexible plastic tube inserted by a surgeon to drain cerebrospinal fluid from the brain and redirect it to another part of the body.

Sickle cell crisis: Sudden onset of pain and organ damage in the chest, bones, abdomen, or joints caused by defective red blood cells blocking blood vessels.

Sleep cycle: A period of NREM sleep followed by a shorter phase of REM sleep. Most adults have four to six sleep cycles per night.

Slit lamp: An instrument that focuses light into a thin slit. It is used by eye doctors to examine eyes for a wide variety of disorders.

Smoking cessation: A term that refers to a product or program to help people quit smoking.

Snellen chart: A series of letters arranged in lines on a chart to be viewed from a distance of 20 feet (6.1 meters) used to measure visual acuity (clearness of vision).

Soft palate: The soft tissue at the back of the roof of the mouth that does not contain bone.

Solar keratoses (singular, keratosis): Rough scaly patches that appear on sun-damaged skin. They are considered precancerous.

Spasticity: Stiffness or spasms in the muscles.

Spectrum disorder: A disorder whose symptoms vary in severity from one patient to the next.

Sphincter: A ring-shaped muscle that can contract to close off a body opening.

Sphygmomanometer: The device used to measure blood pressure. It consists of an inflatable cuff that compresses an artery in the arm. The doctor listens through a stethoscope as the air pressure in the cuff is released in order to measure the blood pressure.

Spirochete: A spiral-shaped bacterium. Lyme disease is caused by a spirochete.

Spirometer: A device that is used to test the air capacity of a person's lungs and the amount of air that enters and leaves the lungs during breathing.

Spleen: An organ located behind the stomach that cleans old blood cells out of the blood and holds a reserve of red blood cells.

Sporadic: Occurring at random.

Spore: The dormant stage of a bacterium.

Sputum: Mucus and other matter that is coughed or brought up from the lungs or throat.

Stacking: Using several different types of steroids at the same time.

Status epilepticus: An ongoing seizure that lasts longer than five minutes; it is a medical emergency.

Stem cell: A type of unspecialized cell that can reproduce itself and differentiate into different types of specialized cells. Stem cells act as a repair system for the body.

Stenosis: The medical term for abnormal narrowing of the opening of a blood vessel.

Stillbirth: The birth of a baby that has died before or during delivery.

Stimulant: Any drug or chemical that temporarily increases the user's awareness or alertness.

Stoma: An opening made in the abdomen following surgery for digestive disorders, including colon cancer, that allows wastes to pass from the body.

Stomatitis: The medical term for an inflammation of the mouth.

Strabismus: A condition in which the eyes are not properly aligned with each other.

Strain: A genetic variant or subtype of a bacterium.

Strawberry tongue: A swollen and intensely red tongue that is one of the classic signs of scarlet fever.

Stress management: Any set of techniques intended to help people deal more effectively with stress in their lives by analyzing specific stressors and taking positive actions to minimize their effects.

Stressor: Any event or stimulus that provokes a stress response in a human or animal.

Stricture: The medical term for an abnormal narrowing of a hollow organ like the bowel.

Substance P: A chemical in the central nervous system that transmits pain signals back and forth between the brain and the rest of the body.

Sulcus (plural, sulci): The space or crevice between a tooth and the surrounding gum tissue.

Sun poisoning: A term sometimes used to refer to a severe reaction to sunburn, consisting of fever, chills, fluid loss, dizziness, and nausea.

Sunsetting: A term used to describe a downward focusing of the eyes.

Surfactant: A protein-containing substance secreted by cells in the lungs that helps to keep them properly inflated during breathing.

Surveillance: Monitoring of infectious diseases by public health doctors.

Synapse: The medical term for specialized connections between nerve cells.

Syndrome: A group of signs or symptoms that occur together and characterize or define a particular disease or disorder.

Synovium: A type of tissue lining the joints that ordinarily secretes a fluid that lubricates the joints.

Systemic: Referring to a disease or disorder that affects the entire body.

Systolic blood pressure: The blood pressure at the peak of each heartbeat.

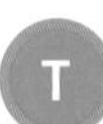

Targeted therapy: A newer type of cancer treatment that uses drugs to target the ways cancer cells divide and reproduce or the ways tumors form their blood supply.

Tartar: Hardened plaque.

Tendon: A thick band or cord of dense white connective tissue that attaches a muscle to a bone.

Teratogen: Any substance that causes birth defects in children. Alcohol is a teratogen.

Testosterone: The principal male sex hormone.

Thalassemia trait: A condition in which a person is missing one or two genes required to make the proteins in the alpha chains of the hemoglobin molecule. The person does not have the symptoms of thalassemia but can pass the genetic deficiency to their children.

THC: The abbreviation for delta-9-tetrahydrocannabinol, the main mind-altering chemical in marijuana.

Thrombus: A blood clot that forms inside an intact blood vessel and remains there.

Thymus: A small organ located behind the breastbone that is part of the lymphatic system and produces T cells.

Thyroid storm: A medical emergency marked by a rise in body temperature as well as other symptoms caused by untreated hyperthyroidism.

Thyroiditis: Inflammation of the thyroid gland.

Tic: A sudden repetitive movement or utterance. Tourette syndrome is considered a tic disorder.

Tick: A small bloodsucking parasitic insect that carries Lyme disease and several other diseases.

Tinnitus: The medical term for ringing in the ears.

Tolerance: The need for greater and greater amounts of a drug to get the desired effects.

Tonometer: An instrument used by an ophthalmologist to measure the pressure of the fluid inside the eye.

Tonsillectomy: Surgical removal of the tonsils.

Topical: Referring to a type of medication applied directly to the skin or outside of the body.

Tourette syndrome: A neurological disorder characterized by recurrent involuntary body movements and repeated words or grunts.

Toxin: A poisonous substance produced by a living cell or organism.

Trachoma: An infectious disease of the eye caused by chlamydia bacteria that can lead to blindness if untreated.

Traction: The use of braces, casts, or other devices to straighten broken bones and keep them aligned during the healing process.

Transdermal: Referring to a type of drug that enters the body by being absorbed through the skin.

Transient ischemic attack (TIA): A brief stroke lasting from a few minutes to twenty-four hours. TIAs are sometimes called mini-strokes.

Translocation: A genetic error in which a part of one chromosome becomes attached to another chromosome during cell division.

Trauma: A severe injury or shock to a person's body or mind.

Tremor: Trembling or shaking caused by a physical disease.

Triglyceride: A type of fat made in the body.

Triplet: In genetics, a unit of three nucleotides that starts or stops the production of a specific protein. Triplets are also called codons.

Trismus: The medical name for the spasms of the jaw muscles caused by tetanus.

Trisomy: A type of genetic disorder in which a cell contains three copies of a particular chromosome instead of the normal two.

Triticale: A grain that is a cross between wheat and rye, first grown in Scotland and Sweden in the nineteenth century.

T-score: The score on a bone density test, calculated by comparing the patient's bone mineral density to that of a healthy thirty-year-old of the same sex and race.

Tumor: An abnormal mass or growth of tissue that may be either cancerous or noncancerous.

Tumor markers: Substances found in blood, urine, or body tissues that can be used to detect cancer.

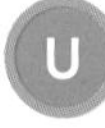

Ureter: A muscular tube that carries urine from the kidney to the bladder.

Urethra: The tube that allows urine to pass from the bladder to the outside of the body.

Urologist: A doctor who specializes in diagnosing and treating disorders of the kidneys and urinary tract.

Urticaria: The medical term for hives.

Uveitis: Inflammation of the interior of the eye.

Uvula: A triangular piece of soft tissue located at the back of the soft palate.

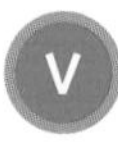

Vasoconstriction: A narrowing of the blood vessels in response to cold or certain medications.

Vector: An insect or other animal that carries a disease from one host to another.

Ventricle (brain): One of four hollow spaces or cavities in the brain that hold cerebrospinal fluid.

Ventricle (heart): One of the two lower chambers of the heart.

Verruca (plural, verrucae): The medical term for a wart.

Vertebra (plural, vertebrae): One of the segments of bone that make up the spinal column.

Vesicle: A small blister or sac containing fluid.

Vestibular system: The group of organs in the inner ear that provide sensory input related to movement, orientation in space, and balance.

Villi (singular, villus): Small finger-like projections along the walls of the small intestine that increase the surface area of the intestinal wall.

Viral load: A measure of the severity of HIV infection, calculated by estimating the number of copies of the virus in a milliliter of blood.

Virilization: The development of male sexual characteristics in females.

Vital signs: Measurements taken to evaluate basic body functions. They are temperature, pulse rate, blood pressure, and breathing rate.

Vocal folds: Twin folds of mucous membrane stretched across the larynx. They are also known as vocal cords.

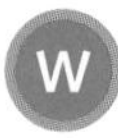

Wasting: Loss of lean muscle tissue.

Werner syndrome: A genetic disease characterized by accelerated aging.

Wheal: A suddenly formed flat-topped swelling of the skin; a welt.

Wheezing: A continuous harsh whistling sound produced by the airways of an asthma patient when the air passages are partly blocked.

Whipple triad: A group of three factors used to diagnose hypoglycemia: symptoms; blood sugar measuring below 45 mg/dL for a woman and 55 mg/dL for a man; and rapid recovery following a dose of sugar.

Window period: The period of time between a person's getting infected with HIV and the point at which antibodies against the virus can be detected in a blood sample.

Withdrawal: A collection of signs and symptoms that appear when a drug (including alcohol, caffeine and nicotine) that a person has used for a long time is suddenly discontinued.

With-the-rule astigmatism: A type of astigmatism in which the eye sees vertical lines more clearly than horizontal lines.

Wood's lamp: A special lamp that uses ultraviolet light to detect certain types of skin infections and infestations.

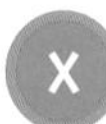

Xerostomia: The medical term for dry mouth.

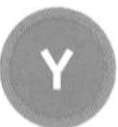

Yaws: A tropical, bacterial infection of the skin, bones, and joints.

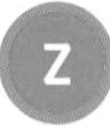

Zoonosis (plural, zoonoses): A disease that can be transmitted from animals to humans.

H

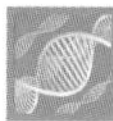 Genetic

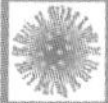 Infection

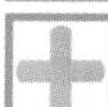 Injury

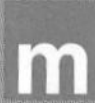 Multiple

 Other

 Unknown

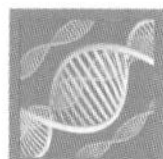

Hand-Foot-and-Mouth Disease

Definition

Hand-foot-and-mouth disease (HFMD) is a contagious virus infection most likely to affect children below the age of ten. Its most noticeable symptoms are sores in the mouth and a rash on the hands, soles of the feet, and sometimes the buttocks. HFMD should not be confused with foot-and-mouth (sometimes called hoof-and-mouth) disease, which is a virus infection that affects cattle, pigs, and sheep. Humans cannot get the animal disease, and they cannot transmit HFMD to household pets or other animals.

Also Known As
HFMD, enterovirus infection, coxsackievirus infection

Cause
Virus

Symptoms
Fever, mouth ulcers, blisters on the hands, feet, and buttocks

Duration
A week to ten days

Description

Hand-foot-and-mouth disease is largely a disease of young children in the United States. It often spreads rapidly in schools, day care centers, and other places where large numbers of children may be in close contact. The viruses that cause HFMD belong to a group of viruses called enteroviruses, which get their name from the fact that they are commonly found in the human digestive tract. The two most common enteroviruses that cause HFMD are called enterovirus 71 (EV71) and coxsackievirus A16, named for the town in New York where it was first identified in 1948.

The enteroviruses that cause HFMD are spread by contact with the mucus, tears, saliva, blister fluid, or feces of an infected person. The most

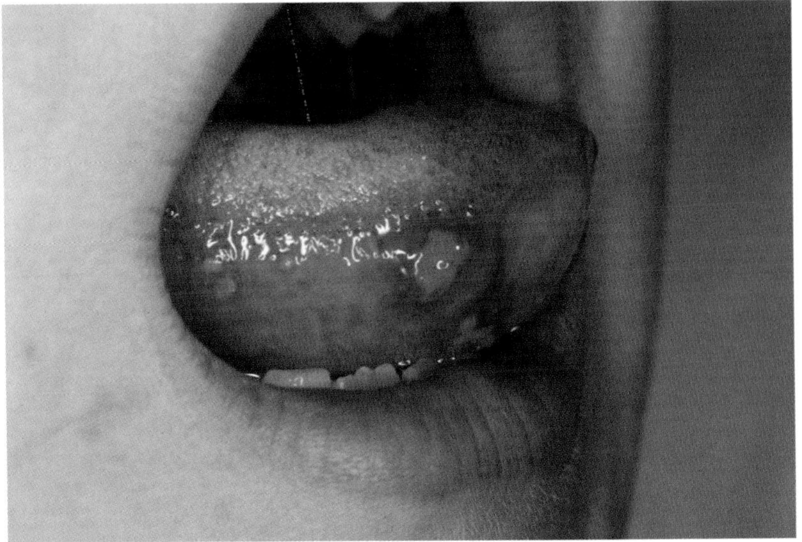

Child with a sore on the tongue from hand-foot-and-mouth disease. © HERCULES ROBINSON/ ALAMY.

common methods of transmission are contact with the unwashed hands of a person with HFMD or with a toy, drinking glass, or other object the infected person has touched. Infected children and adults are most contagious during the first week of illness; the virus can, however, remain in the intestines for about a month after the illness.

HFMD has an incubation period of three to seven days. The first symptoms of illness are usually fever and a sore throat, followed by loss of appetite. About two days after the fever begins, the patient develops painful sores in the mouth. A rash with blisters also appears on the palms of the hands, the soles of the feet, and sometimes on the buttocks or genitals. Some people have only the rash and some have only the mouth sores. The rash and mouth sores last for about a week or ten days and then clear completely.

Children and adults who have been infected with HFMD are immune to the specific virus that caused their symptoms after they recover. They can, however, develop a second case of HFMD if they are infected with a different enterovirus known to cause the disease.

Demographics

Hand-foot-and-mouth disease is a common disease around the world, with millions of cases each year. It is primarily a disease of young children, although young adults sometimes get infected. Older adults rarely get HFMD unless they have weakened immune systems.

There are epidemics of HFMD in the United States about every three years, most often in late summer or early fall. The disease affects both sexes and all racial and ethnic groups equally.

Causes and Symptoms

Hand-foot-and-mouth disease is caused by at least fourteen different enteroviruses, the two most common in the United States being enterovirus 71 and coxsackievirus A16.

The most common symptoms of HFMD include:

- Low-grade fever (101°F [38.3°C])
- Sore throat
- Loss of appetite
- Painful reddish ulcers or blisters around or in the mouth or on the soles of the feet and palms of the hands
- Headache
- Tiring easily or sleeping more than usual
- Crankiness in infants and toddlers

Some children may also:

- Drool
- Develop muscle aches
- Have pains or cramping in the abdomen

Diagnosis

The diagnosis of hand-foot-and-mouth disease is usually based on the doctor's observation of the patient's age, history, and visible symptoms. Blood tests or other laboratory studies are rarely done because the illness is usually mild. It is possible to identify the viruses that cause HFMD by taking stool samples or by swabbing the patient's mouth and throat and culturing the virus in the laboratory, but these tests can take between two and four weeks to yield results.

Treatment

There is no specific medication that can cure hand-foot-and-mouth disease, as antibiotics are not effective against virus infections. Treatment is intended to ease the pain and discomfort of the fever, mouth sores, and other symptoms of HFMD. To bring down the fever and relieve muscle pain, children can be given acetaminophen, ibuprofen, or another non-aspirin fever reducer or pain reliever. The doctor may recommend a mouthwash, throat lozenge, or throat spray that contains a mild anesthetic to relieve pain caused by blisters inside the mouth or throat. Another treatment that can help to ease throat pain is to gargle with a salt water rinse made by adding half teaspoon of salt to an 8-ounce glass of warm water.

It is important to make sure that the patient drinks plenty of fluids. Children with HFMD sometimes become dehydrated because the sores inside the mouth and throat hurt when the child tries to drink fruit juice, soft drinks, tea, or other drinks that contain acid. Milk-based drinks or cold foods like ice cream or popsicles are often less painful for the child to swallow. Children who do become dehydrated may need to be taken to the hospital for treatment with intravenous fluids.

Children with blisters on the hands and feet should keep the areas clean by washing gently with soap and water, then patting the skin dry to avoid breaking the blister and spreading the infection. If the blister does open, it should be covered with a small bandage.

Prognosis

Most people in any age group with HFMD recover completely in about a week. In a few cases, children have developed encephalitis, meningitis, or pneumonia; in rare cases, HFMD can cause death. An epidemic in Taiwan in 1998 that affected 1.5 million children resulted in 405 severe complications and seventy-eight deaths. An outbreak of HFMD in China that began in the spring of 2008 led to 25,000 reported cases and twenty-two deaths by early May.

Pregnant women who become infected with HFMD are at increased risk of losing the baby.

Prevention

There is no vaccine against HFMD. The most effective preventive measure is frequent and thorough hand washing, particularly after using the toilet, changing a diaper, before meals, and before preparing food. Another preventive measure is routinely cleaning shared toys in day care centers as well as in the home with a disinfectant, because the viruses that cause HFMD can live on objects for several days. The Centers for Disease Control and Prevention (CDC) recommends washing toys (or soiled countertops and other surfaces) with soap and water, followed by using a solution of one tablespoon of chlorine bleach added to four cups of water.

Children with HFMD should stay home from child care or school until the fever has gone and the mouth sores and other blisters have healed. Adults with the disease should stay home from work.

The Future

Hand-foot-and-mouth disease is likely to continue to be a common infection because there are so many different enteroviruses that can cause it, and because these viruses are the second most common family of viruses—only the viruses that cause the common cold are more widespread.

Researchers are presently working on a rapid diagnostic test that would allow doctors to distinguish quickly between coxsackievirus A16 and enterovirus 71 in patients with symptoms of HFMD. Such a test would be helpful during epidemics because EV71 infections are more likely to lead to complications than coxsackievirus infections.

SEE ALSO Encephalitis; Meningitis; Pneumonia

For more information

BOOKS

Litin, Scott C., ed. *Mayo Clinic Family Health Book*. 3rd ed. New York: HarperResource, 2003.

PERIODICALS

Jacobs, Andrew. "Virus Kills 22 Children in Eastern China." *New York Times*, May 3, 2008. Available online at http://www.nytimes.com/2008/05/03/world/asia/03china.html?_r=1&oref=slogin (accessed October 20, 2008).

WEB SITES

Centers for Disease Control and Prevention (CDC). *Hand, Foot, and Mouth Disease (HFMD): Fast Facts*. Available online at http://www.cdc.gov/ncidod/dvrd/revb/enterovirus/hfhf.htm (accessed October 20, 2008).

Mayo Clinic. *Hand-Foot-and-Mouth Disease*. Available online at http://www.mayoclinic.com/health/hand-foot-and-mouth-disease/DS00599 (accessed October 20, 2008).

Nemours Foundation. *Hand, Foot, and Mouth Disease*. Available online at http://kidshealth.org/parent/infections/bacterial_viral/hfm.html (accessed October 20, 2008).

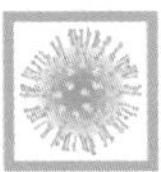

Hantavirus Infection

Definition

Hantavirus infection is more commonly called hantavirus pulmonary syndrome or HPS in the United States. It is a rare but potentially fatal disease that people get by breathing in the virus from the dried urine, feces, or saliva of its vectors —infected mice or rats. Hantavirus infection is classified as both an emerging infectious disease and a zoonosis (disease transmitted from animals to humans).

Description

The most distinctive symptom of hantavirus infection is its effect on the patient's lungs and breathing. After an incubation period of several days to several weeks, the infected person develops symptoms that can easily be mistaken for the flu or food poisoning. In the second phase, however, the patient has trouble breathing and may die as the lungs fill up with fluid and other body organs begin failing.

Demographics

Anyone can get hantavirus infection from infected mice. However, most reported cases are in middle-aged adults. People of both sexes and all races can get the infection. Men are at somewhat greater risk than women, however, because they are more likely to be employed in occupations that expose them to infected mice. Hantavirus infection had been reported in thirty states in the United States as of 2008. It is most likely to occur in the spring and summer as the weather warms and people spend more time outdoors. It can also occur in the fall, when the rodents that carry the virus seek shelter from the cold weather in houses or barns.

Some people are at greater risk of hantavirus infection:

- People who live in New Mexico, Colorado, Arizona, California, Utah, Texas, Washington, Idaho, and Montana.
- Farmers, ranchers, and field hands
- Field biologists and veterinarians
- People who work in grain elevators, feed lots, or feed mills

Also Known As
Hantavirus pulmonary syndrome, HPS, Sin Nombre virus, SNV, Four Corners disease

Cause
RNA virus

Symptoms
Fever, chills, headache, difficulty breathing, cough, death

Duration
Four to ten days

- Utility workers, plumbers, and electricians
- Construction workers and building contractors
- Hikers and campers

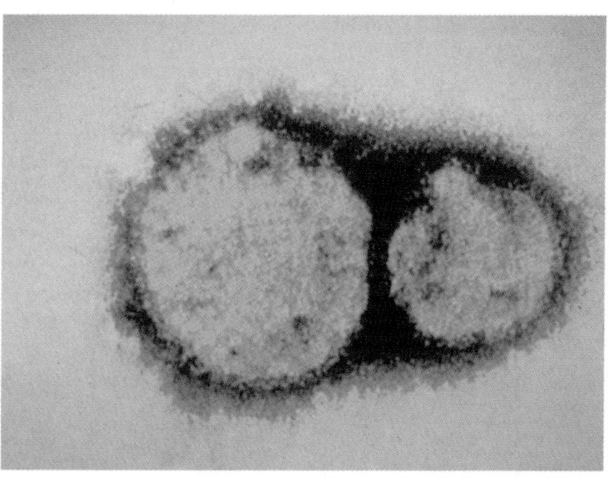

Image of a hantavirus splitting.
© PHOTOTAKE INC. / ALAMY.

Causes and Symptoms

Hantaviruses are RNA viruses that enter the body when people breathe dust contaminated by the urine, feces, or saliva of rodents. They sometimes breathe in this contaminated dust while working in a mouse-infested building, cleaning out a barn or shed, or hiking or camping in an area where infected mice build their burrows. When a person breathes in the dust, the virus particles enter the tissues lining the nose, throat, and lungs.

People can also take in the virus if they touch an object that has been contaminated by rodent droppings and then touch their mouth or nose. It may take anywhere from one week to five weeks for the disease to incubate. In a very few cases, people have been infected with hantavirus after being bitten by an infected mouse, but this method of transmission is unusual. As far as is known, people cannot get hantavirus infection through direct contact with an infected person.

The early stage of the disease is often misdiagnosed as flu or food poisoning because the person may have muscle ache and pains like those of flu or have nausea, vomiting, and diarrhea resembling the signs of food poisoning. This stage of the illness lasts from a few hours to several days. Other early symptoms of hantavirus infection are:

- Fever between 101 and 104°F (38 and 40°C)
- Chills
- A dry cough
- Rattling noises in the lungs
- Fatigue

In the second stage of the disease, the body responds to the virus that is infecting the tissue lining the lungs by secreting large amounts of fluid in order to get rid of the virus. The fluid, however, makes it hard for the person to breathe. Eventually the patient's blood pressure drops, an abnormal heart rhythm may develop, and one's breathing and blood circulation fails.

Discovery of an Emerging Disease

The Indian Health Service and the CDC were puzzled by an outbreak of a new disease in the Four Corners region of the American Southwest in May 1993. A young, healthy Navajo man died shortly after having difficulty breathing. His fiancé had died several days earlier after having similar symptoms. Five other cases followed. The CDC sent special investigators to find the cause. Chief investigator Terry Yates (1950–2007) traced the disease organism to deer mice. An unusually large number of deer mice thrived in spring 1993 due to heavy rains that provided a bumper crop of food for the mice.

The cause of the deaths was a new virus in the hantavirus family called Sin Nombre virus or SNV. Since 1993, several other hantaviruses carried by different species of rats and mice in Florida, Louisiana, Rhode Island, and New York have been identified. The CDC also found that several mysterious deaths in the United States before 1993 had been caused by a hantavirus; the earliest known case concerned a Utah man in 1959.

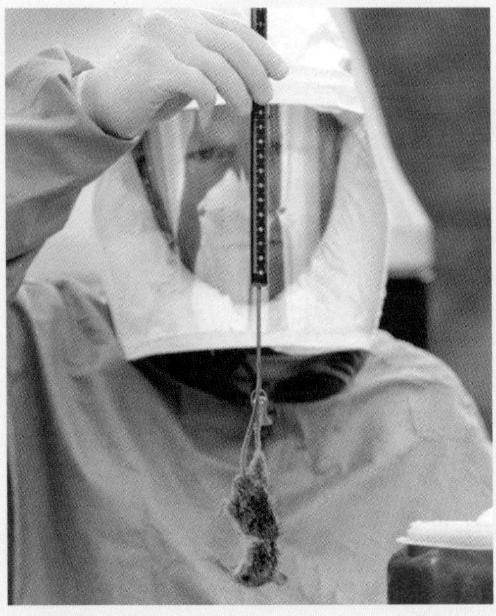

Hantavirus researcher in New Mexico, during a 1996 outbreak. AP IMAGES.

The name "hantavirus" itself comes from the Hantaan River in South Korea, where the first virus in this family was discovered by researcher Dr. Lee Ho-Wang in 1976. Dr. Ho-Wang had been looking for the cause of a hemorrhagic fever that had been killing thousands of people in Siberia, China, and Korea since the 1930s. About 2,300 American soldiers were infected by the hantavirus during the Korean War (1950–1953), and about 800 died as a result.

Diagnosis

The diagnosis of hantavirus infection is based on the patients' history, including their occupational history or other evidence that they were exposed to mice and rats or their droppings. Hantavirus infection can be distinguished from influenza, bubonic plague, and other conditions that may cause painful breathing through a blood test. In most cases the doctor will also order a chest x ray to look for fluid buildup in the lungs.

Treatment

There is no drug that can cure hantavirus infection. The patient's best chance of recovery is being placed on a respirator to help him or her breathe. Another form of treatment that helps some patients is extracorporeal membrane oxygenation, or ECMO. It is a technique in which the patient's blood is pumped through a machine that removes carbon dioxide and adds oxygen to the blood. The oxygenated blood is then returned to the patient's body.

Prognosis

In the early 1990s hantavirus infection was almost always fatal. Better understanding of the disease, however, has reduced the death rate to about 50 percent. Patients who survive, however, recover completely without long-term damage to their lungs.

Prevention

There is no vaccine to prevent hantavirus infection. The risk of hantavirus infection can be lowered considerably, however, by taking proper precautions to keep buildings free of rodents and to minimize exposure to them outdoors. The CDC recommends the following steps:

- Seal up holes, cracks, and other gaps that might allow mice to get into a house or barn.
- Get rid of any food sources (pet food, garbage cans, animal feed) within 100 feet (30 meters) of the house.
- Cut grass short near the house and keep shrubbery trimmed.
- Use mousetraps inside the house; disinfect dead rodents before disposing of them.
- Treat rodent droppings with chlorine bleach or another disinfectant before sweeping or vacuuming them. Wear rubber gloves during cleaning.
- Wear a respirator when cleaning, repairing, or working in a rodent-infested building.

The Future

It is difficult to predict whether hantavirus infection will become more common in the United States and Canada over the next few decades. On the one hand, hantaviruses may spread to parts of North America where the infection has not yet been reported. On the other hand,

WORDS TO KNOW

Emerging infectious disease (EID): A disease that has become more widespread around the world in the last twenty years and is expected to become more common in the future.

RNA virus: A virus whose genetic material is composed of ribonucleic acid (RNA) and does not need DNA to copy itself and multiply.

Vector: An animal that carries a disease from one host to another.

Zoonosis: A disease that can be transmitted from animals to humans.

doctors are now better trained to recognize the disease early and hospitalize patients quickly. It is also possible that an effective vaccine will be developed at some future point.

SEE ALSO Influenza; Plague

For more information

BOOKS

Casil, Amy Sterling. *Hantavirus.* New York: Rosen Publishing Group, 2005.

Leuenroth, Stephanie. *Hantavirus Pulmonary Syndrome.* Philadelphia: Chelsea House Publishers, 2006.

PERIODICALS

Associated Press. "South Dakotans Warned about Hantavirus." *KSFY Sioux Falls*, April 19, 2008. Available online at http://www.ksfy.com/news/local/17942589.html (accessed April 20, 2008).

Shimizu, Masami. "Tenacity Key to Victory over Virus: Researcher's Efforts Reduced by 90 Percent Cases of Hemorrhagic Fever." *Nikkei Net Interactive*, Nikkei Asia Prize Winners 2001. Available online at http://www.nni.nikkei.co.jp/FR/NIKKEI/inasia/prizes/2001/2001lee.html (accessed April 29, 2008). This article is a brief profile of Dr. Lee Ho-Wang, the Korean researcher who gave hantaviruses their name.

Woster, Terry. "Mother of SD Hantavirus Victim Praises Awareness Campaign." *Pierre Argus Leader*, April 18, 2008. Available online at http://www.argusleader.com/apps/pbcs.dll/article?AID=/20080418/UPDATES/80418021 (accessed April 20, 2008).

WEB SITES

Centers for Disease Control and Prevention (CDC). *All about Hantaviruses.* http://www.cdc.gov/ncidod/diseases/hanta/hps/index.htm (updated October 2006; accessed April 18, 2008).

Vogel, Michael, and Jim Knight. "Hantavirus: What Is It and What Can Be Done about It?" *Montana State University Extension Service*, May 2004.

Available online at http://www.montana.edu/wwwpb/pubs/mt9404.html (accessed April 19, 2008). This Web site contains detailed information about mouse-proofing houses and other preventive measures.

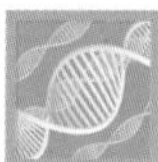

Hashimoto Disease

Definition

Hashimoto disease is an autoimmune disorder in which the body's immune system attacks the cells and tissues of the thyroid gland, a hormone-secreting (also called endocrine) gland resembling a butterfly located at the base of the neck just below the Adam's apple.

Description

Hashimoto disease is caused by autoimmune damage to the thyroid gland at the base of the neck. The gland may become swollen—a condition known as goiter—or it may remain normal in size. In either case it becomes inflamed, and its cells begin to die. This loss of tissue means that the gland no longer produces enough thyroid hormone, a chemical that the body needs to regulate its metabolism. This condition is known as hypothyroidism.

Demographics

Hashimoto disease is the most common cause of hypothyroidism in the United States and Canada in people over six years of age. It is largely a disease of adulthood, with the rate increasing with age. The most commonly affected age group is middle-aged adults between thirty and fifty.

Hashimoto disease is diagnosed in about fourteen women out of every 1,000 and one man in every 2,000. The disorder is estimated to be between ten and twenty times more common in women than in men, for reasons that are not yet known. It appears to be equally frequent in all races and ethnic groups, however.

Also Known As
Hashimoto thyroiditis, chronic lymphocytic thyroiditis

Cause
Autoimmune disorder in which the body's own cells attack the thyroid gland

Symptoms
Fatigue, constipation, dry skin, weight gain, cold intolerance, hair loss

Duration
Lifelong following diagnosis

Causes and Symptoms

Although doctors know that Hashimoto disease is an autoimmune disorder, they do not know what triggers its onset. Some think that the

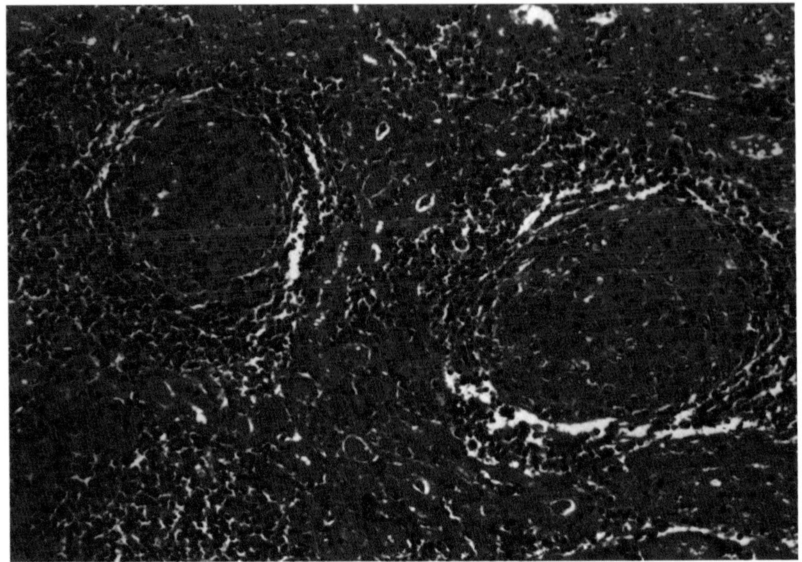

Image of thyroid gland tissue affected by Hashimoto disease. The pink areas have been damaged by the disease. CNRI / PHOTO RESEARCHERS, INC.

disease is related to a gene known as HLA-DR5; however, different genes seem to be related to the appearance of the disease in different ethnic groups. It is known that the disease tends to run in families.

Other researchers think that a bacterium or virus may be the cause of the autoimmune response in Hashimoto's disease. In any case, the autoimmune processes cause the destruction of the cells in the thyroid gland, leading to a drop in the production of thyroid hormone and the characteristic symptoms of hypothyroidism.

The symptoms of Hashimoto disease are not specific to it; that is, they can be caused by other diseases or disorders. In addition, the symptoms typically come on gradually; the person may simply feel tired or less energetic than usual or develop dry, itchy skin and brittle hair that falls out easily. It may take months to years before the person or their doctor begins to suspect a problem with the thyroid gland.

Some patients with Hashimoto disease, however, have an early phase of the disease in which they have too much thyroid hormone in their bloodstream; this temporary hyperthyroidism is caused by the leaking of thyroid hormone from damaged cells in the gland. This condition is called hashitoxicosis and is characterized by anxiety, heavy sweating, restlessness, diarrhea, high blood pressure, and a general feeling of being keyed up. Eventually the damaged thyroid cells die, however, and the level of thyroid hormone in the blood drops below normal.

Typical symptoms of Hashimoto disease include the following:

- Cold, dry skin and increased sensitivity to cold weather
- Dry brittle hair that falls out easily
- Constipation
- Hoarse voice and puffy face
- Unexplained weight gain of 10–20 pounds (4.5–9 kilograms), most of which is fluid
- Sore and aching muscles, most commonly in the shoulders and hips
- In women, extra-long menstrual periods or unusually heavy bleeding
- Weak leg muscles
- Memory loss
- Depression

Diagnosis

The diagnosis of Hashimoto disease is usually made by tests of the patient's thyroid function. The first test is a hormone test for thyroid-stimulating hormone, or TSH. TSH is a hormone produced by the pituitary gland in the brain that stimulates the thyroid gland to produce thyroid hormone. When the thyroid gland is not producing enough hormone, the pituitary gland secretes more TSH; thus a high level of TSH in the blood indicates that the thyroid gland is not as active as it should be. Another type of blood test involves testing for the presence of abnormal antibodies. Because Hashimoto disease is an autoimmune disorder, there will be two or three types of anti-thyroid antibodies in the patient's blood in about 90 percent of cases.

The doctor may also order an ultrasound study of the patient's neck in order to evaluate the size of the thyroid gland or take a small sample of thyroid tissue in order to make sure that the gland is not cancerous. Thyroid tissue that has been affected by Hashimoto's disease has a

Haraku Hashimoto (1881–1934)

Haraku Hashimoto was born into a family of medical doctors in the small village of Midau on the island of Honshu, Japan. He entered the new medical school at Kyushu University at the age of 22, graduating with one of its first classes in 1907. He intended to specialize in surgery, studying under Hayari Miyake (1867–1945), the first Japanese neurosurgeon.

Hashimoto then went to Germany for postgraduate study. He published a paper in 1912 in a German medical journal on four cases of a disorder of the thyroid gland, noting the characteristic abnormalities of the gland's tissue that are still used in diagnosing the disease later named after him. Although Japanese doctors were unaware of Hashimoto's discovery, because it had been published in a German journal, English and American doctors who read the journal recognized that Hashimoto was describing a distinctive disorder, which they named Hashimoto's thyroiditis. Hashimoto himself continued to study in German and English hospitals until 1914, when his father died and he returned to Japan to take up his father's medical practice.

He specialized in major abdominal surgery after his return to Japan rather than continuing to work on disorders of the thyroid. He was only 53 when he died of typhoid fever in 1934.

distinctive pattern of broken cells and other types of tissue damage that will confirm the diagnosis.

Treatment

Treatment for Hashimoto disease consists of a daily dose of a synthetic form of thyroid hormone known as levothyroxine, sold under the trade names of Synthroid, Levothroid, or Levoxyl. The patient is told that the drug must be taken as directed for the rest of his or her life.

In the early weeks of treatment, the patient will need to see the doctor every six to eight weeks to have their TSH level checked and the dose of medication adjusted. After the doctor is satisfied with the dosage level and the patient's overall health, checkups are done every six to twelve months. The reason for this careful measurement of the medication is that too much levothyroxine increases the risk of osteoporosis in later life or abnormal heart rhythms in the present.

Prognosis

The prognosis for patients with Hashimoto disease is excellent, provided they take their medication as directed. They can usually live a normal life with a normal life expectancy.

The chief risks to health with Hashimoto disease are related to lack of treatment for the disorder. If this type of thyroiditis is not diagnosed and treated, patients are at increased risk of goiter, an enlarged heart, and severe depression. In addition, women with untreated Hashimoto disease have a higher risk of giving birth to babies with cleft palate and other birth defects.

Prevention

There is no known way to prevent Hashimoto disease because the cause is not yet completely understood.

The Future

The incidence of Hashimoto disease is not likely to increase in the foreseeable future. Research of the disorder is likely to focus on two questions: tracking down all the specific genes that may be involved in triggering the disorder; and relating Hashimoto disease to other autoimmune disorders that have a high female/male sex ratio. Some researchers think that there may be a common factor linking Hashimoto disease to

WORDS TO KNOW

Autoimmune disease: A disease in which the body's immune system attacks its own cells and tissues.

Goiter: A swelling in the neck caused by an enlarged thyroid gland.

Hashitoxicosis: A temporary phase in some patients with Hashimoto disease in which there is too much thyroid hormone in the blood due to leakage from damaged and dying cells in the thyroid gland.

Hyperthyroidism: A disease condition in which the thyroid gland produces too much thyroid hormone.

Hypothyroidism: A disease condition in which the thyroid gland does not produce enough thyroid hormone.

Levothyroxine: The chemical name for the synthetic thyroid hormone given to treat Hashimoto disease.

Metabolism: The chemical changes in living cells in which new materials are taken in and energy is provided for vital processes,

Thyroiditis: Inflammation of the thyroid gland.

lupus, rheumatoid arthritis, and other autoimmune disorders that disproportionately affect women.

SEE ALSO Graves disease; Hypothyroidism

For more information

BOOKS

Skugor, Mario. *Thyroid Disorders: A Cleveland Clinic Guide*. Cleveland, OH: Cleveland Clinic Press, 2006.

PERIODICALS

Angier, Natalie. "Researchers Piecing Together Autoimmune Disease Puzzle." *New York Times*, June 19, 2001. Available online at http://query.nytimes.com/gst/fullpage.html?res=9502E3DD1031F93AA25755-C0A9679C8B63&sec=&spon=&pagewanted=all (accessed April 4, 2008).

Pérez-Peña, Richard. "Cases: Heeding Thyroid's Warnings." *New York Times*, October 7, 2003. Available online at http://query.nytimes.com/gst/fullpage.html?res=980DE0D6133CF934A35753C1A9659C8B63 (accessed April 4, 2008).

WEB SITES

American Thyroid Association (ATA). *Thyroiditis.* http://www.thyroid.org/patients/patient_brochures/thyroiditis.html (accessed April 4, 2008).

Hormone Foundation. *Hormones and You: Hashimoto's Disease.* http://www.hormone.org/Resources/Thyroid/upload/Bilingual_Hashimotos_Disease.pdf (accessed April 4, 2008).

National Women's Health Information Center. *Hashimoto's Thyroiditis.* http://womenshealth.gov/faq/hashimoto.htm (accessed April 4, 2008).
Nemours Foundation. *Thyroid Disorders.* http://kidshealth.org/kid/health_problems/glandshoromones/thyroid.html (accessed April 4, 2008).

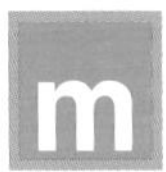

Hay Fever

Definition

Hay fever is a form of allergic rhinitis, or inflammation of the soft tissues lining the nose. It is triggered by plant pollen, most commonly ragweed, tree, or grass pollen in the United States. Hay fever can be either seasonal, meaning that the person has symptoms only during certain periods of the year, or perennial, which means that the person has symptoms all year long. Children are more likely than adults to have perennial hay fever.

Hay fever is often grouped together with eczema and asthma as an atopic disease. Atopy is the medical term for the tendency to develop an allergy. About 20 percent of people with hay fever eventually develop asthma, and some develop eczema as well.

Description

Hay fever is an allergic reaction to tree, grass, or weed pollen that is characterized by a stuffy or runny nose, sneezing, and teary or watery eyes. Some patients also complain of coughing, headaches, fatigue, and drowsiness. Although some patients have relatively mild symptoms that last for only a few weeks and are controlled by medications, others may suffer year round from symptoms and may develop such complications as ear infections or chronic inflammation of the sinuses. The National Institutes of Health (NIH) estimates that hay fever costs the United States about $5.3 billion each year in terms of missed school and work days as well as the direct expenses of diagnosis and treatment.

Also Known As
Allergic rhinitis, rose fever, grass fever

Cause
Allergic reaction to plant or tree pollen

Symptoms
Sneezing, itchy or runny eyes, stuffy nose, coughing

Duration
May be seasonal (a few months per year) or year-round

Demographics

It is estimated that between 20 and 25 percent of Americans have some form of hay fever, although the severity and the specific triggers vary

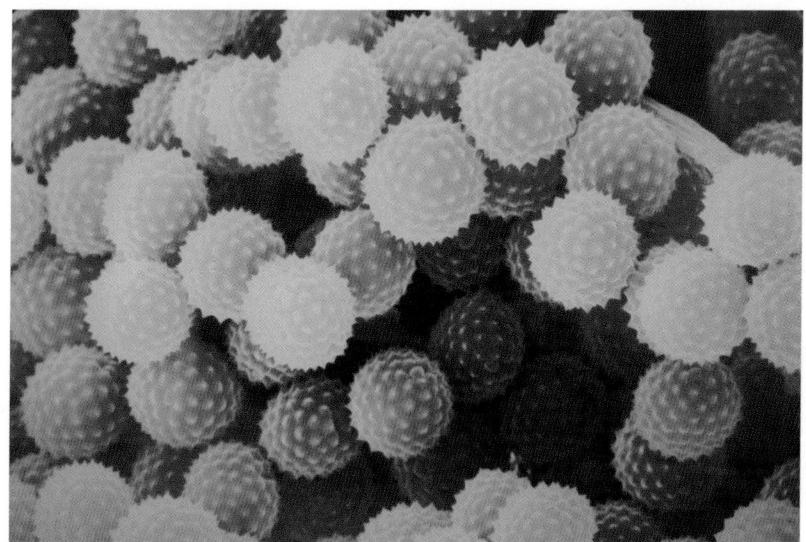

Magnified image of ragweed pollen, a major cause of hay fever. © PHOTOTAKE INC. / ALAMY.

from region to region across the United States. It is difficult to determine whether various races or ethnic groups have different rates of sensitivity to pollen because of the variations in climate across the country and the different types of trees and grasses that are present. In general, the hay fever season is shorter in the northern states and longer in the South, particularly along the East Coast.

About 80 percent of people with hay fever develop it before age twenty, with the average age at onset being eight to eleven years. Some doctors think that as many as 40 percent of children may suffer from hay fever at some point in childhood. The symptoms typically become less severe in adult life and may go away completely in some cases.

Boys are more likely than girls to suffer from hay fever. Among adults, however, men and women are equally likely to have symptoms.

Causes and Symptoms

The basic cause of hay fever is exposure to plant pollen. The most common sources are plants or trees that are pollinated by the wind rather than by bees or other insects. The reason for this difference is that wind-borne pollen particles are lighter and more likely to remain in the air than the heavier pollen grains produced by flowering plants that depend on insects to carry the pollen from one plant to another. For example, ragweed pollen has been found as high as 2 miles (3.2 kilometers) in the

Tips for Minimizing Pollen Exposure

Although it is impossible to avoid airborne pollen completely, people who suffer from hay fever may be helped by the following suggestions:

- Check local news sources for the daily pollen count, and stay indoors during the early morning and evening hours; pollen levels are higher at those times.
- Use a face mask designed to filter out pollen if it is necessary to go outdoors.
- Do not dry clothes outdoors.
- Keep windows closed in the house and car; use the air conditioner to control temperature.
- Take a shower after outdoor activity; wash hair each night to remove pollen before going to bed.
- Minimize exposure to other substances that irritate the nasal passages, including cigarette smoke, chlorine bleach and other household chemicals, insect sprays, wet paint, and strong perfumes.
- Have someone who does not get hay fever do yard work.
- Avoid large fields and grassy areas if possible.
- Consider vacationing at the beach or on a cruise rather than in an inland area.

One approach that usually does not work, however, is relocating to a different part of the country. People who move to get away from a specific type of pollen often develop new allergies within a few years in the new location.

atmosphere and as far as 400 miles (644 kilometers) out to sea. Common sources of airborne pollen include:

- Trees: birch, alder, willow, oak, ash, elm, poplar, olive, hazel, mountain cedar, and horse chestnut.
- Grasses: ryegrass, Kentucky bluegrass, redtop grass, Johnson grass, Bermuda grass, and timothy.
- Weeds: ragweed, sorrel, mugwort, sagebrush, plantain, and nettle.

Hot, dry, and windy days are more likely to trigger the symptoms of hay fever than cool or rainy days. The pollen count is also likelier to be higher early in the morning than later in the day.

When the pollen from these plants enters the patient's airway and the tissues that line the eyelids, immune system reacts to the pollen as an allergen, a substance that triggers an allergy. The process releases a compound called histamine. Histamine is responsible for the runny nose, itchy and watery eyes, and sneezing that characterize hay fever.

Diagnosis

The diagnosis of hay fever is based on a combination of the patient's history and skin tests for specific allergens. It is sometimes difficult to tell at first whether a person has hay fever or the common cold, but in general, the symptoms of a cold get better in a few days or a week. When taking the patient's history, the doctor will ask when the symptoms began; whether the symptoms appear during the same time of the year; whether the symptoms are continuous or off and on; and whether they are worse at specific times of day. In some cases the patient has already noticed that certain activities or places seem to trigger the symptoms.

To perform a skin test, the doctor takes a small amount of material extracted from a specific type of pollen and injects it under the patient's skin or applies it to a tiny scratch on the arm or upper back. If the patient is allergic to the material, his or her skin will develop a wheal, or flat-topped reddish swelling. The skin test cannot be used on patients with eczema, however. These patients can be tested for plant allergies by a type of blood test called a radioallergosorbent test (RAST).

Treatment

Treatment of hay fever has three parts: avoiding the specific trigger(s); using medications to relieve such symptoms as itching eyes and a runny nose; and taking allergy shots to reduce one's sensitivity to triggers.

Medications that are often recommended for hay fever include:

- Antihistamines. These are drugs that counteract the effects of histamine in causing the watery eyes and runny nose associated with hay fever. Some are available over the counter, while others require a prescription. The older antihistamines often make people drowsy. Thus, patients who use these should not drive or operate machinery while taking them. The newer antihistamines are more expensive but do not make people drowsy as a side effect.
- Decongestants. These are sprays or tablets that clear up congestion in the nose. Most can be purchased over the counter while others require a prescription. People with high blood pressure should avoid oral decongestants because they can raise blood pressure.
- Nasal corticosteroids. These are sprays that reduce the inflammation of tissues associated with hay fever. They may take about a week to start to work but are safe for long-term use.
- Gargling and rinsing out the nasal passages with salt water. There are over-the-counter nasal sprays available for his purpose, or patients can make their own rinse by adding one-quarter teaspoon of salt to two cups of warm water. Salt water works well to relieve nasal congestion in many people.

Prognosis

The prognosis for hay fever varies. People with mild symptoms usually do well with a combination of antihistamines and decongestants used as needed during pollen season. Between 85 and 90 percent of patients who are treated by desensitization (allergy shots) benefit from this type of therapy. Some patients continue to do well after the shots are stopped but others find that their symptoms return with the next pollen season. In addition, desensitization carries some risk of a severe allergic reaction.

People with hay fever are at increased risk of chronic sinus disorders, nosebleeds, asthma, or ear infections.

Prevention

The best way to prevent hay fever is to avoid things that trigger it. Some techniques for avoiding or minimizing exposure to ragweed and other pollens are listed in the sidebar. Another preventive approach is desensitization, which is also called immunotherapy. In desensitization, patients are given a series of injections of their specific allergen under the skin, with the concentration of allergen in the shots being gradually increased. It takes an average of eight to twelve months for the patient to see results, however, and the injections must be taken for at least three years and sometimes closer to five years.

The Future

Hay fever appears to be increasing in frequency among adults in developed countries, although the reasons for the rise are not yet known. One theory is that adults who get hay fever for the first time were either not exposed to common allergens as children or that they become sensitized to allergens when their immune systems are weakened by a viral infection or pregnancy.

A newer form of treatment for hay fever that shows promise is a vaccine called Pollinex Quattro that was developed in the United Kingdom. Instead of receiving desensitization shots for three to five years, patients using the new vaccine get only four shots—one per week for a month. The vaccine was tested on patients in the United States and Canada as well as Europe in the summer of 2007. Researchers hope that the vaccine could be available as early as 2010 following further clinical trials.

SEE ALSO Asthma; Common cold; Eczema

For more information

BOOKS

Brostoff, Jonathan, and Linda Gamlin. *Hay Fever: The Complete Guide.* Rochester, VT: Healing Arts Press, 2002.

Parker, Steve. *Allergies.* Chicago, IL: Heinemann Library, 2004.

WORDS TO KNOW

Allergen: Any substance that causes an allergic reaction. Pollen is the allergen that triggers hay fever attacks.

Atopy: The medical term for an allergic hypersensitivity that affects parts of the body that are not in direct contact with an allergen. Hay fever, eczema, and asthma are all atopic diseases.

Chronic: Long-term or recurrent.

Desensitization: A form of treatment for hay fever that involves a series of shots containing the allergen to reduce the patient's sensitivity to that particular trigger. Desensitization is also called immunotherapy.

Histamine: A compound that is released during an allergic reaction.

Rhinitis: The medical term for inflammation of the mucous tissues lining the nose. It can be caused by infections or chemical irritants as well as by allergies.

Wheal: A suddenly formed flat-topped swelling of the skin; a welt.

PERIODICALS

Devlin, Kate. "Hayfever Sufferers Given Hope by Vaccine." *Telegraph (UK)*, June 5, 2008. Available online at http://www.telegraph.co.uk/news/uknews/2075443/Hayfever-sufferers-given-hope-by-vaccine.html (accessed June 7, 2008).

Tarkan, Laurie. "For Adults, Allergies Bring a Surprising Twist." *New York Times*, April 18, 2006. Available online at http://query.nytimes.com/gst/fullpage.html?res=9F04E2DB173FF93BA25757C0A9609C8B63&sec=&spon=&pagewanted=2 (accessed June 7, 2008).

WEB SITES

American Academy of Allergy, Asthma, and Immunology (AAAAI). *Tips to Remember: Rhinitis*. Available online at http://www.aaaai.org/patients/publicedmat/tips/rhinitis.stm (updated 2007; accessed June 7, 2008).

American Academy of Family Practice (AAFP). *Allergies: Things You Can Do to Control Your Symptoms*. Available online at http://familydoctor.org/online/famdocen/home/common/allergies/basics/083.html (updated March 2007; accessed June 7, 2008).

American Academy of Otolaryngology—Head and Neck Surgery. *Allergies and Hay Fever*. Available online at http://www.entnet.org/HealthInformation/allergiesHayFever.cfm (accessed June 7, 2008).

LungUSA. *Allergy Map*. Available online at http://www.lungusa.org/site/pp.asp?c=dvLUK9O0E&b=22911 (accessed June 7, 2008). This is a map of the United States (except for Alaska and Hawaii) with colored zones showing when ragweed, tree, and grass pollens are most likely to trigger hay fever.

National Institute of Allergy and Infectious Diseases (NIAID). *Airborne Allergens: Something in the Air*. Available online in PDF format at http://www3.niaid.nih.gov/healthscience/healthtopics/allergicDiseases/PDF/airborne_allergens.pdf (updated April 2003; accessed June 7, 2008).

Nemours Foundation. *All about Allergies*. Available online at http://www.kidshealth.org/parent/medical/allergies/allergy.html (updated May 2007; accessed June 7, 2008).

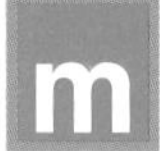

Headache

Definition

A headache is a disorder in which a person feels pain or discomfort somewhere in the face, neck, or scalp. The brain and the skull are not the sources of headache pain because they do not contain pain-sensitive nerve endings. The sources of headache pain are nerve endings in the scalp, face, throat, the muscles of the head, and blood vessels at the base of the brain. When any of these nerve endings are triggered by stress, tension in the muscles, inflammation, or dilation of the blood vessels in the head, the person may experience pain.

Doctors have described over 130 different types of headaches. They can be classified into primary and secondary headaches. Primary headaches are those in which the headache is not caused by an injury, infection, or other disorder, but rather by some type of disturbance in the brain's relationship to the body. They include migraine headaches, tension headaches, cluster headaches, and so-called ordinary headaches.

Secondary headaches are caused by an injury or some other illness. There are at least 300 known causes of secondary headaches. The major types of secondary headaches are post-traumatic headaches, sinus headaches, reactive headaches, and rebound headaches.

It is possible for a person to suffer from more than one type of headache.

Also Known As
Cephalagia, head pain

Cause
Muscle tension, infections, spasms in arteries around the brain, tumors, stroke, injury

Symptoms
Pain in various parts of the scalp, face, or neck; nausea and vomiting; visual disturbances

Duration
Minutes to days

Description

Headache pain can vary in location, severity, duration, and quality (dull, piercing, throbbing, etc.) depending on the cause or type of the headache. The main characteristics of the major types of headaches are described below.

Primary headaches:

- Migraine headaches: Migraine headaches are caused by disturbances in the central nervous system leading to swelling of the blood vessels in the brain and severe pain. The pain affects only one side of the head in 60 percent of cases, and is often accompanied by nausea, vomiting, and extreme sensitivity to light. There are two basic types of migraine: migraine with aura (visual disturbances preceding the pain of the headache) and migraine without aura. The person may be sick for one to two full days.

- Tension headaches: These are characterized by a sensation of tightness or pressure in the head and are often accompanied by muscle tension in the neck. Tension headaches may occur on a daily basis or only at random. They usually last for several hours.
- Cluster headaches: Cluster headaches are sharp and extremely painful headaches that tend to occur several times per day for months and then go away for long periods of time. They are the rarest type of primary headache.
- Ordinary headaches: Some doctors think that ordinary headaches are actually a mild form of migraine. These headaches usually occur at random, are not associated with a head injury or other illness, and usually go away with rest and mild pain relievers.

Secondary headaches:

- Post-traumatic headaches: Post-traumatic headaches occur in as many as 88 percent of people with a closed head injury and 60 percent of people with a whiplash injury. This type of headache is accompanied by pain in the neck and shoulders, dizziness, mood or personality changes, and sleep disturbances.
- Sinus headaches: These are associated with post-nasal drip, sore throat, and a discharge from the nose. The pain of a sinus headache is usually experienced in the front of the face and head, and is usually worse in the morning than later in the day.

When to See the Doctor

Most headaches go away by themselves or with over-the-counter pain relievers in a few hours. Some headaches, however, indicate a serious health problem. Anyone with any of the following symptoms should see their doctor or go to the emergency room at once:

- The headache comes on suddenly and has a violent or explosive quality.
- The headache feels like the worst one the person has ever had.
- The person is experiencing slurred speech, change in vision, problems moving arms or legs, loss of balance, confusion, or memory loss along with the headache.
- The headache is getting worse over a twenty-four-hour period.
- The person has fever, stiff neck, nausea, and vomiting along with the headache.
- The person is over age fifty and the headaches just began.
- The person is losing consciousness or is having convulsions.
- The person suffered a head injury before the headache.
- The headache is so severe that it wakes the person from sleep.
- The headache has lasted longer than a few days.

- Reactive headaches: Reactive headaches are triggered by an irritant in the environment or another illness. There are hundreds of possible triggers, ranging from the weather, pollen, dust, and other allergens, to colds, flu, eyestrain, and stomach upsets.
- Rebound headaches: Rebound headaches are a reaction to overuse of over-the-counter medications for pain relief, decongestants, or muscle relaxants. They can also be caused by withdrawal from caffeine or alcohol.

Demographics

Headaches are a very common problem in the general population. Almost everyone gets an occasional headache, particularly when they are short on sleep, emotionally stressed, have skipped a meal, or are suffering from flu or a cold. Children can get headaches as well as adults; by age six, 31 percent of children have had at least one headache; by the time a child is fifteen, the number has risen to 70 percent. Between 60 and 80 million Americans suffer from frequent headaches but only 30 percent of these people consult a doctor for treatment.

According to the National Institutes of Health (NIH), children in the United States miss 1 million days of school each year because of headaches while adults miss 160 million days of work. Headaches cost the economy an estimated $30 billion each year in medical expenses.

Headaches affect people of all races equally; however, the gender ratio varies depending on the type of headache. Women are three times as likely as men to suffer from migraine headaches, but men are ten times as likely as women to get cluster headaches.

Causes and Symptoms

The basic causes of headaches include disturbances in the central nervous system leading to irritation of the blood vessels in the head; tension in the muscles of the head and neck; infections; allergens and other environmental triggers; overuse of or withdrawal from drugs; lack of sleep; clenching or grinding the teeth; menstruation; depression or anxiety; certain foods; and head injuries.

Less common but dangerous causes of headaches include:

- Brain tumors
- Stroke

- An infection of the brain (encephalitis or meningitis)
- Bursting of a blood vessel in the brain

In addition to the pain of a headache, people may experience nausea, vomiting, diarrhea and other digestive symptoms; dizziness, loss of balance, and visual disturbances; mood and personality changes; extreme tiredness; muscle cramps in the neck and shoulders; inability to concentrate; and extreme sensitivity to light or noise.

Diagnosis

Diagnosing headaches can be complicated because there are so many potential causes and because some people have more than one type of headache. In addition to examining the patient's head, neck, mouth, and throat in the office, most doctors will ask the patient to keep a headache diary, noting the time when a headache occurs, how long it lasts, other symptoms that accompany the headache, the quality and location of the pain, possible triggers, and other illnesses that the patient had at the time.

In some cases the doctor will order a computed tomography (CT) scan or a magnetic resonance imaging (MRI) of the patient's head. If encephalitis or meningitis are suspected, the doctor may order a spinal tap.

Treatment

Treatment depends on the type of headache. Secondary headaches are treated by removing or avoiding the underlying cause, whether a head or whiplash injury, environmental trigger, food allergy, overuse of alcohol or medications, sinus infection, eyestrain, or other problem.

Primary headaches are usually treated by appropriate medications:

- Migraine headaches can be treated either by medications taken before an attack to stop it or reduce its severity, or by medications taken to relieve the headache after it begins. Preventive medications include a group of drugs called triptans; certain antidepressants; and antiepileptic drugs. After the headache starts, the patient may be treated with over-the-counter pain relievers like acetaminophen, naproxen, or ibuprofen, or prescription medications like ergotamine. Most patients with migraine are helped by resting in a quiet darkened room.
- Tension headaches: Usually respond well to over-the-counter pain relievers or to prescription pain relievers containing codeine. Hot showers and rest are also recommended for self-care at home. Some

patients are also helped by biofeedback, relaxation training, yoga, or massage therapy. In some cases the doctor may recommend psychotherapy if the patient's headaches are related to emotional stress.

- Cluster headaches: The triptans are effective in treating cluster headaches in many patients, as is oxygen inhalation. Because cluster headaches often come on very quickly, the triptans are usually given by injection rather than by mouth.
- Ordinary headaches: Usually treated in the same way as tension headaches.

Prognosis

The prognosis for a headache depends on whether it is primary or secondary and its underlying cause or causes. Most ordinary headaches can be treated at home with few long-term side effects or complications. Cluster headaches, recurrent tension headaches, and migraines require long-term follow-up with a doctor. Cluster headaches are more difficult to treat successfully than either migraines or recurrent tension headaches.

Prevention

People can lower their risk of headaches in several ways:

- Getting enough rest, eating a healthful diet without skipping meals, and exercising regularly.
- Taking occasional work or study breaks, particularly if working at a computer or reading for long periods of time.
- Having the eyes checked regularly, particularly if the person wears prescription eyeglasses or contacts.
- Avoiding overuse of over-the-counter pain relievers, decongestants, caffeine, or alcohol.
- Quitting smoking.
- Practicing relaxation techniques, yoga, meditation, or other approaches to stress management.
- Avoiding allergens, foods, or other factors known to trigger headaches whenever possible.

The Future

Headaches are likely to be an ongoing health problem in the general population, if only because they have so many possible causes and

WORDS TO KNOW

Aura: A symptom that precedes migraine headaches in some people. The person may see flashing or zigzag lights, or have other visual disturbances.

Biofeedback: An alternative treatment for headaches (and other conditions) that consists of teaching patients to consciously control their blood pressure, muscle tension, temperature, and other body processes.

Migraine: A type of primary headache characterized by severe pain, nausea and vomiting, and sensitivity to light. It may occur on only one side of the head.

Withdrawal: A collection of signs and symptoms that appear when a drug (including caffeine and nicotine) that a person has used for a long time is suddenly discontinued.

environmental triggers. Research into the causes of migraine headaches has yielded new insights since the late 1990s. Clinical trials include research into the causes of cluster headaches, which are still not well understood; evaluations of newer triptan drugs in treating migraine and cluster headaches; studies of the factors that affect the prognosis for recovery from headaches; studies comparing different types of treatment for rebound headaches; and studies of yoga, acupuncture, massage therapy, and other alternative treatments.

SEE ALSO Alcoholism; Allergies; Brain tumors; Common cold; Concussion; Encephalitis; Influenza; Meningitis; Stroke; Whiplash

For more information

BOOKS

Diamond, Seymour, and Merle Lea Diamond. *A Patient's Handbook of Headache and Migraine.* Newtown, PA: Handbooks in Health Care Co., 2001.

Forshaw, Mark. *Understanding Headaches and Migraines.* Hoboken, NJ: John Wiley and Sons, 2004.

Robbins, Lawrence D., and Susan S. Lang. *Headache Help: A Complete Guide to Understanding Headaches and the Medicines that Relieve Them*, rev. ed. Boston: Houghton Mifflin Co., 2000.

PERIODICALS

Jaret, Peter. "A Hidden Cause of Headache Pain." *New York Times*, May 24, 2008. Available online at http://health.nytimes.com/ref/health/healthguide/esn-headache-ess.html (accessed on August 15, 2008). This is an article about the rebound effect.

WEB SITES

American Academy of Family Physicians (AAFP). *Headaches.* Available online at http://familydoctor.org/online/famdocen/home/tools/symptom/502.html (reviewed 2008; accessed on August 15, 2008). This is a flow chart or diagram intended to help the reader evaluate the symptoms and possible causes of their headache.

National Headache Foundation (NHF). *Headache Topic Sheets*. Available online at http://www.headaches.org/education/Headache_Topic_Sheets (accessed on August 15, 2008). This is a page with links to over a hundred specific topics related to headaches.

National Institute of Neurological Disorders and Stroke (NINDS). *Headache: Hope through Research*. Available online at http://www.ninds.nih.gov/disorders/headache/detail_headache.htm (updated July 31, 2008; accessed on August 15, 2008).

National Pain Foundation. *Help for Headaches*. Available online at http://www.nationalpainfoundation.org/MyTreatment/articles/Headache_Overview.asp (updated March 28, 2008; accessed on August 15, 2008).

Nemours Foundation. *Headaches*. Available online at http://kidshealth.org/parent/general/aches/headache.html (updated March 2006; accessed on August 15, 2008).

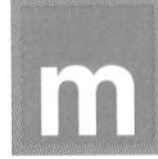

Hearing Loss

Definition

Hearing loss is a disorder in which a person begins to lose the ability to hear in one or both ears. It may come on suddenly or develop slowly over a period of years; it may be temporary or permanent, and vary in severity from mild hearing loss to total deafness. There are many possible causes of hearing loss ranging from birth defects and ear infections (common causes in children) to exposure to high levels of noise in the workplace and the aging process (common causes in adults).

There are two major categories of hearing loss, defined by whether the loss results from problems in the structures of the outer or middle ear or whether it results from damage to the hair cells of the inner ear. The first type is called conductive hearing loss (CHL) and the second type is called sensorineural hearing loss (SNHL). CHL is often reversible while SNHL is not. People who have both CHL and SNHL are said to have mixed hearing loss.

Also Known As
Deafness, hearing impairment, being hard of hearing

Cause
Head injuries, birth defects, infections, long-term noise exposure, medications, aging

Symptoms
Difficulty hearing conversations, radio, or television; difficulty learning to talk (children)

Duration
Days to years

Description

Conductive hearing loss occurs when sound waves cannot move through the structures of the outer and middle ear. Ordinarily, sound

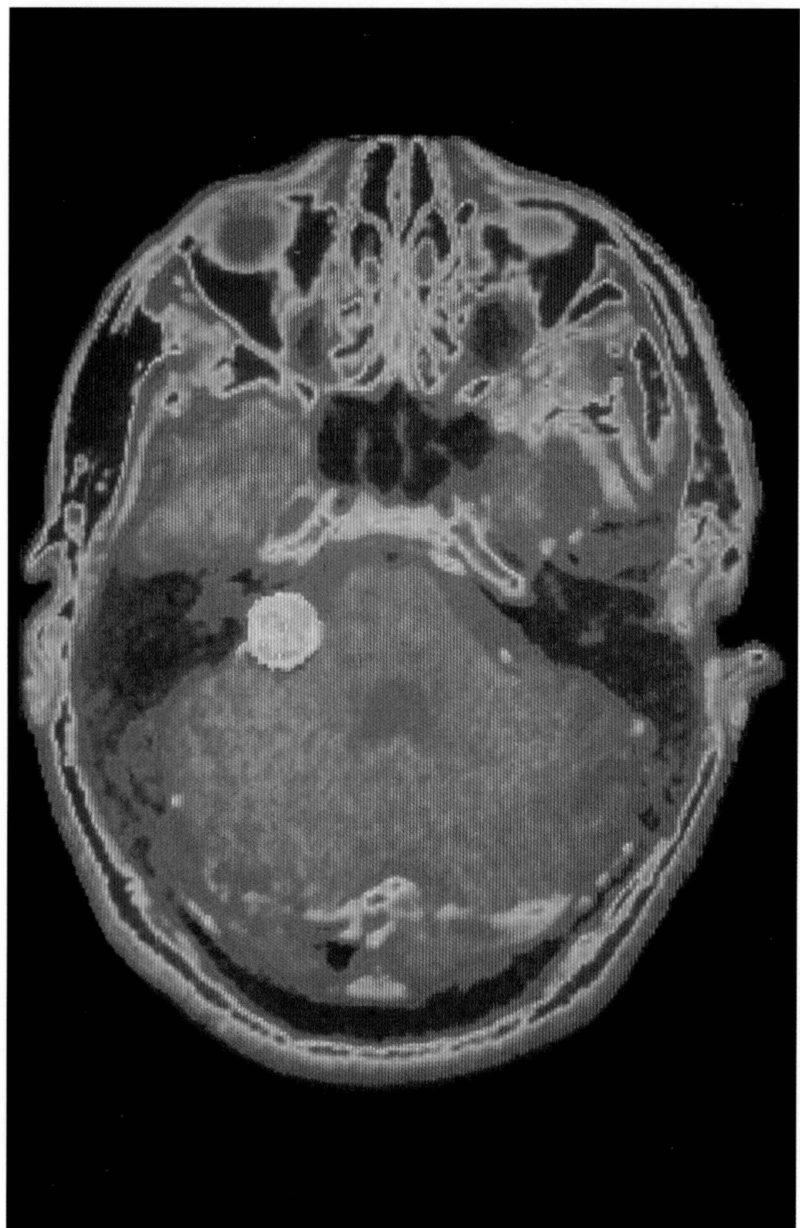

Brain image of a patient with benign tumor (green circle) that results in progressive deafness. MEHAU KULYK / PHOTO RESEARCHERS, INC.

waves are funneled into the ear by the pinna, the visible part of the outer ear. The sound waves then pass through the ear canal, where they cause the eardrum and three tiny bones called ossicles to vibrate. The vibrations of the ossicles cause the liquid inside a snail-shaped structure

Did You Know?

Doctors have found that unprotected exposure to sounds above 85–90 decibels (dB) for long periods of time can harm a person's hearing. Here is a list of the decibel levels of various common sounds:

- Weakest sound that can be heard: 0 dB.
- Soft whisper: 30 dB.
- Normal conversation: 60–70 dB.
- Piano music: 60–70 dB.
- Telephone dial tone: 80 dB.
- Freeway traffic: 85–90 dB.
- Trombone or French horn music: 90–110 dB.
- Subway train 200 feet away: 95–100 dB.
- Power saw: 110 dB.
- Rock music: 115–120 dB.
- Pneumatic drill: 125 dB. This is the level at which most people feel pain in the ear.
- Gun blast, jet engine: 140 dB. This is the loudest recommended noise level even with hearing protection. Even short-term exposure can cause permanent hearing loss.
- Loud rock concert: 150 dB.
- Death of nerve endings and other hearing-related tissues: 180 dB.
- Loudest possible sound: 194 dB.

called the cochlea to move. The movement of the liquid in turn causes hair cells inside the cochlea to respond. The hair cells convert movement into electrical signals that are then relayed to the brain via the auditory nerve. Conductive hearing loss can occur when the ear canal is blocked by wax or a foreign object, the ear drum is punctured, the ossicles are dislocated, or the ear canal is swollen shut due to infection.

Sensorineural hearing loss is caused by damage to the hair cells in the cochlea or to the nerves that conduct hearing signals to the brain. This damage can be caused by infections (measles, mumps, rubella, influenza, or mononucleosis); by trauma; by diabetes and other disorders that affect the circulatory system; by cancer drugs and some other medications; or by a tumor affecting the auditory nerve. SNHL is sometimes associated with such problems as tinnitus (ringing in the ears) or dizziness.

Demographics

Hearing loss is a common problem in the general American population, particularly in older adults. According to the Centers for Disease Control and Prevention (CDC), most people over the age of twenty begin to develop a mild hearing loss. A third of adults over the age of seventy have trouble hearing. Hearing loss is more common in older men than in older women.

About 24,000 children (three in every 1,000) are born with hearing loss in the United States each year. Causes include genetic disorders, infections before birth (particularly rubella), absence of ossicles or other abnormalities in the shape or inner structures of the ear, or low birth weight.

Hearing loss is equally common in all racial and ethnic groups, as far as is known.

Causes and Symptoms

The most common causes of conductive hearing loss are infections, trauma to the outer or middle ear, a buildup of earwax in the ear canal, foreign bodies in the ear, or dislocation of the ossicles caused by a blow to the ear.

The causes of sensorineural hearing loss include noise-induced hearing loss (NIHL), which causes trauma to the acoustic nerve; changes in atmospheric pressure inside the ear during deep-sea diving; fracture of the bone at the side and base of the skull; drugs that damage the nerves involved in hearing (cancer drugs, some antibiotics, diuretics, and aspirin or ibuprofen); diabetes; tumors on the auditory nerve; infectious diseases (mumps, measles, syphilis, meningitis, mononucleosis, and herpes); and aging.

The symptoms of hearing loss depend partly on the person's age. A baby who has not yet learned to talk or a child with hearing problems may have the following symptoms:

- Not responding to cooing or conversation from the parents or other family members
- Does not react to sudden loud noises
- Has trouble with certain word sounds
- Does not repeat words or phrases used by others
- Uses gestures to communicate with others
- Seems to watch people's faces for clues to understanding what they are saying
- Has trouble paying attention in school
- Turns up the radio or television louder than other members of the family

In adults, the symptoms of hearing loss may include:

- Problems hearing over the telephone
- Having trouble following conversations, particularly if two or more people are talking
- Having to ask others to repeat what they have just said
- Having difficulty hearing higher-pitched sounds, such as the voices of women and children
- Failing to hear the doorbell or telephone ring
- Having difficulty telling the direction of a sound

Diagnosis

Diagnosing hearing problems in babies or toddlers is critical because the period from birth to three years of age is when children learn to use language. Hearing difficulties during this period can affect a child's ability to speak normally. To test hearing in infants and small children, an audiologist (hearing professional) can perform a variety of tests.

In adults, the doctor will examine the ear canal for signs of infection, a foreign object, or damage to the ear drum. A primary care doctor can test each ear separately with a tuning fork to check for conductive hearing loss, but the patient may be referred to an audiologist for more detailed measurement of the type and extent of hearing loss.

Treatment

Treatment for hearing loss depends on the cause. Infections of the outer and middle ear can be treated with medicated ear drops or oral antibiotics. Earwax and foreign bodies in the ear are removed by suction, forceps, or flushing the ear canal with water. If the earwax has hardened, the doctor may use special drops to soften it and have the patient return a few days later to have it removed. Hearing loss caused by medications is treated by discontinuing the medication.

A tumor of the auditory nerve will usually be removed by a neurosurgeon or an otolaryngologist (a doctor who specializes in ear, nose, and throat disorders). Patients with sensorineural hearing loss are also usually referred to ear, nose, and throat specialists for evaluation and treatment.

Patients whose hearing loss is caused by exposure to high levels of noise in their workplace will be advised to wear earplugs or other protective equipment. Well-fitted ear plugs can reduce noise level by about 25 dB. In extreme cases, the patient may be advised to switch jobs.

Conductive hearing loss can be treated by hearing aids, which are electronic devices that fit in or behind the ear and amplify sounds. A recent variation on traditional hearing aids is the bone-implanted hearing aid or BAHA. A BAHA is implanted in the patient's skull by a neurosurgeon. It consists of a titanium post that allows a sound processor to be attached outside the skull. The processor transmits sound waves to the titanium implant, which transfers the sound vibrations to the skull and inner ear. BAHAs are recommended for patients who cannot wear hearing aids inside the ear or for those with one-sided hearing loss.

Another newer treatment for severe sensorineural hearing loss is the cochlear implant. A cochlear implant is an electronic device that is inserted in the inner ear by a surgeon and connected to a device worn outside the ear. Unlike a traditional hearing aid, a cochlear implant does not make sounds louder or clearer. Instead it works by stimulating the auditory nerve directly and bypassing damaged hair cells in the cochlea. Cochlear implants can be used only in adults or children over the age of twelve.

Prognosis

The prognosis of hearing loss depends on the cause and type. CHL is often reversible; typically, patients who suffer conductive hearing loss as a result of a plug of earwax or a foreign body in the ear, an infection of the outer or middle ear, or a ruptured eardrum will find that their hearing returns to normal after treatment.

Hearing loss caused by a medication may or may not improve after the drug is stopped. There is no proven treatment that can restore hearing other than discontinuing the drug.

Hearing loss caused by meningitis, tumors of the auditory nerve, and aging is usually permanent.

Prevention

Hereditary hearing loss cannot be prevented, but there are ways that other people can lower their risk of hearing loss as they get older:

- Avoid using several noisy machines at the same time.
- Learn to enjoy music, television, or radio programs at a moderate sound level.
- Avoid going to loud rock concerts on a frequent basis. Listening to rock music is a common cause of sensorineural hearing loss in teenagers and young adults.
- Wear earplugs when operating noisy equipment or when exposed to loud background noise for long periods of time. Earplugs can mean the difference between a safe and a dangerous level of noise.
- If work or commuting involves exposure to high noise levels, choose quiet activities for recreation or leisure time.
- See a doctor if hearing is lost suddenly or if there is pain, dizziness, or ringing in the ears.

WORDS TO KNOW

Audiologist: A health care professional who is specially trained to evaluate hearing disorders.

Cochlea: A snail-shaped fluid-filled chamber in the inner ear.

Decibel (dB): A unit of measurement for expressing the relative intensity of sounds.

Hair cells: Special cells in the cochlea that convert the movement of the fluid inside the cochlea into electrical signals that travel to the brain via the auditory nerve.

Ossicles: A group of three small bones in the middle ear that transmit sound waves to the cochlea.

Pinna: The visible part of the outer ear.

Tinnitus: The medical term for ringing in the ears.

The Future

Hearing loss is a growing concern to public health doctors because there is evidence that it is a growing problem in the United States, particularly among younger adults. One study completed in 2008 estimated that as many as 29 million Americans have at least partial hearing loss.

SEE ALSO Brain tumors; Ear infection; Measles; Rubella

For more information

BOOKS

Olsen, Wayne, ed. *Mayo Clinic on Hearing*. Rochester, MN: Mayo Clinic, 2003.

Pryor, Kimberley Jane. *Hearing*. Philadelphia: Chelsea Clubhouse Books, 2004.

Waldman, Debby. *Your Child's Hearing Loss: What Parents Need to Know*. New York: Perigee Books, 2005.

PERIODICALS

"Aiding Hearing Loss." *New York Times*, September 26, 2006. Available online at http://video.on.nytimes.com/index.jsp?fr_story=22877bf669006281649b8d4ccaeed977b66fa46b (accessed on August 18, 2008). This is a three-minute video about the technological advances in hearing aids since the 1990s.

WEB SITES

American Academy of Otolaryngology—Head and Neck Surgery. *Hearing Loss*. Available online at http://www.entnet.org/HealthInformation/Hearing-Loss.cfm (updated January 2008; accessed on August 18, 2008). This page includes a brief 15-item questionnaire to help readers evaluate their need for a professional hearing test.

Centers for Disease Control and Prevention (CDC). *Hearing Loss*. Available online at http://www.cdc.gov/ncbddd/dd/hi3.htm (updated October 29, 2004; accessed on August 18, 2008).

How Stuff Works. *Hearing*. Available online at http://www.howstuffworks.com/hearing.htm# (accessed on August 18, 2008). This is a short animation that describes the basic structures of the ear and how they work.

KidsHealth. *What's Hearing Loss?* Available online at http://kidshealth.org/kid/health_problems/sight/hearing_impairment.html (updated June 2006; accessed on August 18, 2008).

National Institute on Deafness and Other Communication Disorders (NIDCD). *Noise-Induced Hearing Loss*. Available online at http://www.nidcd.nih.gov/health/hearing/noise.asp (updated May 2007; accessed on August 18, 2008).

National Institutes of Health Senior Health. *Hearing Loss*. Available online at http://nihseniorhealth.gov/hearingloss/toc.html (updated March 13, 2007; accessed on August 18, 2008).

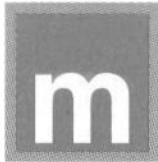

Heart Attack

Definition

A heart attack, also called a myocardial infarction or MI, is a potentially fatal health crisis caused by a loss of blood supply to the heart muscle. If normal blood flow is not restored within a few minutes, the tissue begins to die from lack of oxygen. Treatment should be started as soon as possible to prevent permanent damage to the heart.

Heart attacks are not the same thing as heart failure. Heart failure is a condition in which the heart cannot pump enough blood to meet the needs of the rest of the body. It usually develops slowly over a period of years and produces early symptoms like loss of energy or fluid buildup in the feet and ankles rather than sudden chest pain. A heart attack can, however, lead to heart failure.

Also Known As
Myocardial infarction, MI

Cause
Death of heart tissue due to loss of blood supply

Symptoms
Chest pain, shortness of breath, sweating, nausea

Duration
Several hours

Description

The classic symptoms of a heart attack are pain in the chest, shortness of breath, nausea, and breaking out in a cold sweat. The patient may feel the pain as pressure or squeezing, a sensation of fullness or tightness, a heavy weight on the chest, or a mild or strong ache in the center of the

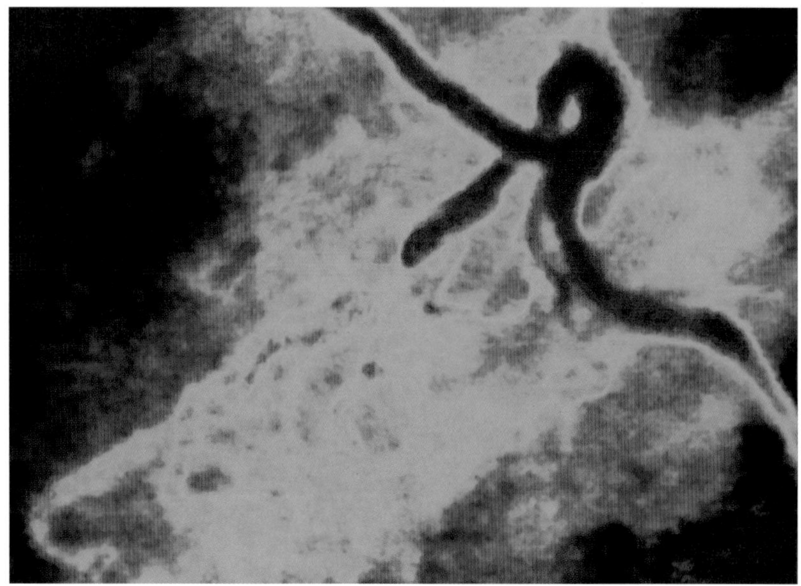

Image showing a blockage in a coronary artery, which resulted in a heart attack. JAMES CAVALLINI / PHOTO RESEARCHERS, INC.

chest. The pain may move from one part of the body to another, or extend from the chest to the jaw, arms, neck, or back. The person may also feel dizzy or lightheaded. The pain lasts for twenty minutes or longer, or it goes away briefly and then returns.

Not everyone with an MI has these classic symptoms. Some people may have a tight feeling only in the arms or upper back, feel mild indigestion or clammy skin, or may have trouble breathing. Women, people with diabetes, and the elderly are more likely than men to have mild or vague symptoms that can be easily missed; these are sometimes called silent heart attacks. Silent heart attacks are particularly dangerous because they are easy to ignore.

Demographics

Heart attacks primarily affect adults. About 1.5 million Americans have heart attacks each year, and about half of them die within a year. Coronary artery disease, the major cause of heart attacks, is the leading killer of both men and women in the United States. Heart attacks are increasing worldwide, including the developing countries.

In the United States, heart attacks affect all races and ethnic groups equally.

Risk factors for heart attacks include:

- Lifestyle issues. People who smoke, consume large amounts of alcohol, or are physically inactive are at increased risk of heart attacks.
- Cocaine use. Cocaine causes blood vessels to tighten, thus potentially cutting off blood supply to the heart. Heart attacks in young adults are often caused by cocaine abuse.
- Family history of heart disease.
- Age. The risk of a heart attack increases after age sixty.
- Sex. Men are more likely to have heart attacks than women up to age seventy, when both sexes have an equal risk.
- High blood pressure and high blood cholesterol levels.
- Obesity.
- Diabetes.
- High levels of emotional stress.

What to Do about a Heart Attack

A person having a heart attack needs to get help *as soon as possible*. If someone is having the symptoms of a heart attack:

- Call 911 *within five minutes* if possible.
- Call the doctor even if the symptoms go away in five minutes.
- Call for an ambulance to go to the hospital; do not take a private car because that will delay treatment.
- Take a nitroglycerin pill (or give one to the patient) if the doctor has prescribed this type of medicine.

Many people put off seeking help when they notice the warning signs because they are embarrassed to ask for help, do not want to cause trouble for other family members, or do not think their symptoms are serious. Doctors agree that it is much better to go to the hospital and find out that the symptoms have another cause than to wait too long and risk dying of a heart attack. According to the National Heart, Lung, and Blood Institute (NHLBI), about half the people who die from heart attacks die within an hour of their first symptoms and before they reach the hospital.

Causes and Symptoms

Heart attacks are caused by the loss of blood supply to the heart muscle, a condition known as ischemia. In about 90 percent of cases, blockage of the arteries that carry blood to the heart results from atherosclerosis, hardening of the arteries due to the formation of plaques along the walls of the blood vessel. Plaques are composed of a fatty material made up of dead white cells and cholesterol. If a plaque in one of the arteries supplying the heart ruptures, it can cause a blood clot to form in the artery and block it, thus starving the heart of blood.

The remaining 10 percent of heart attacks are caused by sudden spasms in the coronary arteries that shut down the flow of blood to the heart muscle. These spasms may result from cocaine use, a sudden emotional shock, or an abnormality in the shape of the coronary artery.

The major symptoms of a heart attack are:

- Pain in the chest, which may be experienced as an ache, tightness, weight, or a squeezing sensation. The pain may move to the back, neck, arms, or jaw
- Nausea and vomiting
- Shortness of breath
- Breaking out in a heavy cold sweat

Other symptoms of a heart attack may include lightheadedness or dizziness, intense anxiety, coughing, or a feeling that the heart is racing.

Diagnosis

Most people having a heart attack will be taken to a hospital emergency room, where they will be asked to describe their symptoms. These questions help the doctor to rule out panic disorder, which is a type of anxiety disorder that can cause people to think they are having a heart attack. In addition to taking the patient's personal and family history of risk factors for a heart attack, the doctor will also take the patient's temperature, blood pressure, and pulse. Listening to the patient's lungs and heartbeat through a stethoscope can help to rule out pneumonia or other diseases that might cause chest pain or difficulty breathing.

The next step is diagnostic tests, which include:

- Electrocardiogram (ECG or EKG). An ECG or EKG measures the heart's electrical activity. Injured heart muscle makes unusual patterns or tracings on the paper printout produced by the ECG machine. If only a small amount of the heart muscle has been affected, the ECG may not show any abnormal patterns.
- Blood tests. These are done to confirm the diagnosis of a heart attack or to make sure that the electrocardiogram did not miss a small heart attack. Injured heart muscle leaks small amounts of enzymes into the bloodstream, which can be detected in a blood test. The emergency room doctor may repeat this blood test after several hours because it takes time for these enzymes to show up in the patient's blood.
- Chest x ray. A chest x ray may be done to see whether the patient's lungs are normal.
- Coronary angiography. Coronary angiography is a type of x-ray study in which the doctor threads a long thin tube called a catheter

into the heart through an artery in the arm or upper thigh. A dye that will show up on x ray is injected into the bloodstream through the catheter. This test allows the doctor to find the location of the blockage in the coronary artery.

Treatment

Treatment of a heart attack begins before the diagnosis is confirmed. The emergency room doctor will give the patient oxygen to help with breathing, aspirin to prevent further blood clotting, nitroglycerin to speed up the blood flow through the coronary arteries, and morphine or another pain reliever to make the patient comfortable.

The next step is the administration of clot-busting and blood-thinning drugs. These drugs can improve the patient's chances of survival and reduce the long-term damage to the heart. The patient may also be given beta-blockers, a group of drugs that slow down the heart rate and lower blood pressure; statins, drugs that lower blood cholesterol levels; or medicines to treat abnormal heart rhythms, which often develop after a heart attack.

In some cases the patient may need surgery. The two operations that are most commonly performed are coronary artery bypass surgery and coronary angioplasty. In bypass surgery, the surgeon takes a piece of a healthy artery from another part of the patient's body and sews it in place to go around a blocked coronary artery. This procedure will restore normal blood flow to the heart. In a coronary angioplasty, the surgeon inserts a catheter with a special balloon tip into the coronary artery. When the catheter is in the proper position, the balloon is expanded, which reopens the blocked artery. The surgeon will then insert a stent, which is a tube made of metal mesh, to keep the artery open.

Patients who survive their heart attack usually undergo rehabilitation after they leave the hospital. Rehabilitation includes lifestyle changes and psychological counseling as well as medications to keep the heart healthy.

Prognosis

The prognosis for recovery from a heart attack depends on how quickly the patient is diagnosed and treated as well as his or her age and overall health. About 30 percent of people do not survive their first heart attack; another 5–10 percent die within a year after the event. About half of patients diagnosed with a heart attack will need to be rehospitalized within a year.

A person who lives through the first two hours after the attack is likely to survive but may have complications like heart failure or blood clots in the lungs. Patients who do not have complications may recover completely.

Prevention

People who have already had a heart attack can lower their risk of a second by taking a daily aspirin, other blood-thinning medications, cholesterol-lowering medications, beta-blockers, or other drugs that the doctor may prescribe to lower the strain on their heart muscle.

People who have not yet had a heart attack can lower their risk by:

- Quitting smoking or not starting in the first place.
- Getting regular medical checkups. This precaution is important because risk factors for heart attacks like high blood pressure, high cholesterol levels, and diabetes have no symptoms in their early stages.
- Avoiding using cocaine and drinking large quantities of alcohol.
- Keeping one's weight at a healthy level and getting regular exercise.
- Controlling blood pressure.
- Learning how to manage emotional stress.
- Eating a low-fat diet rich in fruits and vegetables.

The Future

People are much more likely to survive heart attacks than they were in the 1960s because of the introduction of clot-busting drugs and improvements in heart surgery. New drugs to treat heart attacks are currently being studied as well as the effectiveness of using bone marrow or stem cells to help repair injured heart tissue.

SEE ALSO Coronary artery disease; Hypercholesterolemia; Hypertension; Panic disorder; Stroke

For more information

BOOKS

Chung, Edward K. *100 Questions and Answers about Heart Attack and Related Cardiac Problems*. Boston: Jones and Bartlett Publishers, 2004.

WORDS TO KNOW

Atherosclerosis: Stiffening or hardening of the arteries caused by the formation of plaques within the arteries.

Cholesterol: A fatty substance produced naturally by the body that is found in the membranes of all body cells and is carried by the blood.

Ischemia: Loss of blood supply to a tissue or organ resulting from the blockage of a blood vessel.

Plaque: A deposit of cholesterol along the inside wall of an artery.

Stem cell: A type of unspecialized cell that can reproduce itself and differentiate into different types of specialized cells. Stem cells act as a repair system for the body.

Phibbs, Brendan. *The Human Heart: A Basic Guide to Heart Disease*, 2nd ed. Philadelphia: Lippincott Williams and Wilkins, 2007.

Rimmerman, Curtis Mark. *Heart Attack: A Cleveland Clinic Guide*. Cleveland, OH: Cleveland Clinic Press, 2006.

PERIODICALS

Farrell, Patrick, Gina Kolata, and Erik Olsen. "Heart Disease, the No.1 Killer." *New York Times*, March 2007. Available online at http://video.on.nytimes.com/index.jsp?fr_story=691db69642099ef35fdca7aa0d9a8bc7365db79e (accessed on September 17, 2008). This is an online video that takes about four and a half minutes to play.

WEB SITES

American Heart Association HeartHub. *Heart Attack*. Available online at http://www.hearthub.org/hearthub/hc-heart-attack.htm (accessed on September 17, 2008).

eMedicine Health. *Heart Attack*. Available online at http://www.emedicinehealth.com/heart_attack/article_em.htm#Heart%20Attack%20Causes (accessed on September 16, 2008).

KidsHealth. *Heart Disease*. Available online at http://kidshealth.org/kid/grownup/conditions/heart_disease.html (updated February 2007; accessed on September 17, 2008).

National Heart, Lung, and Blood Institute (NHLBI). *Act in Time to Heart Attack Signs*. Available online at http://www.nhlbi.nih.gov/actintime/video.htm (accessed on September 17, 2008). This is a 13-minute video about the warning signs of a heart attack and the importance of getting help quickly.

National Heart, Lung, and Blood Institute (NHLBI). *What Is a Heart Attack?* Available online at http://www.nhlbi.nih.gov/health/dci/Diseases/HeartAttack/HeartAttack_WhatIs.html (updated March 2008; accessed on September 16, 2008).

Heart Diseases

Heart diseases are a group of disorders that affect the heart's ability to pump enough oxygenated blood to the rest of the body to meet its needs. Some heart diseases are caused by birth defects that slow down the flow of blood or change the path of the blood's flow between the heart and the lungs. Other heart diseases are caused by infectious diseases like rheumatic fever, which can cause an inflammation of the valves in the heart. Still others are caused by lifestyle choices like alcoholism, smoking, or failure to get treated for such conditions as diabetes or high blood pressure.

Heart diseases may involve damage to the heart muscle itself, damage to the valves inside the heart, or damage to the arteries that supply the heart. Partial or complete blockage of one of these arteries is the most common heart disease in the United States and can lead to a heart attack.

Heart diseases are the leading cause of death in North America and a major cause of disability. Almost 700,000 people die of heart disease in the United States each year, according to the Centers for Disease Control and Prevention (CDC). That figure represents 29 percent of all American deaths.

SEE ALSO Congenital heart disease; Coronary artery disease; Heart attack; Heart failure; Hypercholesterolemia; Hypertension; Rheumatic fever

Heart Failure

Definition

Heart failure is a condition in which the heart cannot pump enough blood to meet the body's needs. A healthy heart can pump out 60 percent of the blood it receives in one beat; a failing heart pumps only 40 percent or less. Heart failure is not the same thing as a heart attack or cardiac arrest. Heart failure may develop either suddenly, in which case it is called acute heart failure, or slowly over a period of time, in which case it is called chronic heart failure.

Though most cases of heart failure involve both sides of the heart, it can be classified as left-sided or right-sided heart failure, depending on which side of the heart is affected. Left-sided heart failure is more common. In left-sided heart failure, the heart cannot pump enough oxygenated blood from the lungs to the rest of the body, leading to fluid buildup in the lungs. This buildup is called congestion, which is why heart failure is sometimes called congestive heart failure. The patient typically feels short of breath with left-sided heart failure. He or she may tire easily with even small amounts of exercise and have trouble breathing at night when lying flat.

In right-sided heart failure, the heart does not pump enough blood to the lungs to be oxygenated. As a result, fluid may collect in the patient's feet, ankles, and abdomen, causing swelling in the feet and ankles. In some cases the liver also becomes enlarged, and the veins in the patient's neck swell up.

Description

Heart failure can occur in children or adolescents but is usually a disorder of adults. In most cases the symptoms develop slowly over a period of months and years and are often attributed to aging. As the heart muscle gradually weakens—often as the result of a disease like diabetes or long-term high blood pressure, damage caused by a heart attack, or a congenital abnormality of one of the heart valves—the heart works harder to meet the body's needs for the oxygen and nutrients carried by the blood. As the heart becomes less efficient, the person often feels tired or lacking in energy. Heart failure is often not diagnosed until the person begins to develop fluid buildup in their feet or legs, lungs, abdomen, or liver.

As the heart muscle is weakened, the heart tries to make up for its loss of strength in one or more of three ways. It may enlarge, which allows it to fill with more blood and so have more blood to pump to other parts of the body. Second, it may acquire more muscle mass, which allows it to pump blood more forcefully, at least for a time. Third, the heart may simply speed up and pump faster.

In addition to the heart's attempts to make up for its growing weakness, the body may also respond, either by narrowing its veins and arteries in order to maintain blood pressure, or by redirecting blood away

Also Known As
Congestive heart failure, cardiac failure, CHF

Cause
Inability of the heart to pump enough blood to supply the rest of the body

Symptoms
Swelling of feet, ankles, or abdomen; shortness of breath; weakness; rapid or irregular heartbeat

Duration
Months to years

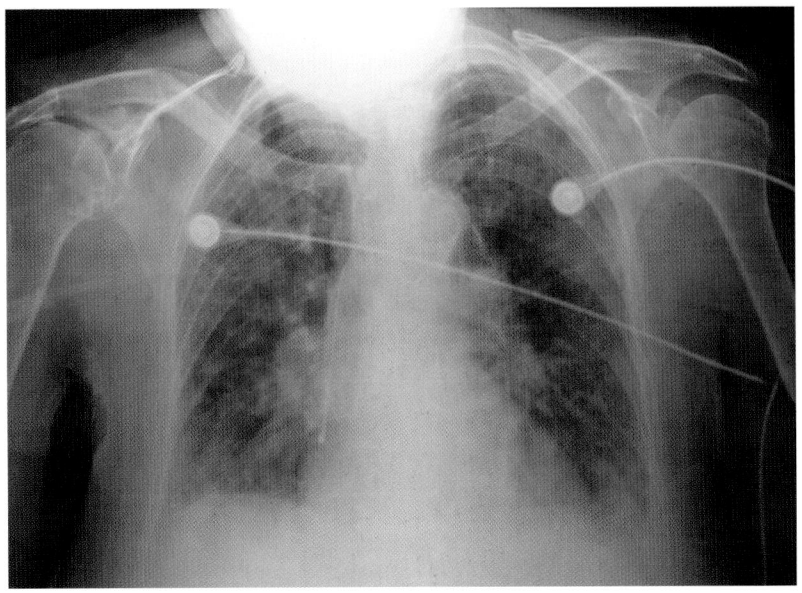

X ray showing congestive heart failure. The heart is enlarged, and there is excess fluid in the lungs. © PHOTOTAKE INC. / ALAMY.

from less vital parts of the body to the brain and heart, which are the most vital organs. These responses help to explain why some people can go on for years without being aware that their heart has lost some of its ability to function.

Demographics

Heart failure is a common disorder in the general American population, particularly among older adults. According to the Centers for Disease Control and Prevention (CDC), about 5 million people in the United States were living with heart failure in 2008, with about 550,000 new cases diagnosed annually. More than 287,000 people die each year from heart failure in the United States. The disorder costs the country $30 billion each year in direct health care costs.

Heart failure is more common among people over 65 than among younger adults. It is the most common reason for hospitalization for patients on Medicare. Among children, congenital (inborn) heart defects are the most common reason for heart failure.

Other risk factors for heart failure include:

- Sex. Men are more likely than women to develop heart failure; however, among adults over the age of 75, more women than men have the condition.

- Race. African Americans are more likely than members of other races to develop heart failure, to develop it at younger ages, to get worse faster, and to die from heart failure.
- Obesity. Excess weight puts a strain on the heart muscle.
- Diabetes. Diabetes increases a person's risk of coronary artery disease and high blood pressure.
- History of coronary artery disease (narrowing of the arteries) or high blood pressure. Coronary artery disease lowers the supply of oxygen to the heart muscle.
- Virus infections that may have weakened the heart.
- Heart attack. A heart attack weakens the heart's ability to pump blood. According to the CDC, 22 percent of men with heart attacks and 46 percent of women will develop heart failure within six years of the heart attack.
- Alcohol abuse. Too much alcohol can weaken the heart muscle.
- Sleep apnea. Sleep apnea lowers the supply of oxygen to the blood during the person's sleep time and increases the risk of developing irregular heart rhythms as well as weakening the heart muscle.
- Kidney disease. Disorders of the kidneys increase the risk of heart failure because they lead to fluid retention and high blood pressure.

Causes and Symptoms

The causes of heart failure include a number of factors that can weaken the heart's ability to pump blood, ranging from congenital defects in the structure of the heart to infections, lifestyle choices, or other diseases and disorders in later life.

The most common symptoms of heart failure are:

- Shortness of breath. The person may have trouble sleeping unless propped up on pillows, or may wake up suddenly feeling short of breath.
- Persistent coughing or wheezing, or coughing up bloody mucus. This symptom is caused by fluid building up in the lungs.
- Swelling of the feet, ankles, or abdomen. The patient may gain several pounds of weight very suddenly or notice that their shoes feel tight.

- Tiredness and fatigue. The person may find that even minor tasks or chores, such as shopping or carrying a small bag of groceries, leave them unusually tired.
- Nausea and loss of appetite. Fluid building up in the abdomen affects the digestive tract, causing the person to feel full or sick.
- Memory loss and confusion.
- Rapid heartbeat. The patient may notice that the heart is beating faster and experience it as a racing or throbbing sensation.
- Need to urinate at night. In some people with swollen feet or ankles, the body is able to dispose of some of the fluid at night through the urine.

Diagnosis

The diagnosis of heart failure is complicated because many of the symptoms of the disorder are not unique. The doctor will usually begin with the patient's history and note such risk factors as a previous heart attack, diabetes, or high blood pressure. The doctor will then listen to the patient's heart and lungs with a stethoscope to detect evidence of congestion in the lungs or abnormal heart sounds.

If the doctor suspects that the patient has heart failure, he or she will order one or more laboratory or imaging tests:

- Blood test. This may be done to rule out kidney disease as the cause of fluid retention or to test for the presence of a hormone that is found in the blood when the heart is overworked.
- Electrocardiogram (ECG). This test measures the electrical activity of the heart.
- Chest x ray. This imaging test can identify fluid in the lungs and enlargement of the heart.
- Echocardiogram. This is an important test that uses sound waves to produce an image of the heart on a video monitor. It can be used to measure the percentage of blood pumped out by the left ventricle—the heart's main pumping chamber—with each beat.
- Stress tests. In these tests, the patient is either asked to exercise on a treadmill or is given a medication that stresses the heart to determine whether there are blockages in the heart's arteries.
- Computed tomography (CT) or magnetic resonance imaging (MRI) scans of the heart.

- Cardiac catheterization. In this type of test, the doctor inserts a thin tube called a catheter into a blood vessel in the groin or arm and threads it through the aorta into the coronary arteries. Radioactive dye injected through the catheter makes the arteries and the left ventricle of the heart visible on an x ray.

Treatment

Except for cases of heart failure caused by damaged heart valves (which can be corrected by surgery), heart failure cannot be cured but only controlled. Patients may be given one or more medications or surgical treatments to control their symptoms and prevent further damage to the heart.

Medications that may be prescribed to treat heart failure include:

- Diuretics. Sometimes called water pills, these are drugs that help the body get rid of excess fluid through the urine.
- ACE inhibitors. These are medications that lower blood pressure, improve blood flow, and decrease the workload on the heart.
- Digoxin. Also known as digitalis, this drug increases the strength of the heart's contractions and slows down the heartbeat.
- Beta blockers. These medications slow heart rate, lower blood pressure, and reduce the risk of abnormal heart rhythms.
- Aldosterone antagonists. These drugs enable the body to get rid of salt and water through the urine, which lowers the volume of blood that the heart must pump.

Patients with acute heart failure may require treatment in a hospital. Hospital care usually includes oxygen therapy and medications (most commonly diuretics and drugs to relax the blood vessels) given intravenously.

Severe heart failure that cannot be controlled by medications requires surgical treatment:

- Implantable cardioverter defibrillator (ICD). ICDs are devices that surgeons implant beneath the skin and attach to the heart with small wires. They monitor the heart rate and correct heart rhythms that are too fast.
- Cardiac resynchronization therapy (CRT). In this type of treatment, a pacemaker sends timed electrical impulses to both ventricles of the heart to coordinate their rhythm.
- Heart pump. A heart pump, sometimes called a left ventricular assist device or LVAD, is a device implanted in the abdomen and

attached to a weakened heart to help it pump blood more efficiently. Originally used to keep candidates for heart transplants alive while they waited for a donor heart, LVADs are now thought of as alternatives to transplantation for some patients.

- Heart transplant.

Prognosis

The prognosis of heart failure depends on the person's age, sex, race, lifestyle, and other diseases they may have that affect the heart. Heart failure usually shortens a person's life expectancy by several years. Between 5 and 20 percent of people hospitalized for acute heart failure die in the hospital.

Prevention

Some causes of heart failure, such as congenital malformations, cannot be prevented. People can, however, lower their risk of heart failure in adult life by watching their weight, avoiding heavy drinking or the use of illegal drugs, getting regular exercise, and eating a diet focused on fruits, vegetables, whole grains, low-fat diary products, and lean meat.

People being treated for diabetes, high blood pressure, or coronary artery disease can lower their risk of heart failure by taking all medications prescribed by their doctor, following their doctor's recommendations about diet and exercise, and having regular checkups.

The Future

Heart failure is expected to continue to be a common disease of older adults in developed countries because of increasing life expectancy. Until the 1990s, doctors focused on controlling patients' symptoms. More recently, however, doctors are recommending preventive health care and lifestyle changes in the early adult years, before people develop the symptoms of heart failure or other disorders that increase the risk of heart failure.

SEE ALSO Coronary artery disease; Diabetes; Heart attack; Hypertension; Sleep apnea

For more information

BOOKS

American Heart Association. *To Your Health! A Guide to Heart-Smart Living.* New York: Clarkson Potter, 2001.

WORDS TO KNOW

Cardiac arrest: Heart attack; a condition in which the circulation of the blood stops abruptly because the heart stops beating.

Congenital: Present at birth.

Ventricles: The two lower chambers of the heart.

WEB SITES

American Heart Association. *Heart Failure.* Available online at http://www.americanheart.org/presenter.jhtml?identifier=1486 (updated December 6, 2007; accessed July 21, 2008).

Centers for Disease Control and Prevention (CDC). *Heart Failure Fact Sheet.* Available online at http://www.cdc.gov/dhdsp/library/fs_heart_failure.htm (updated August 30, 2006; accessed July 21, 2008).

Heart Failure Society of America. *What You Should Know about Heart Failure.* Available online at http://www.abouthf.org/questions_about_hf.htm (updated September 29, 2006; accessed July 21, 2008).

HeartFailureMatters.org. *Heart Failure Animations.* Available online at http://www.heartfailurematters.org/English_Lang/Single/Pages/Animations.aspx (accessed July 21, 2008). Sponsored by the European Society of Cardiology, these are nine animations, each taking about two minutes to play, that demonstrate the working of a normal heart, the causes of heart failure, and the effects of various medications and devices in treating heart failure.

National Heart, Lung, and Blood Institute (NHLBI). *Heart Failure.* Available online at http://www.nhlbi.nih.gov/health/dci/Diseases/Hf/HF_WhatIs.html (updated December 2007; accessed July 21, 2008).

National Library of Medicine (NLM). *Congestive Heart Failure.* Available online at http://www.nlm.nih.gov/medlineplus/tutorials/congestiveheartfailure/htm/index.htm (accessed July 20, 2008). This is an online tutorial with voiceover; viewers have the option of a self-playing version, a text version, or an interactive version with questions.

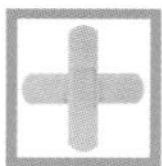

Heat Cramps

Definition

Heat cramps are the mildest of the three forms of heat illness that can develop when the body is exposed to heat. They are defined as brief, involuntary painful muscle spasms in the legs or other parts of the body involved in work or exercise outdoors in hot weather.

Description

Heat cramps are painful but brief muscle cramps that occur during exercise or work in a hot environment. The muscles may twitch or jerk involuntarily. The cramping sensations may also be delayed and occur a few hours after the work or exercise.

Demographics

Heat cramps can affect people of all ages who are not used to hot weather, are not drinking enough fluid, sweat heavily, or have not been properly conditioned (improved their level of physical fitness). The cramps are most likely to affect the parts of the body involved in heavy work, such as the calves, thighs, shoulders, and upper arms.

Causes and Symptoms

Heat cramps result when a person sweats heavily during work or exercise in hot weather. Sweating is the body's way of regulating its internal temperature to get rid of heat. As sweat evaporates, it cools the body. In addition to losing water through sweating, however, the body also loses electrolytes, which are minerals that are necessary for the body to function properly. When the levels of sodium and other electrolytes in the blood fall too low, the painful sensations of heat cramps occur.

Conditioning (improved physical fitness) reduces the risk of heat cramps by increasing blood volume; causing people to sweat more quickly, which helps the body get rid of heat; and making the sweat more dilute, so that fewer electrolytes are lost from the body in the sweat.

Also Known As
Heat-related muscle cramps

Cause
Heat exposure followed by loss of water and minerals through sweating

Symptoms
Painful muscle spasms in the legs, arms, or other muscles involved in exercise

Duration
A few minutes

Diagnosis

Diagnosis of heat cramps is usually based on their characteristics: the cramps are painful; they are involuntary; they come and go; they are brief; and they usually go away on their own. There are no blood tests or other diagnostic studies that can detect heat cramps.

Treatment

Heat cramps are not usually considered a serious health problem even though the muscle cramps may be temporarily painful. They can be treated at home by stopping exercise or work; resting for a few minutes; and drinking fluids mixed with salt to replace the fluids and electrolytes lost through perspiration. People can have either a sports drink like

Gatorade or clear fruit juice, or mix their own salt solution by adding one-fourth to one-half teaspoon of table salt to a quart of water. Salt tablets should not be taken because they upset the stomach.

To ease the cramping sensations, a person can practice gentle stretching or range-of-motion exercises to relax the muscles, or gently massage the affected parts of the body.

A doctor should be consulted when:

- The muscle cramps last longer than an hour.
- The affected person cannot drink the needed fluids because of nausea and vomiting.
- The person has more serious symptoms of heat-related illness, including dizziness, headache, shortness of breath, extreme tiredness, and a temperature higher than 104°F (40°C).

The doctor may administer intravenous fluids and check the affected person for signs of heat exhaustion or heat stroke.

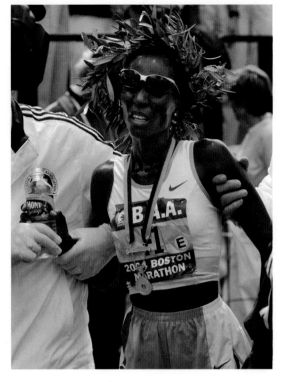

Catherine Ndereba of Kenya suffering from heat cramps after winning the women's 2004 Boston Marathon. AP IMAGES.

Prognosis

Heat cramps usually go away by themselves once the person has cooled off and replaced fluids lost through sweating.

Prevention

Preventing heat cramps is largely a matter of taking time to adjust to hot weather or visiting a hot climate and dressing sensibly for local weather conditions:

- Most people in temperate climates need time to acclimate, or adjust to seasonal temperature changes. People should work up gradually to outdoor activities during the first few warm days of summer rather than overdoing it. The same is true of visiting a country with a tropical or hot climate. It is best to keep one's activity level moderate for a few days rather than crowding in too many activities. It can take people between seven and fourteen days to adjust to a hot climate. Marathon runners generally take two weeks to acclimate to training in the heat.

- Wear loose-fitting and light-colored clothing; choose fabrics that absorb sweat, such as cotton; wear a hat outdoors.
- Drink some fluids before exercising or working outside in hot weather. The American College of Sports Medicine recommends drinking about 20 ounces (0.6 liter) of water or a sports drink two to three hours prior to exercise, and 10 ounces (0.3 liter) of water or a sports drink ten to twenty minutes before exercise. It is important to *not* use thirst as a guide to fluid intake; a person can become dehydrated before feeling thirsty enough to want a drink.
- Use sunscreen generously, as sunburn lowers the body's ability to get rid of excess heat.
- Avoid caffeinated beverages and alcohol; they cause the body to lose additional fluid through the urine.
- Exercise during the early morning or late evening, when the temperature is cooler and the humidity lower.
- Consult a heat stress index like the one printed in the American Council on Exercise fact sheet listed below to help decide whether it is safe to exercise outdoors. There are times when the heat and humidity are so high that exercise should be avoided. Heat cramps are likely to occur when the heat stress index (the apparent temperature) is between 90–105°F (32–40.5°C).

The Future

Heat cramps are a common consequence of exercising or working outdoors without proper conditioning or precautions. They are not dangerous by themselves, however. They can be prevented by dressing appropriately for hot weather, drinking enough fluids, and consulting the local heat index before outdoor activity.

SEE ALSO Heat exhaustion; Heat stroke

For more information

BOOKS

Dvorchak, George. *The Pocket First-Aid Field Guide: Treatment and Prevention of Outdoor Emergencies*. Accokeek, MD: Stoeger Publishing Company, 2007.

Isaac, Jeff. *Outward Bound Wilderness First-Aid Handbook*, revised and updated. Guilford, CT: Falcon Guides, 2008.

WORDS TO KNOW

Acclimation: The process of adjusting to seasonal climate changes or to a new climate.

Conditioning: The process of becoming physically fit through a program of diet, exercise, and rest.

Electrolytes: Minerals that are essential for proper body functioning. They include potassium, sodium, calcium, and magnesium.

Heat illness: A general term for heat-related disorders, ranging from heat cramps (the mildest) to heat stroke (the most serious).

Involuntary: Not under the control of the will.

PERIODICALS

Comeau, Matthew. "A Hot Issue for Summer Exercisers." *American College of Sports Medicine Fitness Page*, Summer 2001, p. 4. Available online in PDF format at http://www.acsm.org/AM/Template.cfm?Section=Search §ion=20015&template=/CM/ContentDisplay.cfm&ContentFileID=22 (accessed May 2, 2008).

WEB SITES

American Council on Exercise (ACE). *Fit Facts: Beat the Heat before It Beats You.* Available in PDF format at http://www.acefitness.org/fitfacts/pdfs/fit-facts/itemid_35.pdf (accessed May 2, 2008). This is a one-page fact sheet on heat stress that contains a useful temperature/humidity index to evaluate the risk of heat cramps.

Nemours Foundation. *Heat Illness.* http://www.kidshealth.org/parent/fitness/problems/heat.html (updated March 2007; accessed May 2, 2008).

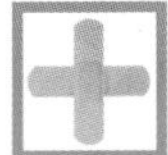

Heat Exhaustion

Definition

Heat exhaustion is a condition in which the body is overwhelmed by exercising or working in a hot environment; it produces more heat than it can get rid of through evaporation of sweat or moving into cooler surroundings. Heat exhaustion is the intermediate form of heat-related illness, heat cramps being the mildest and heat stroke the most serious.

Description

Heat exhaustion is characterized by thirst, headaches, muscle cramps, shortness of breath, and nausea. Most patients with heat exhaustion have a normal level of alertness, although some people become slightly confused or feel anxious.

Demographics

Heat exhaustion is the most common form of heat-related illness seen by physicians, although the exact number of people affected every year is not known because people can be treated for heat exhaustion outside a hospital or doctor's office. According to the Centers for Disease Control and Prevention (CDC), Arizona has the highest rate of cases of heat exhaustion in the United States.

Heat exhaustion affects people from all races and ethnic groups. It affects males and females equally.

Some groups of people have a greater risk of heat exhaustion:

- Newborn infants. A baby cannot adjust to changes in temperature as efficiently as an adult can. In addition, babies have only a limited ability to get out of a hot environment.
- Elderly people. As with infants, the bodies of elderly people do not regulate internal temperature as effectively as those of younger adults. In addition, elderly people may have underlying illnesses that make them more vulnerable to heat stress.
- Workers whose jobs require working outdoors in hot weather or near ovens, blast furnaces, or other sources of heat.
- People who are not physically fit or have not undergone conditioning to get their bodies used to work or exercise in the heat.
- People who take certain types of medications, including diuretics, drugs that regulate blood pressure, tranquilizers, antihistamines, and drugs given to treat people with schizophrenia.
- Homeless people.
- Obese people.

Also Known As
Heat illness, heat stress, hyperthermia

Cause
Overworking the body in hot and humid weather

Symptoms
Heavy sweating, fainting, nausea and vomiting, headache, dark urine

Duration
Two to three hours with treatment

Causes and Symptoms

Like heat cramps, heat exhaustion is caused by the loss of water and salt from the body due to sweating during exposure to heat or vigorous physical exercise in hot conditions. High humidity makes it harder for the body to regulate its internal temperature through sweating, which is its normal way to get rid of heat when the outside temperature is 95°F (35°C) or higher. As sweat evaporates, it carries body heat with it. In addition to losing water through sweating, however, the body also loses electrolytes, which are minerals that are necessary to proper body functioning.

Other factors that can affect the body's ability to regulate its temperature in hot, humid weather include drinking alcohol, which leads to losing more water through the urine, and wearing tight clothes or clothes made of fabrics that do not allow sweat to evaporate easily.

The symptoms of heat exhaustion are more severe than those of heat cramps; they may come on either gradually or suddenly. People suffering from heat exhaustion may feel dizzy and faint as a result of the loss of body fluids and minerals.

- Skin is hot and moist; the person may develop goose bumps.
- Body temperature may be normal or a few degrees above normal.
- Nausea and vomiting.
- Rapid heartbeat and weak pulse.
- Blood pressure is low or drops lower if the person tries to stand up.
- Patient's legs may be swollen.
- Urine is darker than normal.

Diagnosis

In most cases the diagnosis is obvious from the weather conditions and the person's level of activity before feeling ill. People can take care of heat exhaustion themselves by moving into a cooler location; by drinking cool (not cold) water or sports drinks; and by lying down with the legs propped on a pillow or cushion to raise them above heart level.

If the person does not feel better in about half an hour; if they start to lose consciousness; or if their temperature goes above 104°F (40°C), they should be taken to an emergency room as soon as possible.

Treatment

The most important aspect of treating heat exhaustion is to keep it from getting worse. Untreated heat exhaustion can develop into heat stroke, which is a much more serious condition. In some cases a doctor may give the patient intravenous fluids if he or she appears to be severely dehydrated and is vomiting or otherwise unable to take fluids by mouth.

Prognosis

Most people recover from heat exhaustion within two to three hours with no long-term effects.

Prevention

Preventing heat exhaustion is largely a matter of taking time to adjust to hot weather or visiting a hot climate and dressing sensibly for local weather conditions:

- Most people in temperate climates need time to acclimate, or adjust, to seasonal temperature changes. People should work up gradually to outdoor activities during the first few warm days of summer rather than overdoing. The same is true of visiting a country with a tropical or hot climate; it is best to keep one's activity level moderate for a few days rather than crowding in too many activities. It can take people between seven and fourteen days to adjust to a hot climate; marathon runners generally take two weeks to acclimate to training in the heat.
- Wear loose-fitting and light-colored clothing; choose fabrics that absorb sweat, such as cotton; wear a hat outdoors.
- Drink some fluids before exercising or working outside in hot weather. The American College of Sports Medicine recommends drinking about 20 ounces (0.6 liter) of water or sports drink two to three hours prior to exercise, and 10 ounces (0.3 liter) of water or a sports drink ten to twenty minutes before exercise. It is important to *not* use thirst as a guide to fluid intake; a person can become dehydrated before feeling thirsty enough to want a drink.
- Use sunscreen generously, as sunburn reduces the body's ability to get rid of excess heat.
- Avoid caffeinated beverages and alcohol; they cause the body to lose additional fluid through the urine.
- People who must take prescription medications for allergies, high blood pressure, heart conditions, or certain types of mental disorders should ask their doctor whether any of their medications affect their response to heat.

WORDS TO KNOW

Acclimation: The process of adjusting to seasonal climate changes or to a new climate.

Conditioning: The process of becoming physically fit through a program of diet, exercise, and rest.

Electrolytes: Minerals that are essential for proper body functioning. They include potassium, sodium, calcium, and magnesium.

Heat illness: A general term for heat-related disorders, ranging from heat cramps (the mildest) to heat stroke (the most serious).

- Exercise during the early morning or late evening, when the temperature is cooler and the humidity lower. Workers in occupations that require them to work in hot environments are often encouraged to take rest breaks during periods of hot weather. Some companies also provide rest areas where workers can cool off.
- Consult a heat stress index like the one printed in the American Council on Exercise fact sheet listed below or the National Weather Service's heat index to help decide whether it is safe to exercise outdoors. There are times when the heat and humidity are so high that exercise should be avoided. Heat exhaustion is likely to occur when the heat stress index (the apparent temperature) is over 105°F (40.5°C).
- People with elderly friends or relatives should check on them during summer heat waves to make sure that they are in good health. Heat waves that last longer than two days put the elderly at risk of heat exhaustion.

The Future

Heat exhaustion is a common hot-weather health problem or a consequence of exercising or working outdoors without proper conditioning or precautions. It is dangerous only if it progresses to heat stroke, however. Heat exhaustion can be prevented by dressing appropriately for hot weather, drinking enough fluids, consulting the local heat index before outdoor activity, and knowing when to slow down and cool off.

SEE ALSO Heat cramps; Heat stroke

For more information

BOOKS

Dvorchak, George. *The Pocket First-Aid Field Guide: Treatment and Prevention of Outdoor Emergencies.* Accokeek, MD: Stoeger Publishing Company, 2007.

Isaac, Jeff. *Outward Bound Wilderness First-Aid Handbook*, revised and updated. Guilford, CT: Falcon Guides, 2008.

PERIODICALS

Comeau, Matthew. "A Hot Issue for Summer Exercisers." *American College of Sports Medicine Fitness Page*, Summer 2001, p. 4. Available online in PDF format at http://www.acsm.org/AM/Template.cfm?Section=Search§ion=20015&template=/CM/ContentDisplay.cfm&ContentFileID=22 (accessed May 2, 2008).

WEB SITES

American Council on Exercise (ACE). *Fit Facts: Beat the Heat before It Beats You.* Available in PDF format at http://www.acefitness.org/fitfacts/pdfs/fitfacts/itemid_35.pdf (accessed May 2, 2008). This is a one-page fact sheet on heat stress that contains a useful temperature/humidity index to evaluate the risk of heat exhaustion.

Mayo Clinic. *Heat Exhaustion.* Available online at http://www.mayoclinic.com/health/heat-exhaustion/DS01046 (updated February 8, 2008; accessed May 7, 2008).

National Institute for Occupational Safety and Health (NIOSH). *Working in Hot Environments.* Available online at http://www.cdc.gov/niosh/hotenvt.html (updated 1992; accessed May 7, 2008).

National Oceanic and Atmospheric Administration (NOAA), National Weather Service. *Heat Safety Heat Index.* Available online at http://www.nws.noaa.gov/om/heat/index.shtml (accessed December 9, 2008).

National Weather Service and the American Red Cross. *Heat Wave: A Major Summer Killer.* Available online at http://www.nws.noaa.gov/om/heat/heat_wave.shtml (updated June 8, 2007; accessed May 8, 2008). This is a guide to prevention of and basic first aid for heat-related illness.

Nemours Foundation. *Heat Illness.* http://www.kidshealth.org/parent/fitness/problems/heat.html (updated March 2007; accessed May 2, 2008).

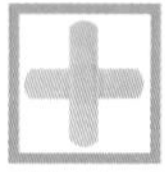

Heat Stroke

Definition

Heat stroke is the most severe of the three forms of heat-related illness. In heat stroke, a person's body temperature rises to 104°F (40°C) or higher. Unlike heat cramps and heat exhaustion, however, heat stroke

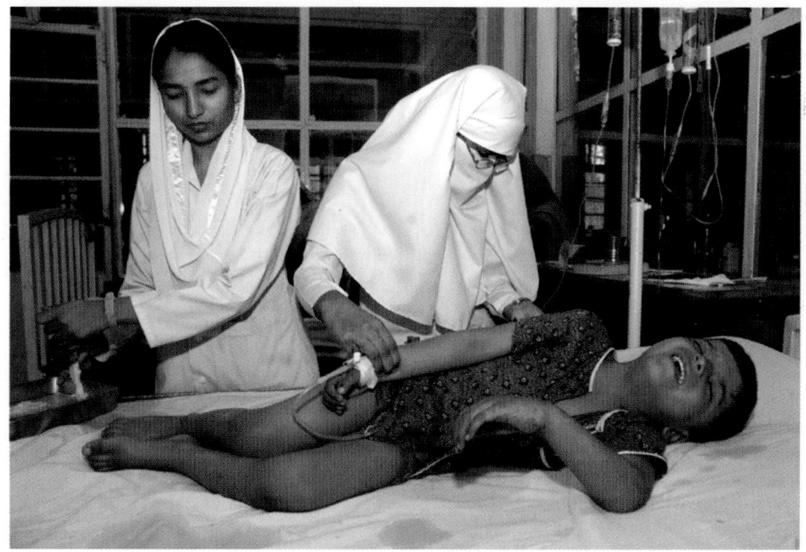

Pakistani child being treated for heat stroke at a local hospital during a 2005 heat wave. AP IMAGES.

is a life-threatening condition. It has two forms: exertional heat stroke (EHS), related to work or exercise in the heat; and nonexertional heat stroke (NEHS), which is not caused by working or exercising outside and primarily affects the elderly, chronically ill persons, and infants during heat waves.

Description

Heat stroke is a medical emergency that develops when a person's body can no longer get rid of excess heat through sweating and evaporation of the sweat. As a result, the body's core temperature rises, damaging the proteins and cell membranes in the body tissues and leading to organ failure, destruction of muscle tissue, the collapse of the cardiovascular system, and eventually death.

Also Known As
Hyperthermia

Cause
Exposure to hot weather and high humidity

Symptoms
Body temperature of 104°F (40°C) or higher; hot, dry skin; nausea; loss of consciousness

Duration
Minutes to hours

Demographics

According to the CDC, over 8,000 people died in the United States from heat-related illness between 1979 and 2003. People over the age of sixty-five account for 44 percent of heat-related deaths.

Heat stroke affects people from all races and ethnic groups. Men and women are equally affected by heat stroke; however, men are twice as likely as women to die from heat stroke because more men than women

First Aid for Heat Stroke

The Centers for Disease Control and Prevention (CDC) give the following instructions for treating someone with heat stroke:

- Have someone call 911 while the person is being cooled as rapidly as possible.
- Depending on what is available nearby, the affected person can be cooled by putting him or her in a tub with cool water; spraying the person with a garden hose; putting the person in the shower and running cool water over them; or sponging the person with a damp cloth dipped in cool water.
- Take the person's temperature from time to time if a thermometer is available, and keep cooling them until it drops to 101–102°F (38.3–38.8°C).
- Call a hospital for further instructions if rescue workers are delayed.
- Do *not* give the person water to drink.
- If possible, loosen or remove some of the person's clothing.

are employed in occupations that require working outdoors in hot weather.

Some groups of people have a greater risk of heat stroke:

- Newborn infants. The body of a baby cannot adjust to changes in temperature as efficiently as an adult's. In addition, babies have a limited ability to exit a hot environment.
- Elderly people. As with infants, the bodies of elderly people do not regulate internal temperature as effectively as those of younger adults. In addition, elderly people may have underlying illnesses or take medications that make them more vulnerable to heat stress.
- Workers whose jobs require working outdoors in hot weather or near ovens, blast furnaces, or other sources of heat.
- People who are not physically fit or have not undergone a conditioning program to get their bodies used to work or exercise in the heat.
- People who take certain types of medications, including diuretics, drugs that regulate blood pressure, tranquilizers, antihistamines, and drugs given to treat people with schizophrenia.
- Homeless people.
- Obese people.

Causes and Symptoms

Like heat exhaustion, heat stroke is caused by the loss of water and salt from the body due to sweating during exposure to heat or vigorous physical exercise in hot conditions. High humidity makes it harder for the body to regulate its internal temperature through sweating, which is its normal way to get rid of heat when the outside temperature is 95°F (35°C) or higher. As sweat evaporates, it carries body heat with it.

In addition to losing water through sweating, however, the body also loses electrolytes, which are minerals that are necessary to proper body functioning. In heat stroke, the body's cooling mechanisms are overwhelmed, and the body's internal temperature starts to rise uncontrollably.

Other factors that can impair the body's ability to regulate its temperature in hot, humid weather include drinking alcohol, which leads to losing more water through the urine, and wearing tight clothes or clothes made of fabrics that do not allow sweat to evaporate easily.

Heat stroke is often preceded by the symptoms of heat exhaustion, which include nausea and vomiting, headache, muscle cramps, dizziness, and difficulty breathing. The symptoms of heat stroke itself usually include:

- Hot, flushed, dry skin
- Changes in level of consciousness, including hallucinations, confusion, and irrational behavior
- Rapid heartbeat, sometimes as high as 130 beats per minute
- Rapid, shallow breathing
- Blood pressure may be either normal or low
- Body temperature above 104°F (40°C) or rectal temperature above 106°F (41.1°C).

Diagnosis

The diagnosis of heat stroke is usually obvious from the patient's situation and previous activities. In addition to taking the patient's temperature, doctors in the emergency room may also take a urine sample to check kidney function or a blood sample to check the level of the patient's electrolytes and blood sugar. A blood test can also be used to evaluate whether the patient's liver has been damaged. In addition to these laboratory tests, the doctor may also order a muscle function test to see whether the patient's muscle tissue has begun to break down.

Treatment

Immediate treatment for heat stroke is essential as death or permanent brain damage can occur within minutes. Emergency treatment is focused on cooling the patient as quickly as possible to a core body temperature of 102°F (38.9°C). Cooling may be done by spraying water on the body, covering the patient with sheets soaked in ice water, or placing ice packs in the patient's armpits and groin area. The patient's temperature is not lowered further because they may start to shiver, and shivering will raise their internal temperature again.

If the patient is conscious, they may be given additional oxygen to breathe and intravenous fluids to restore their blood volume. In most cases these fluids will contain sugar in order to lower the risk of liver failure. Patients who are having muscle cramps or convulsions are usually given benzodiazepine tranquilizers, which relax the muscles and reduce the risk of damage to muscle tissue.

The patient will be kept in the hospital for at least forty-eight hours after emergency treatment and monitored for brain damage, signs of liver failure, or other complications. This period of observation is necessary because heat stroke can damage almost all major body systems.

Prognosis

Although people have survived body temperatures as high as 114.8°F (46°C), any temperature above 106°F (41.1°C) is potentially fatal. People who receive prompt treatment for heat stroke have a 90 percent chance of survival; without prompt treatment, 80 percent will die.

Prevention

Heat stroke is largely preventable by taking time to adjust to hot weather and dressing sensibly for local weather conditions:

- Most people in temperate climates need time to acclimate to seasonal temperature changes. People should work up gradually to sports and other outdoor activities during the first few warm days of summer rather than overdoing. The same is true of visiting a country with a tropical or hot climate; it is best to keep one's activity level moderate for a few days rather than crowding in too many activities. It can take people between seven and fourteen days to adjust to a hot climate; marathon runners generally take two weeks to acclimate to training in the heat.
- Wear loose-fitting and light-colored clothing; choose fabrics that absorb sweat, such as cotton; wear a hat outdoors.
- Drink fluids before exercising or working outside in hot weather. The American College of Sports Medicine recommends drinking about 20 ounces (0.6 liter) of water or sports drink two to three hours prior to exercise, and 10 ounces (0.3 liter) of water or a

sports drink ten to twenty minutes before exercise. Do *not* use thirst as a guide to fluid intake; a person can become dehydrated before feeling thirsty enough to want a drink.

- Use sunscreen generously, as sunburn lowers the body's ability to get rid of excess heat.
- Avoid caffeinated beverages and alcohol; they cause the body to lose additional fluid through the urine.
- People who must take prescription medications for allergies, high blood pressure, heart conditions, or certain types of mental disorders should ask their doctor whether any of their medications affect their response to hot weather.
- Exercise during the early morning or late evening, when the temperature is cooler and the humidity lower. Workers in occupations that require them to work in hot environments should take rest breaks during periods of hot weather. Some companies also provide rest areas where workers can cool off.
- Consult a heat stress index like the one printed in the American Council on Exercise fact sheet listed below or the National Weather Service's heat index to help decide whether it is safe to exercise outdoors. There are times when the heat and humidity are so high that exercise should be avoided. Heat stroke is likely to occur when the heat stress index (the apparent temperature) is over 105°F (40.5°C) and the person is exposed to it for a long period of time; if the heat index is 130°F (54.4°C) or higher, heat stroke is highly likely even with short exposure.
- People with elderly friends or relatives should check on them during summer heat waves. Heat waves that last longer than two days put the elderly at risk of heat exhaustion.
- People who do not have air conditioning in their homes should go to a library, shopping mall, or other public building that is air-conditioned during a heat wave. Even a few hours in a cooler location can help to lower the risk of heat stroke.

The Future

Heat stroke is a common hot-weather disorder; it is often a consequence of exercising or working outdoors without proper conditioning or precautions. Heat stroke can be prevented in normally healthy individuals by

WORDS TO KNOW

Acclimation: The process of adjusting to seasonal climate changes or to a new climate.

Conditioning: The process of becoming physically fit through a program of diet, exercise, and rest.

Electrolytes: Minerals that are essential for proper body functioning. They include potassium, sodium, calcium, and magnesium.

Heat illness: A general term for heat-related disorders, ranging from heat cramps (the mildest) to heat stroke (the most serious).

dressing appropriately for hot weather, drinking enough fluids, consulting the local heat index before outdoor activity, and knowing when to slow down and cool off.

It is possible that heat stroke may become more common in some parts of the United States in the summer time because of the growing size of the elderly population and others who do not tolerate heat well because of chronic illness. One problem is geography: most parts of the United States have uncomfortably high temperatures for at least part of the summer, and some areas have temperatures at or above 90°F (32.2°C) for weeks on end. In addition, large cities tend to be hotter than the surrounding areas.

SEE ALSO Heat cramps; Heat exhaustion

For more information

BOOKS

Armstrong, Lawrence E., ed. *Exertional Heat Illnesses*. Champaign, IL: Human Kinetics, 2003.

Dvorchak, George. *The Pocket First-Aid Field Guide: Treatment and Prevention of Outdoor Emergencies*. Accokeek, MD: Stoeger Publishing Company, 2007.

Isaac, Jeff. *Outward Bound Wilderness First-Aid Handbook*, revised and updated. Guilford, CT: Falcon Guides, 2008.

PERIODICALS

Comeau, Matthew. "A Hot Issue for Summer Exercisers." *American College of Sports Medicine Fitness Page*, Summer 2001, p. 4. Available online in PDF format at http://www.acsm.org/AM/Template.cfm?Section=Search§ion=20015&template=/CM/ContentDisplay.cfm&ContentFileID=22 (accessed June 9, 2008).

WEB SITES

Centers for Disease Control and Prevetion (CDC). *Extreme Heat: A Prevention Guide to Promote Your Personal Health and Safety*. Available online at http://

emergency.cdc.gov/disasters/extremeheat/heat_guide.asp (updated August 15, 2006; accessed June 9, 2008).

Mayo Clinic. *Heatstroke*. Available online at http://www.mayoclinic.com/health/heat-stroke/DS01025 (updated September 7, 2007; accessed June 9, 2008).

National Institute for Occupational Safety and Health (NIOSH). *Working in Hot Environments*. Available online at http://www.cdc.gov/niosh/hotenvt.html (updated 1992; accessed May 7, 2008).

National Oceanic and Atmospheric Administration (NOAA), National Weather Service. *Heat Safety Heat Index*. Available online at http://www.nws.noaa.gov/om/heat/index.shtml (accessed December 9, 2008).

National Weather Service and the American Red Cross. *Heat Wave: A Major Summer Killer*. Available online at http://www.nws.noaa.gov/om/heat/heat_wave.shtml (updated June 8, 2007; accessed June 9, 2008). This is a guide to prevention of and basic first aid for heat-related illness.

Nemours Foundation. *Heat Illness*. http://www.kidshealth.org/parent/fitness/problems/heat.html (updated March 2007; accessed May 2, 2008).

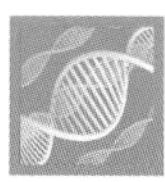

Hemophilia

Definition

Hemophilia is the name of a group of hereditary blood disorders characterized by deficiencies in the blood's ability to form clots. Although hemophilia varies in severity from person to person, all patients with the disease bruise easily and bleed for abnormally long periods of time when cut.

There are two major forms of hemophilia: hemophilia A, sometimes called classic hemophilia, which accounts for about 80 percent of cases; and hemophilia B, called Christmas disease, which accounts for the remaining 20 percent. Both types are caused by gene mutations, hemophilia A by a mutation of the F8 gene and hemophilia B by a mutation of the F9 gene. Both genes are located on the X chromosome, which means that females (who have two X chromosomes) can transmit the mutations that cause hemophilia, but males (who have only one X chromosome) get the disease.

There is a very rare form of hemophilia called acquired hemophilia, which means that the disease is not genetic but develops later in life. It results from an autoimmune reaction in which the body attacks its own production of coagulation factor VIII, one of the blood factors required for normal clotting.

Also Known As
Bleeder's disease, royal disease, Christmas disease

Cause
Genetic mutations on the X chromosome; in rare cases, autoimmune disorders

Symptoms
Prolonged bleeding from minor cuts; excessive bruising; nosebleeds; blood in urine or stool

Duration
Lifelong

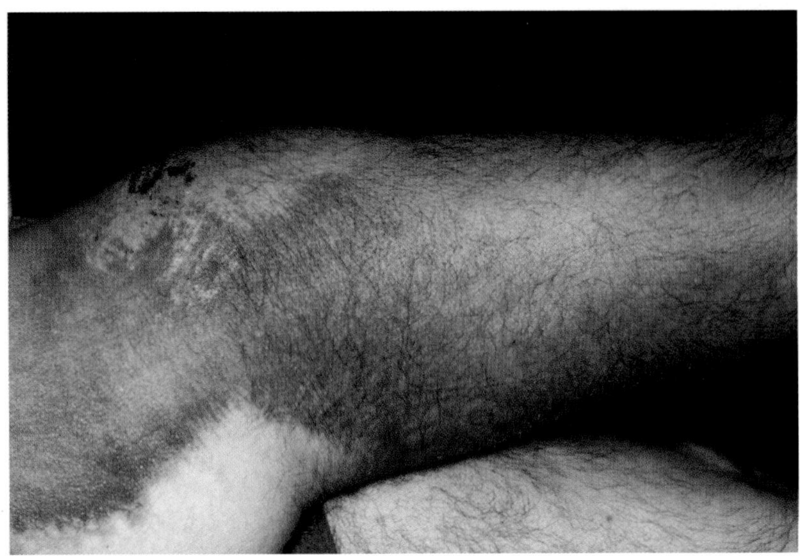

Bruised leg of a hemophiliac, a week after falling from a bike. DR P. MARAZZI / PHOTO RESEARCHERS, INC.

Description

Hemophilia is a disease that has been known for centuries, although ancient doctors could do little to treat it. It was not until 1803 that John Otto, a doctor in Philadelphia, noted that the disease ran in families but that only males suffered from it. Hemophilia became known as the royal disease in the later nineteenth century, when several descendants of Queen Victoria (1819–1901)—including the queen's youngest son, Leopold—died young from brain hemorrhages. Two of Victoria's daughters were carriers of the defective F8 gene and passed on the disease to the royal houses of Spain, Russia, and Germany.

It was not until the twentieth century that doctors were able to understand the cause of hemophilia. At first they thought that it resulted from unusually fragile blood vessels. In the 1920s, doctors thought that defective platelets, cells in the blood involved in clot formation, were to blame. By 1937, however, it was found that substances dissolved in blood plasma, the liquid part of blood, were a necessary part of the normal clotting process. These proteins in the plasma were called coagulation factors. By 1944, a doctor in Argentina found that there are two distinct forms of hemophilia, each caused by a deficiency of a specific coagulation factor. It was not until 1965, however, that another doctor discovered a way to separate the protein factors from the liquid part of blood plasma by a freeze-drying process. This method made it possible for people with hemophilia to be treated without frequent high-volume blood transfusions, previously the only method of treatment.

To understand the significance of these advances and discoveries, it helps to understand how blood clots are usually formed. When a blood vessel is cut, it contracts to slow down the bleeding. Platelets in the blood go to the break or cut and form a clump or plug to patch the hole. The coagulation factors in the blood interact with the platelets and other chemicals in the blood to form a network or web that holds the clot in place. This complicated series of chemical reactions is called the coagulation cascade. People with hemophilia, however, have low amounts of coagulation factors. The severity of hemophilia depends on the level of the coagulation factors. A person with mild hemophilia has between 5 and 40 percent of normal coagulation factor activity; a person with moderate hemophilia has between 1 and 5 percent; a person with severe hemophilia has less than 1 percent of normal coagulation factor activity.

Demographics

Hemophilia A is the more common form of the disorder, occurring in about one in every 4,000 male infants around the world. Hemophilia B affects about one in every 20,000 newborn boys. Girls who carry a defective F8 or F9 gene usually do not suffer from the disease; however, about 10 percent of girls with one abnormal copy of either defective gene will experience heavy menstrual periods and other mild problems with bleeding.

As far as is known, both hemophilia A and hemophilia B are equally common in all racial and ethnic groups around the world. About 60

Safety of the Blood Supply

The discovery of freeze-drying techniques to separate clotting factors from whole blood in the 1960s reduced hemophiliacs' need for periodic visits to a hospital for long and costly transfusions of whole blood. Clotting factors that could be infused at home as well as in a doctor's office lengthened the life spans of hemophiliacs and also gave them more independence to lead relatively normal lives.

The situation changed abruptly in the early 1980s with the discovery of the AIDS virus. Although human blood in the United States was screened for syphilis after 1948 and hepatitis B after 1971, the blood supply had been contaminated with AIDS before screening was available. By the fall of 1982, only a few months after the Centers for Disease Control and Prevention (CDC) had issued its first bulletin about AIDS, hemophiliacs who had received clotting factors derived from human blood were being diagnosed with it. By 1985, when effective tests to screen donated blood for HIV had been developed and were in use, about 30,000 Americans, including 9,500 hemophilia patients, had already been infected via contaminated blood. Many hemophiliacs subsequently died from AIDS rather than hemophilia.

The development of genetically engineered clotting factors, made by using recombinant DNA technology without involving human blood or cells, later virtually eliminated the possibility of disease transmission. Two of the products are BeneFIX, designed to supply coagulation factor IX in patients with hemophilia B, and ReFacto, which supplies coagulation factor VIII in patients with hemophilia A.

percent of persons diagnosed with hemophilia A and 44 percent of persons with hemophilia B have severe disease.

Causes and Symptoms

Both hemophilia A and B are caused by genetic mutations that affect the blood's ability to clot normally. Without enough factor VIII (in the case of hemophilia A) or factor IX (in the case of hemophilia B), the platelets that move to the cut or break in a blood vessel are not held securely within a network of protein fibers. They cannot form a clot strong enough to effectively stop the bleeding, which continues for a longer period of time than in normal people.

The symptoms of hemophilia may include:

- Large or deep bruises, or unexplained bruises
- Nosebleeds that start suddenly without any obvious injury
- Tightness in the joints from blood collecting in the joint spaces
- Blood in the stools or urine
- Prolonged bleeding after minor cuts or injuries, or after routine dental work, tooth extractions, or minor surgical procedures

Patients with severe hemophilia may develop symptoms that indicate a medical emergency. These include sudden severe headache, neck pain, seeing double, repeated vomiting, or sudden pain, swelling, and warmth in the large joints (knees, elbows, hips and shoulders) or in the muscles of the arms and legs.

Diagnosis

The diagnosis of hemophilia depends in part on its severity. Male babies with severe hemophilia are often diagnosed shortly after birth, particularly if they are circumcised. In some cases the disorder is diagnosed when the toddler begins to walk, bruises easily, or starts having nosebleeds. Patients with milder hemophilia may not be diagnosed until they are older and have prolonged bleeding following dental work or minor surgery.

The most common test used to diagnose hemophilia is a blood test. A sample of the patient's blood is analyzed for the amount of clotting factor activity that is present. Genetic testing can also be used to diagnose people who have only mild symptoms of hemophilia A or B, as well as identify women who are carriers of hemophilia gene mutations before they become pregnant.

Treatment

There is no cure for hemophilia. Treatment is directed at preventing severe bleeding episodes and managing symptoms when they do occur.

Patients with mild hemophilia A may be treated with injections of a hormone called desmopressin or DDAVP, which stimulates the patient's body to release more of its own clotting factor. Patients with hemophilia B or moderate to severe hemophilia A are treated with clotting factors derived from donated human blood or from genetically engineered blood products called recombinant clotting factors.

Patients with hemophilia can be taught to inject themselves with desmopressin or clotting factors at home two or three times a week as a form of prophylaxis, or preventive measure.

Patients with severe hemophilia whose joints have been damaged by bleeding usually need physical therapy to restore range of motion and strength in the damaged joints. They may eventually need to have the joints replaced with artificial joints in adult life.

Prognosis

The life expectancy and quality of life for males with hemophilia have increased dramatically since the 1950s. Before 1960, the average life expectancy of a boy with hemophilia was 11 years. Early death was often preceded by severe pain from bleeding into the joints. As of the early 2000s, life expectancy has increased to fifty-five to sixty years. Older men with severe hemophilia who were treated in the late 1970s or early 1980s are still at risk of death from AIDS; 90 percent of these patients are HIV-positive. About 8 percent of patients with hemophilia eventually die from bleeding into the brain.

About 25 percent of children between six and eighteen years of age with severe hemophilia have below-normal academic skills and an increased risk of emotional and behavioral problems.

Prevention

Hemophilia can be prevented in part by genetic testing of prospective parents. Although males with hemophilia cannot pass the disease on to sons, they can father daughters who will carry the disease to the next

WORDS TO KNOW

Coagulation cascade: The complex process in which platelets, coagulation factors, and other chemicals in the blood interact to form a clot when a blood vessel is injured.

Coagulation factors: Proteins in blood plasma involved in the chain of chemical reactions leading to the formation of blood clots. They are also called clotting factors.

Gene therapy: An approach to treating disease by inserting healthy genes into a person's genetic material or by inactivating defective genes.

Plasma: The liquid part of blood, about 55 percent of blood by volume.

Platelets: Specialized cells in the blood that are involved in forming blood clots. Platelets are also called thrombocytes.

Prophylaxis: The use of a medication or other therapy to maintain health and prevent disease.

generation. Hemophilia cannot be completely eliminated by family planning, however, as 34 percent of all hemophilia A cases and 20 percent of all hemophilia B cases are caused by spontaneous mutations in each generation.

The Future

Hemophilia will always be rare, but it is unlikely to ever be completely eliminated for two reasons. One is the role of spontaneous mutations in producing defective F8 and F9 genes in each new generation. The other reason is that most men with hemophilia now live long enough to father children and pass on the defective genes. Because of this change in life expectancy, researchers are presently concentrating on gene therapy as a possible cure for hemophilia. In gene therapy, a normal gene to replace the defective gene is inserted into the patient's genetic material by using a virus as a carrier. Research on gene therapy for hemophilia A is being conducted as of 2008.

SEE ALSO AIDS; Hepatitis A

For more information

BOOKS

Britton, Beverly. *Hemophilia.* San Diego, CA: Lucent Books, 2003.

Raabe, Michelle. *Hemophilia.* New York: Chelsea House, 2008.

Sherman, Irwin W. *Twelve Diseases That Changed Our World.* Washington, DC: ASM Press, 2007. Chapter 1 is about hemophilia.

WEB SITES

Biology Animations. *Blood Clotting Animation.* Available online at http://biology-animations.blogspot.com/2008/01/for-detailed-information-httpen.html (accessed July 22, 2008). The animation describes the process of normal blood clotting. It takes about a minute to play.

Genetics Home Reference. *Hemophilia.* Available online at http://ghr.nlm.nih.gov/condition=hemophilia (updated March 2007; accessed July 21, 2008).

National Heart, Lung, and Blood Institute (NHLBI). *What Is Hemophilia?* Available online at http://www.nhlbi.nih.gov/health/dci/Diseases/hemophilia/hemophilia_what.html (updated June 2007; accessed July 21, 2008).

National Human Genome Research Institute (NHGRI). *Learning about Hemophilia.* Available online at http://www.genome.gov/20019697 (updated February 15, 2008; accessed July 21, 2008).

World Federation of Hemophilia. *Hemophilia in Pictures.* Montréal, Canada: World Federation of Hemophilia, 2005. Available online in PDF or slideshow format at http://www.wfh.org/index.asp?lang=EN (accessed July 22, 2008). This is an easy-to-understand 41-page illustrated explanation of hemophilia, also available in French, Spanish, Russian, Chinese, and Arabic.

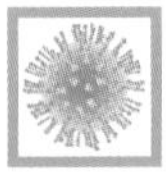

Hepatitis A

Definition

Hepatitis A is an infectious disease of the liver caused by the HAV virus. The disease is usually transmitted by food or water contaminated by human wastes containing the virus or by close human contact. As far as is known, only humans and some primates can get hepatitis A; it is not carried by other animals.

Also Known As
Infectious hepatitis, viral hepatitis

Cause
Virus

Symptoms
Nausea, vomiting, jaundice, fever, fatigue, abdominal pain, dark-colored urine

Duration
A few weeks to six to nine months

Description

Hepatitis A is an inflammation of the liver caused by the HAV virus. It differs from hepatitis B and hepatitis C in that it does not cause long-term liver damage. Even though people can take several weeks or months to recover completely from hepatitis A, they have lifelong immunity afterward. Complications from hepatitis A are rare and usually limited to people with chronic liver disease or who have received a liver transplant.

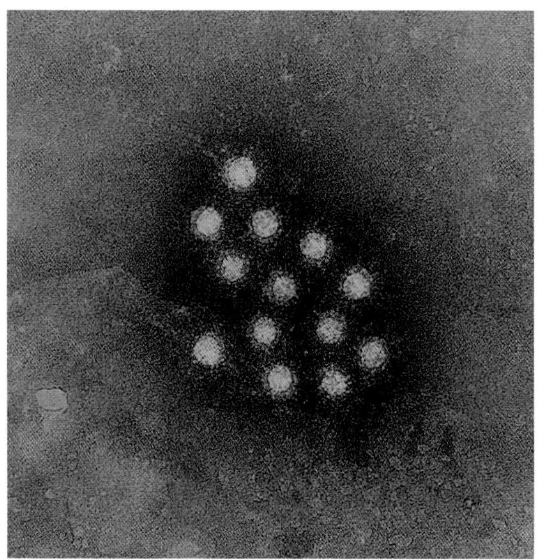

Magnified image of the hepatitis A virus. © PHOTOTAKE INC. / ALAMY.

Hepatitis A varies in severity. Children and younger adults may have no symptoms at all, although they can still spread the disease. In general, adults are more likely to have noticeable symptoms than children or teenagers. The symptoms begin between two and six weeks after the person has been infected with HAV. The most common symptom is loss of energy and overall tiredness. Some people develop a mild flu-like illness with diarrhea, low-grade fever, nausea, vomiting, and muscle cramps. People with more severe symptoms may have pain in the abdomen in the area of the liver (below the rib cage on the right side of the body); they may notice that their urine has turned dark brown or that they have jaundice—yellowing of the skin and the whites of the eyes. Some have itchy skin.

Most people feel better within four to six weeks after the symptoms begin, although about 15 percent of patients may take up to nine months to completely regain their energy and feel normal again.

Demographics

Hepatitis A is much more common in Africa, Asia, and South America than in the United States. The rates of hepatitis A in North America have been steadily dropping since the 1980s. In 1988 the Centers for Disease Control and Prevention (CDC) reported 32,000 cases in the United States; in 2003, 7,653 cases were reported. In developing countries, children below the age of two account for most new cases of hepatitis A; in the United States, the age group most often affected is children between the ages of five and fourteen.

Males and females are equally likely to get hepatitis A, as are people from all races and ethnic groups in the United States.

Some groups of adults are at increased risk of hepatitis A:

- People who travel to parts of the world with high rates of the disease and poor sanitation
- Male homosexuals
- People who use illicit drugs, whether injected or taken by mouth

- Medical researchers and laboratory workers who may be exposed to HAV
- Child care workers
- Homeless people

Causes and Symptoms

Hepatitis A is caused by a virus that is transmitted by close personal contact with an infected person, by needle sharing, and by eating food or drinking water contaminated by fecal matter. After the virus enters the body, it multiplies in the cells of the liver, causing inflammation of the liver and a general response from the immune system that leads to most of the symptoms of the illness.

The HAV virus is shed from the liver into the bile (a digestive fluid secreted by the liver) and then into the person's stools between fifteen and forty-five days before symptoms appear. That means that people can spread the virus through their feces before they know that they are sick. In the United States, hepatitis A is most commonly spread by food handlers who do not wash their hands properly after using the bathroom; by childcare workers who do not wash their hands after changing a baby's diaper; by anal sex; and by eating raw shellfish harvested from sewage-polluted waters. In very rare cases the virus can be transmitted through blood transfusions.

In addition to fatigue, the most common symptoms of hepatitis A include:

- Low-grade fever (101°F [38.3°C])
- Nausea, vomiting, and diarrhea
- Loss of appetite and weight loss
- Swelling of the liver and pain in the area of the abdomen over the liver

Hepatitis E

Hepatitis E is an infection of the liver caused by the hepatitis E virus, or HEV, first identified during an outbreak in New Delhi, India, in 1955, when 30,000 cases were reported following river flooding that carried raw sewage into the city's water supply. At first the disease was thought to be hepatitis A, but was later identified as a new virus. In 1990 its genetic material was analyzed and the virus was named hepatitis E.

Hepatitis E is most common in countries with tropical climates, particularly in southeastern Asia, Africa, India, and Central America. Unlike hepatitis A, which seems to affect only humans, hepatitis E has been found in deer, pigs, rats, and other animals, and can be spread by uncooked meat or shellfish. Mortality rates are generally low (around 2 percent) with hepatitis E; however, pregnant women are at high risk of liver failure from the disease. In India as many as 20 percent of pregnant women infected with hepatitis E die of liver failure.

Hepatitis E is rare in the United States, affecting primarily people who travel to countries where it is common. The disease is self-limited and is usually treated with fluid replacement; antibiotics are not effective in treating viruses. The best treatment is prevention—travelers in countries with tropical climates should avoid drinking water that has not been tested for purity and eating uncooked shellfish or raw, unpeeled fruits or vegetables.

- Tea- or coffee-colored urine
- Jaundice
- Generalized sensation of itching
- Pale or clay-colored stools
- Muscle pains

Diagnosis

The doctor may suspect that a patient has hepatitis A during a physical examination by feeling the area over the liver for signs of swelling and pain; and checking the skin and eyes for signs of jaundice. A definite diagnosis is provided by a blood test for certain antibodies to the HAV virus. The doctor will also have the sample of blood checked for abnormally high levels of chemicals produced in the liver.

Treatment

There is no specific drug treatment for hepatitis A, as antibiotics cannot be used to treat virus infections. Most people can care for themselves at home by making sure they get plenty of fluids and adequate nutrition. People whose appetite has been affected may benefit from eating small snacks throughout the day rather than three main meals and eating soft and easily digested foods. Patients with mild vomiting may be prescribed antiemetics (drugs to control nausea). Those with severe vomiting may need to be hospitalized in order to receive intravenous fluids.

Patients with hepatitis A should avoid drinking alcohol or taking acetaminophen (Tylenol), which make it harder for the liver to recover from inflammation. Patients should also tell their doctor about any other over-the-counter or prescription drugs they are taking, because the drugs may need to be stopped temporarily or have the dosages changed.

Prognosis

Most people recover fully from hepatitis A within a few weeks or months. Between 3 and 20 percent have relapses (temporary recurrences of symptoms) for as long as six to nine months after infection.

About 1 percent of patients develop liver failure following HAV infection, mostly those over sixty or those with chronic liver disease. In these cases liver transplantation may be necessary for the patient's survival. There are about 100 deaths from hepatitis A reported each year in the United States.

WORDS TO KNOW

Antiemetic: A type of drug given to control nausea and vomiting.

Bile: A yellow-green fluid secreted by the liver that aids in the digestion of fats.

Hepatitis: The medical term for inflammation of the liver. It can be caused by toxic substances or alcohol as well as infections.

Jaundice: A yellowish discoloration of the skin and whites of the eyes caused by increased levels of bile pigments from the liver in the patient's blood.

Prevention

Hepatitis A can be prevented by a vaccine called Havrix that is given before exposure to the HAV virus. The vaccine is given in two shots, the second given between six and eighteen months after the first. It confers immunity against hepatitis A for at least twenty years. Those who should receive the vaccine include people in the military and those who travel abroad frequently; men who have sex with other men; people who use intravenous drugs; people with hemophilia who must receive human blood products; and people who have chronic hepatitis B or C infection.

People who have been exposed to the HAV virus and children under the age of two should not be given Havrix, but they can be given another type of drug to protect them against HAV.

Everyone can reduce their risk of hepatitis A by observing the following precautions:

- Practice good personal hygiene; wash hands frequently, especially after using the toilet or changing a child's diaper.
- When traveling, drink only bottled water, avoid raw or undercooked meat or shellfish, and avoid eating fresh fruits or vegetables unless you have washed and peeled them yourself.
- Avoid sharing drinking glasses and eating utensils. If someone in the family has hepatitis A, wash their glasses and utensils separately in hot, soapy water.
- Avoid sexual contact with anyone who has hepatitis A.

The Future

The rates of hepatitis A in the United States and other developed countries are likely to continue to drop, given the availability of an effective vaccine against the disease. Hepatitis A is, however, likely to continue to be a major health problem in developing countries, and travelers will need to protect themselves against it for the foreseeable future.

SEE ALSO Alcoholism; Hemophilia; Hepatitis B; Hepatitis C

For more information

BOOKS

Centers for Disease Control and Prevention (CDC). "Surveillance for Acute Viral Hepatitis—United States, 2006." *Morbidity and Mortality Weekly Report*, 57 (March 21, 2008): 1–24. Available online at http://www.cdc.gov/mmwr/preview/mmwrhtml/ss5702a1.htm (accessed July 26, 2008).

National Institute of Allergy and Infectious Diseases (NIAID). "The Story of the Hepatitis E Vaccine." *NIAID Discovery News*, Spring 2007. Available online at http://www3.niaid.nih.gov/healthscience/healthtopics/HepatitisE/storyHepatitisEVaccine.htm (accessed July 26, 2008).

WEB SITES

American Academy of Family Physicians (AAFP). *Hepatitis A*. Available online at http://familydoctor.org/online/famdocen/home/common/infections/hepatitis/897.html (updated October 2007; accessed July 25, 2008).

American Liver Foundation. *Hepatitis A*. Available online at http://www.liverfoundation.org/education/info/hepatitisa/ (updated November 27, 2007; accessed July 26, 2008).

Mayo Clinic. *Hepatitis A*. Available online at http://www.mayoclinic.com/health/hepatitis-a/DS00397 (updated September 7, 2007; accessed July 26, 2008).

National Institute of Allergy and Infectious Diseases (NIAID). *Hepatitis A*. Available online at http://www3.niaid.nih.gov/healthscience/healthtopics/HepatitisA/default.htm (updated December 10, 2007; accessed July 26, 2008).

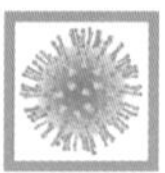

Hepatitis B

Definition

Hepatitis B is a viral infection of the liver transmitted through the blood or body fluids of someone who is infected. It is the most common serious liver infection worldwide. The disease has two forms: an acute form that lasts a few weeks, and a chronic form that can last for years and can lead to cirrhosis, liver failure, liver cancer, and even death. Acute hepatitis B has a 5 percent chance of leading to the chronic form of the infection in adults; however, infants infected during the mother's pregnancy have a 90 percent chance of developing chronic hepatitis B, and children have a 25–50 percent chance.

About two-thirds of people with chronic HBV infection are so-called "healthy" carriers of the virus. They may never get sick themselves but they can transmit the infection to others. The remaining one-third of people with chronic hepatitis B develop liver disease that can lead to permanent scarring of the liver. Between 15 and 25 percent of people with chronic hepatitis B eventually die of liver disease.

Description

Hepatitis B has an incubation period of one to six months. About 50 percent of people with the acute form of the disease have no symptoms at all; the others experience loss of appetite, nausea and vomiting, and jaundice around twelve weeks after getting infected. Some patients may also have joint pain, itchy skin, or abdominal pain. Many of these patients assume that they have influenza.

Patients with chronic hepatitis may have no symptoms at all. The one-third who do eventually fall ill have the same symptoms as patients with the acute form of the disease.

People who have been infected by HBV and have recovered from the infection are protected against hepatitis B for the rest of their lives. People can also be protected by receiving a vaccine against the virus.

Also Known As
HBV infection

Cause
Virus

Symptoms
Loss of appetite, jaundice, fatigue, nausea, vomiting, itchy skin; some patients have no symptoms

Duration
Months to years

Demographics

There are about 200,000 new cases of hepatitis B in the United States each year; it is estimated that 1–1.25 million people carry the disease.

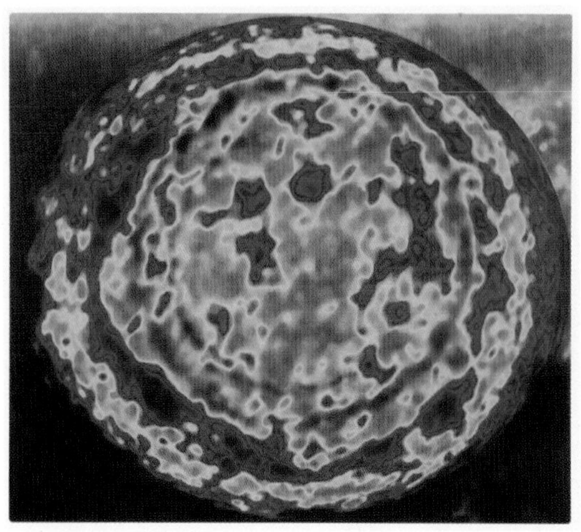

Magnified image of the hepatitis B virus. © PHOTOTAKE INC. / ALAMY.

Hepatitis B causes about 5,100 deaths in the United States each year. In the rest of the world, as many as a third of the population are chronic carriers of the disease.

The age group most commonly affected by hepatitis B in the United States is adults between the ages of twenty and fifty. African Americans are more likely to be infected than either Hispanics or Caucasians; however, Alaskan Eskimos and Pacific Islanders have higher rates of carrier status than members of other racial groups. More males than females are infected with hepatitis B in all races and age groups.

Risk factors for hepatitis B include:

- Having unprotected sex with a partner regardless of sexual orientation.
- Having a large number of sexual partners.
- Being infected with another sexually transmitted disease (STD), particularly gonorrhea or chlamydia.
- Sharing needles with other intravenous drug users.
- Having a family member with chronic HBV infection.
- Having had a blood transfusion or use of blood products before 1972.
- Needing hemodialysis for kidney disease.
- Frequent travels to parts of the world with high rates of hepatitis B. These include the Middle East, southern Africa, Southeast Asia, Brazil, and the Pacific Islands.
- Working in a hospital, clinic, or other facility requiring frequent exposure to blood, open wounds, or other body secretions.

Causes and Symptoms

Hepatitis B is caused by a virus. It is primarily a bloodborne infection, but can also be transmitted through contact with the semen or saliva of an infected person. The virus enters the body through injection, a break in the skin, or contact with the mucous membranes, tissues that line the mouth, genitals, and rectum. People cannot get hepatitis B from food or from shaking hands, sneezing or coughing, breastfeeding, or casual contact with an infected person.

The symptoms of acute hepatitis B infection include:

- Loss of appetite
- Feeling tired
- Muscle and joint aches
- Low-grade fever
- Abdominal pain in the area below the rib cage
- Yellowish discoloration of the skin and whites of the eyes
- Tea- or cola-colored urine
- Grayish or clay-colored stools

A few people develop a severe form of hepatitis B known as fulminant hepatitis. This form of the disease appears rapidly and can cause death. Its symptoms include:

- Sudden collapse
- Mental confusion, hallucinations, or extreme sleepiness
- Jaundice
- Noticeable swelling of the abdomen

Hepatitis D

Hepatitis D, or delta hepatitis, is a liver disease caused by a virus (HDV) unrelated to the viruses that cause hepatitis A, B, and C. HDV is sometimes called the delta agent. Discovered only in 1977, the hepatitis D virus can replicate (multiply) only in patients infected with HBV. As of 2008 HDV infection was found in about 5 percent of patients diagnosed with hepatitis B. Hepatitis D can range from an acute, but limited, infection to a sudden, severe disease that leads to liver failure in 1 percent of patients. Most patients who are infected with hepatitis D alongside hepatitis B eventually get better. Chronic infection with both viruses occurs in only 5 percent of patients.

The World Health Organization (WHO) estimates that there are about fifteen million people worldwide infected with HDV. In the United States, hepatitis D is primarily a disease of adults rather than children. Risk factors include intravenous drug use and coming from southern Italy or other countries around the Mediterranean Sea.

HDV infection produces the same symptoms as hepatitis B. It can be detected by a blood test known as the anti-delta agent antibody test. Treatment is the same as for hepatitis B.

Diagnosis

Hepatitis B is diagnosed by one or more blood tests, since patients may not have any apparent symptoms. In a number of cases, the person is diagnosed following a routine blood test given as part of an annual health checkup. The most common clue is abnormal liver function results.

To confirm the diagnosis, the doctor will take one or more blood samples for testing:

- A test of liver function, if this has not already been done.
- Tests for antibodies to the hepatitis B virus. A positive result means that the person has either been effectively vaccinated against

HBV or has been infected at some point in the past and has recovered.

- Tests for the surface antigen of the hepatitis B virus (HBsAg). The surface antigen is the outer coating of the virus. A positive HBsAg test means that the patient is currently infected and may be able to pass on the virus to others.
- Hepatitis B DNA test. This blood test measures the levels of virus in the patient's blood.

Patients with chronic active hepatitis B may be given a computed tomography (CT) scan or ultrasound of the liver to see whether the liver has been damaged by the infection. The doctor may also perform a liver biopsy. This test involves inserting a long hollow needle into the patient's liver through the abdomen and withdrawing a small amount of tissue for examination under a microscope.

Treatment

Patients who know that they have been exposed to the hepatitis B virus can be treated by administering an immune-boosting injection and three shots of the HBV vaccine to prevent them from developing an active infection. Those who have already developed symptoms of the acute form of the disease may be given intravenous fluids to prevent dehydration or anti-nausea medications to stop vomiting. To date, there is no medication that can prevent acute hepatitis B from becoming chronic once the symptoms begin.

There are few treatment options for chronic hepatitis B. If the patient has no symptoms and little sign of liver damage, the doctor may suggest monitoring the levels of HBV in the patient's blood periodically rather than starting treatment right away. There are five different drugs used to treat hepatitis B, but they do not work in all patients and may produce severe side effects. Most doctors will wait until the patient's liver function begins to worsen before administering these drugs.

If the patient develops fulminant hepatitis B or their liver is otherwise severely damaged by HBV, the only option is a liver transplant. This is a serious operation with a lengthy recovery period; its success also depends on finding a suitable donor liver.

Prognosis

Patients with acute hepatitis B usually recover; the symptoms go away in two to three weeks, and the liver itself returns to normal in about four months. Other patients have a longer period of illness with very slow improvement. Chronic hepatitis leads to an increased risk of cirrhosis and liver cancer, and eventual death in about 1 percent of cases.

Prevention

Hepatitis B can be prevented by vaccination with a vaccine called Engerix-B. The person receives the first two doses of the vaccine a month apart and the third dose six months later. The vaccine is recommended for all persons under the age of twenty; it can be given to newborns and infants as part of their regular vaccination series. Others who should be vaccinated include health care workers, military personnel, firefighters and police, people who travel frequently to countries with high rates of hepatitis B, people with hemophilia, people who must be treated for kidney disease, people who inject illegal drugs, and men who have sex with other men.

Other preventive measures include:

- Practicing safe sex
- Not sharing needles, razors, toothbrushes, or any other personal item that might have blood on it
- Avoiding getting a tattoo or body piercing, as some people who perform these procedures do not sterilize their needles and other equipment properly
- Getting tested for HBV infection if pregnant, as the virus can be transmitted from a mother to her unborn baby
- Consulting a doctor before taking an extended trip to any country with high rates of hepatitis B

The Future

The rate of hepatitis B in the United States began to drop after 1992, when vaccination of infants became routine, followed by vaccination of adolescents in 1995. Public health doctors expect the decline to continue for the foreseeable future.

Researchers at the National Institutes of Health (NIH) are presently looking for medications that will be effective in treating all patients with chronic hepatitis B with fewer side effects.

SEE ALSO Hemophilia; Hepatitis A; Hepatitis C

WORDS TO KNOW

Carrier: A person who is infected with a virus or other disease organism but does not develop the symptoms of the disease.

Chronic: Long-term or recurrent.

Cirrhosis: Disruption of normal liver function by the formation of scar tissue and nodules in the liver.

Fulminant: Referring to a disease that comes on suddenly with great severity.

Hepatitis: A general term for inflammation of the liver. It can be caused by toxic substances or alcohol as well as infections.

Jaundice: A yellowish discoloration of the skin and whites of the eyes caused by increased levels of bile pigments from the liver in the patient's blood.

For more information

BOOKS

Freedman, Jeri. *Hepatitis B.* New York: Rosen Publishing, 2009.

Green, William Finley. *The First Year—Hepatitis B: An Essential Guide for the Newly Diagnosed.* New York: Marlowe and Co., 2002.

PERIODICALS

Bakalar, Nicholas. "Tracking the Response to Hepatitis B Vaccine." *New York Times*, August 14, 2007. Available online at http://query.nytimes.com/gst/fullpage.html?res=990CE3DD133EF937A2575BC0A9619C8B63 (accessed September 15, 2008).

WEB SITES

American Academy of Family Physicians (AAFP). *Hepatitis B.* Available online at http://familydoctor.org/online/famdocen/home/common/infections/hepatitis/032.html (accessed September 15, 2008).

American Liver Foundation. *Hepatitis B.* Available online at http://www.liverfoundation.org/education/info/hepatitisb/ (accessed September 15, 2008).

Centers for Disease Control and Prevention (CDC). *Hepatitis B.* Available online at http://www.cdc.gov/hepatitis/HepatitisB.htm (accessed September 15, 2008).

eMedicine Health. *Hepatitis B.* Available online at http://www.emedicinehealth.com/hepatitis_b/article_em.htm (accessed September 15, 2008).

KidsHealth. *Hepatitis.* Available online at http://kidshealth.org/kid/health_problems/infection/hepatitis.html (accessed September 15, 2008).

National Library of Medicine (NLM). *Hepatitis B.* Available online at http://www.nlm.nih.gov/medlineplus/tutorials/hepatitisb/htm/index.htm (accessed September 15, 2008). This is an online tutorial with voiceover; viewers have the option of a self-playing version, an interactive version with questions, or a text version.

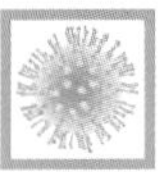

Hepatitis C

Definition

Hepatitis C infection is an inflammatory disease of the liver caused by HCV. HCV is most commonly transmitted from person to person through contaminated blood.

Description

Hepatitis C is an infection that often goes undetected until it has done significant damage to a patient's liver. The infection has two phases, acute (the first six months) and chronic (after the first six months). A minority of patients clear the virus from their bodies during the acute phase, but 60–85 percent have a chronic hepatitis C infection.

People may have no symptoms of illness during the acute phase of hepatitis C infection and possibly only a mild flu-like syndrome later. Symptoms of severe liver damage, such as nausea, vomiting, collection of fluid in the abdomen, and mental changes, may not develop for ten or twenty years after the initial infection.

Demographics

Hepatitis C is the major source of chronic liver infection in North America. There are approximately 30,000 new infections and 8,000–10,000 deaths each year in the United States. It is estimated that 4 million persons in the United States have been infected by HCV and 2.7 million of these have the chronic form. HCV infection presently accounts for 40 percent of referrals to liver clinics.

HCV is more common among Hispanics and African Americans than among Caucasians, Asian Americans, or Native Americans. Sixty-five percent of persons with HCV infection are between thirty and forty-nine years of age.

People who are at increased risk of HCV include:

- Those who abuse intravenous drugs (60 percent of new cases)
- People who have unprotected sex with a large number of partners
- People who require hemodialysis for kidney disorders
- People who need frequent blood transfusions

Also Known As
Non-A, non-B hepatitis

Cause
Bloodborne virus

Symptoms
Fatigue, nausea, vomiting, jaundice, dark urine, liver pain, joint and muscle pains

Duration
May be lifelong after infection

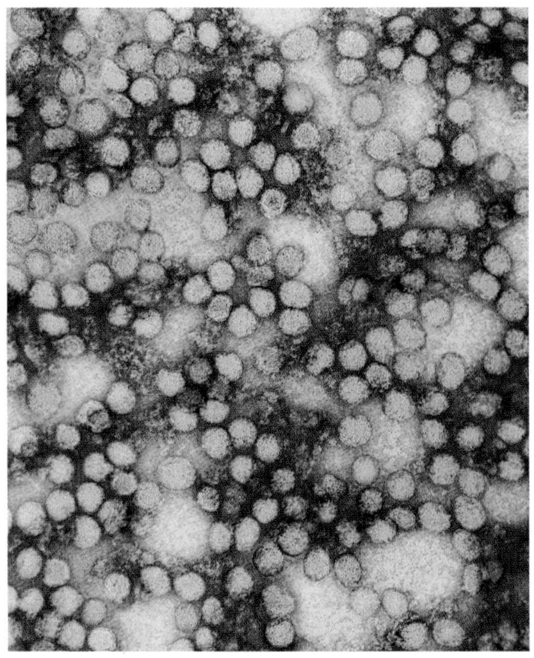

Magnified image of the hepatitis C virus. © PHOTOTAKE INC. / ALAMY

- People who are HIV-positive
- Health care workers who may get needle-stick injuries

Causes and Symptoms

Hepatitis C is caused by HCV. It is most often transmitted from one person to another through infected blood or blood products, but can also be (uncommonly) transmitted from mother to child during childbirth or through sexual intercourse. Before 1992, HCV was sometimes transmitted through blood transfusions, hemodialysis, or transplanted organs from infected donors; these are now rare events. In 1992, researchers invented a new test for checking blood products for HCV; as a result, new infections annually in the United States declined from 240,000 in the 1980s to about 20,000–30,000 in 2007. The most common cause of HCV transmission is intravenous drug use; transfusion-related cases of hepatitis C now occur only once in every 2 million transfused units of blood.

Hepatitis C infection is sometimes divided into an early phase called the acute stage and a later phase called the chronic stage. The acute stage begins when the virus enters the body; it lasts for about six months. Antibodies to the virus can usually be detected between three and twelve weeks after infection. About 15–40 percent of people who are infected clear the virus from their bodies during this phase, while the other 60–85 percent go on to develop chronic hepatitis C infection. It is this second group of patients who run the risk of suffering cirrhosis or other forms of liver or kidney damage years later.

Eighty percent of patients infected by HCV in its early stage do not have any symptoms, or have mild and nonspecific symptoms like fatigue. Others have a flu-like syndrome marked by poor appetite or nausea, soreness in the area of the liver, or pains in the joints and muscles. Some may notice that their urine is dark and looks like tea or cola. If chronic HCV infection leads to liver disease ten to twenty years later, the patient may have the following symptoms:

- Severe loss of appetite
- Nausea and vomiting, with blood in the vomit

- Low-grade fever
- Itchy skin
- Jaundice (This is a yellowish discoloration of the whites of the eyes and the skin caused by an increase in the amount of bile pigments from the liver in the patient's blood.)
- Sleep disturbances
- Swelling of the abdomen caused by fluid retention
- Diarrhea
- Difficulty urinating
- Confusion, hallucinations, difficulty concentrating, or other mental disturbances

Diagnosis

Diagnosis of hepatitis C infection is often delayed for years because many patients with chronic hepatitis C infection do not have noticeable or troublesome symptoms until liver damage has already occurred. In some cases a person with chronic hepatitis C infection is detected through routine blood testing for abnormal liver function or because they have a history of intravenous drug abuse or HIV infection. Testing for chronic infection begins with blood tests that indicate the presence of antibodies to HCV. Since antibody tests cannot tell whether the person is currently infected, however, a second blood test that looks for the virus's characteristic genetic material is performed.

If the results are positive for both tests, the doctor will order a third blood test that determines the virus's specific genotype or genetic makeup. There are six known genotypes of HCV as of 2008, and knowing which type is involved helps to guide the patient's treatment.

An Outbreak in Nebraska

Transmission of hepatitis C virus (HCV) within health care facilities is never supposed to occur. In 2000–2001, however, an outbreak in Nebraska, traced to poor health safeguards at a private cancer clinic, affected almost 100 patients. A physician's wife who began treatment for breast cancer at the clinic in 2001 was surprised to find out in 2002 that she was infected with HCV. Her husband discovered on checking his records that several of his patients were also infected; all were undergoing cancer therapy at the same clinic.

An investigation by the Nebraska Health and Human Services System found that in March 2000 a clinic nurse used a syringe to rinse a known HCV patient's chemotherapy port with saline solution then used the same syringe to draw more saline from a large common container, thus transferring HCV from the infected port into the container. The virus was transmitted to other patients via the saline solution and repeated use of contaminated syringes.

Between March 2000 and June 2001, when the nurse left the clinic, 99 of the clinic's 857 patients were infected with HCV. As of 2008, at least one had died. Disturbingly, the Nebraska case is not alone; the Centers for Disease Control and Prevention (CDC) recorded at least 32 outbreaks of HCV in the United States since 1999. In March–May of 2008, 84 patients contracted HCV at an endoscopy center in Las Vegas, Nevada—again as the result of reusing contaminated syringes.

To determine the extent of damage to the patient's liver, the doctor may order a liver biopsy. In this procedure, a needle is inserted into the patient's liver through the abdomen in order to remove a small sample of tissue for analysis.

Treatment

Not all patients with HCV require therapy, but if treatment is needed, the first line of treatment comprises two medications known as Interferon, a drug that resembles some of the proteins that the body makes naturally to fight viruses, and Virazole, which is an antiviral drug. The combination of these drugs works better than Interferon alone. Interferon is usually given as a shot once a week and Ribavirin is taken as a pill twice a day. The length of treatment depends on the genotype of HCV; patients with genotype 2 or 3 are treated for twenty-four weeks whereas patients with genotype 1 or 4 must undergo forty-eight weeks of treatment. The cure rates for genotypes 1 and 3 are about 75 percent; the cure rate for genotype 1 is 50 percent; and for genotype 4 it is 65 percent. Unfortunately, Interferon and Ribavirin produce unpleasant side effects for patients that range from depression and irritability to weight loss, nausea, and muscle pains. In addition to side effects, Ribavirin cannot be given at all to pregnant women because it can harm the unborn child.

The only treatment for cirrhosis or severe liver disease is liver transplantation. The problem, however, is that there are many more patients waiting for donated livers than there are suitable organs available. In addition, liver transplantation does not cure hepatitis C infection; most people who receive transplanted livers will develop a recurrence of the virus. The effectiveness of medication treatment of hepatitis C following a liver transplant is unclear.

Patients with chronic hepatitis C should stop drinking alcohol, as it can speed up the rate of liver damage. They should also be vaccinated against hepatitis A and hepatitis B.

Prognosis

According to the CDC, between 75 and 85 percent of people infected with HCV will develop chronic hepatitis C infection. Twenty percent of these chronically infected persons will develop cirrhosis of the liver within twenty years of infection; 1–5 percent of chronically infected people will eventually die of liver disease.

WORDS TO KNOW

Chronic: Recurrent or long-term.

Cirrhosis: Liver damage most commonly caused by alcoholism or hepatitis C.

Genotype: The genetic makeup of a cell or organism.

Hepatitis: Inflammation of the liver. It can be caused by toxic substances or alcohol as well as infections.

Jaundice: A yellowish discoloration of the skin and whites of the eyes caused by increased levels of bile pigments from the liver in the patient's blood.

Women with chronic hepatitis C have better outcomes than men, and patients infected at younger ages have better outcomes than those infected in middle age. The reason for these differences is not clear.

Prevention

There is no vaccine that can prevent HCV. Prevention depends on careful observation of good health practices in hospitals and clinics and on individual lifestyle changes. The CDC recommends the following ways that individuals can lower their risk of getting hepatitis C:

- Do not use intravenous drugs. People who cannot quit should never share their needles, syringes, water, or other materials used to inject drugs. They should also get vaccinated against hepatitis A and hepatitis B.
- Do not share personal items (razors, toothbrushes, etc.) that might have blood on them.
- Avoid getting tattoos or body piercing. People who do get a tattoo, however, should at least make sure that the operator who performs the tattoo is using proper sterile procedure.
- Use latex condoms when having sex. Although it is rare for HCV to be transmitted through sexual intercourse, it can happen.
- People who discover that they are infected with HCV should not donate blood, organs, or tissues.

The Future

Researchers expect the number of people who die from hepatitis C in the United States to increase in the following years. One researcher found that the number of deaths due to HCV-related complications rose from fewer than 10,000 in 1992 to almost 15,000 in 1999. This number is expected to rise in the years ahead because of the growing numbers of people with HIV and other chronic infections. These infections increase a person's risk of developing severe liver disease if they do become infected with HCV.

Researchers are continuing to work on an effective vaccine against HCV and more effective medications with fewer side effects for treating the chronic form of the disease.

SEE ALSO Hepatitis A; Hepatitis B

For more information

BOOKS

Fabry, Stephen, and R. Anand Narasimhan. *100 Questions and Answers about Hepatitis C: A Lahey Clinic Guide*. Sudbury, MA: Jones and Bartlett Publishers, 2006.

McKnight, Evelyn V. *A Never Event: The Story of the Largest American Outbreak of Hepatitis C in History*. New York: Arbor Books, 2008.

PERIODICALS

Associated Press. "CDC: Syringe Reuse Linked to Hepatitis C Outbreak." *Las Vegas Sun*, May 19, 2008. Available online at http://www.lasvegassun.com/news/2008/may/19/cdc-syringe-reuse-linked-to-hepatitis-c-outbreak/ (accessed June 11, 2008).

Macedo de Oliveira, Alexandre, Kathryn White, Dennis Leschincky, et al. "An Outbreak of Hepatitis C Infections among Outpatients at a Hematology/Oncology Clinic." *Annals of Internal Medicine* 142 (June 7, 2005): 898–902. Available online at http://www.largestamericanoutbreak.com/ (accessed June 11, 2008). Article about the Nebraska hepatitis C outbreak of 2001, the largest to date in North America.

McKeever, Kevin. "Sharp Rise in Hepatitis C-Related Deaths." *HealthDay*, March 27, 2008. Available online at http://www.nlm.nih.gov/medlineplus/news/fullstory_62713.html (accessed June 11, 2008).

WEB SITES

Centers for Disease Control and Prevention (CDC). *Viral Hepatitis C: Fact Sheet*. Available online at http://www.cdc.gov/ncidod/diseases/hepatitis/c/fact.htm (updated March 6, 2008; accessed June 11, 2008).

Mayo Clinic. *Hepatitis C*. Available online at http://www.mayoclinic.com/health/hepatitis-c/DS00097 (updated September 14, 2007; accessed June 11, 2008).

National Institute of Diabetes and Digestive and Kidney Diseases (NIDDK). *Viral Hepatitis: A through E and Beyond*. Available online at http://digestive.niddk.nih.gov/ddiseases/pubs/viralhepatitis/ (updated February 2008; accessed June 11, 2008).

National Library of Medicine (NLM). *Hepatitis C.* Available online at http://www.nlm.nih.gov/medlineplus/tutorials/hepatitisc/htm/index.htm (accessed June 11, 2008). Online tutorial with voiceover; viewers have the option of a self-playing version, an interactive version with questions, or a text version.

Nemours Foundation. *Hepatitis.* Available online at http://www.kidshealth.org/parent/infections/bacterial_viral/hepatitis.html (updated February 2006; accessed June 11, 2008).

High Cholesterol

See **Hypercholesterolemia.**

HIV Infection

See **AIDS.**

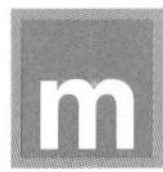

Hives

Definition

Hives refers to an eruption of wheals (flat-topped itching or stinging bumps, welts, or patches) on the skin following contact with an allergen or some other physical agent. It is not a single disease but rather a pattern of reaction to an irritant of some kind. Hives may be caused by infections, medications, insect bites, chemicals, food allergies, underlying medical disorders, or a variety of other causes. Hives that last less than six weeks are defined as acute urticaria; hives that are present for six weeks or longer or that recur frequently are known as chronic urticaria.

Also Known As
Urticaria, nettle rash

Cause
Allergy, exposure to cold or scratching, reaction to medication

Symptoms
Itching, burning, or stinging patches or wheals on the skin

Duration
A few hours to years, depending on type

Description

Hives are pale, itchy, or stinging welts or wheals that form on the skin, most commonly as a reaction to an irritant. Hives located near the mouth, eyes, or genitals may cause the lower layers of nearby skin to swell up or look puffy—this reaction is known as angioedema.

Hives vary in size from about a quarter-inch in diameter to six inches or even larger. They can also join together to form even larger patches of

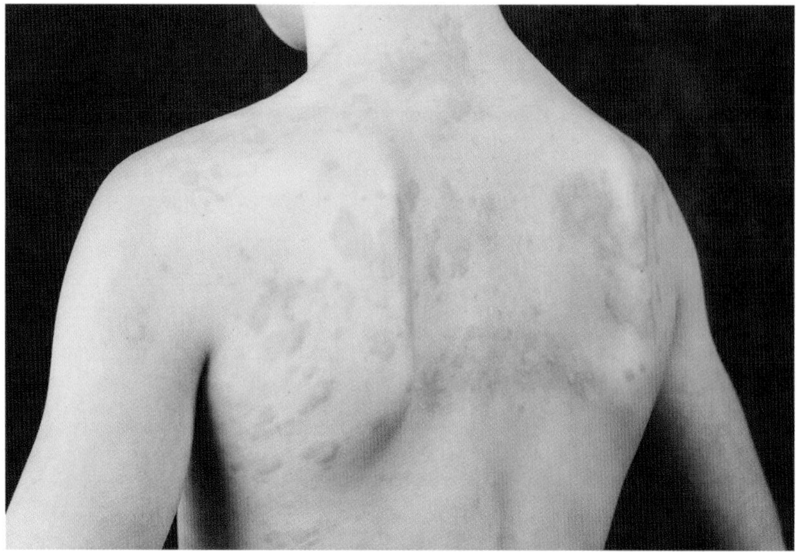

Hives on a patient's back, a result of a strep infection. © PHIL DEGGINGER / ALAMY.

raised skin with clearly defined edges. They will turn white when the center of the wheal is pressed. They may appear suddenly, change shape, and disappear within hours or even minutes. Hives, after disappearing, do not leave scars on the skin.

Acute hives are typically caused by an allergic reaction to foods or medications, fresh foods being more likely to cause hives than cooked foods. The most common "problem" foods are nuts, chocolate, fish and shellfish, tomatoes, eggs, fresh berries, soy, wheat, and milk. Almost any medication can cause hives in a susceptible person. The common offenders are aspirin and ibuprofen; penicillin and other antibiotics; codeine and pain relievers containing codeine; and medications given to treat high blood pressure. Other triggers of acute hives include certain substances, particularly latex; pollen, molds, and animal dander; infections, particularly the common cold; and insect bites.

Some cases of acute hives are triggered by physical causes, such as exposure to sunlight, hot weather, cold water, or exercise. Hives resulting from sun exposure usually fade in one to two hours. Some people who get hives after swimming in cold water may feel faint or dizzy as well. A few people get hives when their skin is scratched or stroked firmly. This condition is called dermatographism and can occur together with hives caused by allergens.

Chronic hives last for longer than six weeks. The causes of chronic urticaria are usually more difficult to identify than the causes of acute hives. They often include autoimmune disorders like lupus or Hashimoto disease, or bacterial or fungal infections. In the majority of cases, however, the cause of chronic hives is never discovered. Chronic hives may last for months or even years and have a severe impact on the patient's quality of life.

Demographics

Hives are a common skin problem in North America, affecting between 20 and 25 percent of people at some point in their lives. As far as is known, hives are equally frequent in all races and ethnic groups, although they are more common in women—there are three females for every two males affected. Chronic urticaria is less common that acute urticaria, affecting between 1 and 3 percent of the population. Dermatographism affects about 5 percent of the general American population.

Acute hives can develop in people of any age, but are most common in teenagers and young adults in their twenties. Chronic hives, on the other hand, are more common in middle-aged adults.

Causes and Symptoms

The basic cause of hives is the release of a chemical called histamine. The histamine causes small blood vessels to leak plasma (the liquid part of blood) into the skin, causing the surface of the skin to rise and form wheals or angioedema.

The symptoms of hives are itching, stinging, and burning on the affected parts of the skin. In some cases, angioedema can affect the tissues that line the throat, causing the airway to swell shut and make it difficult to breathe or swallow. This type of angioedema is a medical emergency and requires immediate treatment in an emergency room.

Home Treatment for Hives

While waiting for antihistamine and other medications to take effect, patients with hives can do the following to relieve itching and speed the healing of their skin:

- Avoid taking hot baths or showers; use lukewarm water instead.
- Avoid using harsh or heavily perfumed soaps.
- Stay out of direct sunlight during the hottest hours of the day; exercise during the early morning or early evening.
- Avoid heavy exercise in hot weather or any activity that might cause sweating, as perspiration can make hives worse.
- Wear light, loose-fitting clothing.
- Apply cool compresses to the affected area.
- Try to work or sleep in a cool room.
- Lower the stress level if possible.

If any of the following symptoms appear with hives, a doctor should be contacted *at once* or the patient taken to an emergency room:

- Dizziness or fainting
- Difficulty in breathing or swallowing
- Wheezing
- Tightness or pain in the chest
- Swelling of the tongue, lips, or entire face
- Nausea, vomiting, abdominal cramps, or diarrhea

Diagnosis

Diagnosis of the cause of acute hives is usually helped by asking patients about their food or medication history, recent exposure to sun or insect bites, recent infections, or their occupation. Patients may be asked to keep a record of the foods they eat, the medications they use, and the types of exercise they do on a regular basis. Doctors may also ask patients to keep a record of the location of the hives when they appear and how long the individual hives last.

Although it is usually not necessary to test for the causes of acute hives in order to treat the problem, the doctor may order skin tests to see whether specific foods, medications, or chemicals are triggering the hives. In some cases the hives may have more than one cause. Blood tests may be ordered to test for the possible causes of chronic hives. A primary care doctor may refer the patient to a dermatologist (a specialist in skin diseases) for more detailed tests or to make sure that the patient does not have a different type of skin disease.

Treatment

Acute hives can often be treated at home by a combination of antihistamine medications prescribed by the doctor, avoiding known triggers, and protecting the skin against further irritation (see sidebar). If the hives are not relieved by antihistamines, the doctor may prescribe cortisone or other steroid medications, but these should be used only for short periods of time.

Patients who have severe attacks of hives or angioedema are usually given an injection of adrenaline to clear the airway and are taken to a hospital emergency room. People who have repeated episodes of angioedema that cause breathing problems are usually given an EpiPen, which is a device that contains adrenaline, so that they can inject themselves in an emergency.

Patients whose hives appear to be triggered by emotional stress may be helped by relaxation techniques or stress management programs.

Prognosis

The prognosis of hives depends on the cause and whether the hives are acute or chronic. Acute hives often clear up rapidly once the allergen or other cause of the skin reaction has been removed. Chronic hives, however, can be difficult to treat or cope with, particularly if the skin eruptions are related to an autoimmune disorder. One study found that

WORDS TO KNOW

Adrenaline: A hormone that can be used in medicine to open the breathing passages in patients with severe angioedema. It is also called epinephrine.

Allergen: Any substance that can provoke an allergic reaction in susceptible individuals.

Angioedema: The medical term for the swelling of tissues around the eyes, lips, and genitals that sometimes accompanies hives.

Chronic: Long-term or recurrent.

Dander: Tiny skin, feather, or fur particles from household pets that cause allergic reactions in some people.

Dermatographism: A type of hives produced by scratching or stroking the skin.

Dermatologist: A doctor who specializes in diagnosing and treating diseases of the skin.

Histamine: A compound that is released during an allergic reaction.

Urticaria: The medical term for hives.

Wheal: A suddenly formed flat-topped swelling of the skin; a welt.

chronic hives lasted a year or longer in more than 50 percent of patients and 20 years or more in 20 percent of them.

Prevention

There is no known way to prevent all possible types of hives, although avoiding foods and medications known to trigger acute hives can help. The limitation of this approach, however, is that specific triggers cannot be identified in about 50 percent of cases.

Another recommendation is to cut down on alcoholic beverages—they can make the itching of hives worse or even trigger hives in some people. Some patients are also advised by their doctors to take antihistamines on a daily basis in order to prevent acute attacks of hives.

The Future

Both acute and chronic hives are likely to be common skin problems for the foreseeable future. It may be that further research will shed light on the causes of chronic hives so that more effective treatments can be developed.

SEE ALSO Allergies; Anaphylaxis; Hashimoto disease; Lupus

For more information

BOOKS

Wanderer, Alan A. *Hives: The Road to Diagnosis and Treatment of Urticaria: A Workbook and Resource for Healthcare Professionals and Patients.* Bozeman, MT: Anson Publishing, LLC, 2004.

PERIODICALS

Roth, Sharon. "A Shot in Time." *New York Times*, May 14, 2006. Available online at http://query.nytimes.com/gst/fullpage.html?res=9C0DE5DA173EF937A25756C0A9609C8B63&sec=&spon=&pagewanted=all (accessed May 12, 2008). This is an article about the use of the EpiPen to treat emergency episodes of angioedema.

WEB SITES

American Academy of Dermatology (AAD). *Urticaria—Hives.* Available online at http://www.aad.org/public/publications/pamphlets/skin_urticaria.html (updated September 2005; accessed May 12, 2008).

Mayo Clinic. *Chronic Hives (Urticaria).* Available online at http://www.mayoclinic.com/health/chronic-hives/DS00980 (updated June 22, 2007; accessed May 11, 2008).

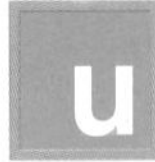

Hodgkin Disease

Definition

Hodgkin disease, also known as Hodgkin lymphoma or HL, is a cancer of the blood and lymphatic system. It is the most common type of blood cancer and the third most common childhood cancer. The disease is named for Thomas Hodgkin (1798–1866), the British doctor who first described it in 1832.

Also Known As
Hodgkin lymphoma, HL

Cause
Unknown

Symptoms
Swollen lymph nodes, night sweats, fever, weight loss, lack of energy

Duration
Lifelong unless treated

Description

Hodgkin disease is one of the two major types of lymphoma, a form of cancer that originates in lymphocytes, which are a specific type of white blood cells in the immune system. It is unusual in that it primarily affects two different age groups, adolescents and young adults between the ages of fifteen and thirty-five, and older adults over age fifty-five. Hodgkin begins in the lymphatic system, a group of organs and tissues that are part of the immune system and also help to form new blood cells. The lymphatic system includes lymph nodes, small organs composed of

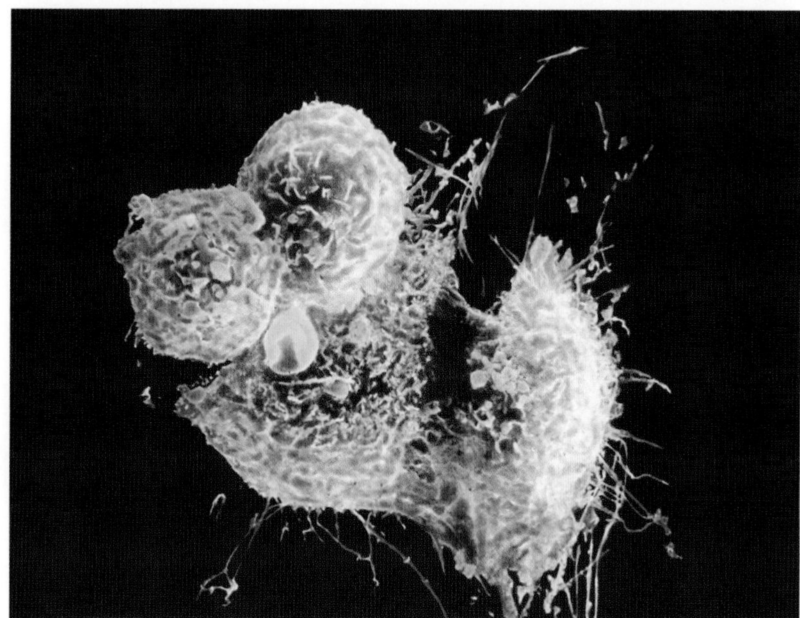

Image of cancer cells dividing in Hodgkin disease. © DR. ANDREJS LIEPINS/SPL/ PHOTO RESEARCHERS, INC.

lymphoid tissue located at various points throughout the body that are joined by lymphatic vessels; the spleen, a small organ on the left side of the abdomen; the bone marrow; and the thymus gland, which is just below the neck.

Hodgkin disease begins when a type of lymphocyte called a B cell turns into an abnormal form called a Reed-Sternberg cell. These abnormal cells continue to reproduce themselves until they form a tumor. In most cases this first tumor develops in one of the lymph nodes above the diaphragm (the thin sheet of muscle that divides the chest cavity from the abdominal cavity); however, the tumor can develop in a group of lymph nodes or elsewhere in the lymphatic system. The disease usually spreads from lymph node to lymph node along the lymphatic vessels rather than skipping around the body. In the later stages of the disease, it spreads outside the lymphatic system to other organs.

There are two basic subtypes of Hodgkin disease: classic, which accounts for 95 percent of cases, and nodular lymphocyte predominant Hodgkin disease (NLPHD), which accounts for the remaining 5 percent. NLPHD differs from classic Hodgkin diseae in that it occurs primarily in lymph nodes in the neck and armpits, and its large abnormal cells are known as "popcorn" cells because they look like pieces of popped popcorn under the microscope.

Demographics

Hodgkin lymphoma is a relatively rare form of cancer, affecting two or three people in every 100,000. It accounts for less than 1 percent of cancers worldwide. As of 2008, there were about 500,000 people in the United States with some form of lymphoma, but only 143,000 had Hodgkin disease. According to the National Cancer Institute (NCI), about 8,200 new cases of HL are diagnosed in the United States each year, and 1,350 people die from the disease annually.

The rates for Hodgkin disease vary according to race and sex. The highest rates are in Caucasian males (3.2 cases per 100,000), followed by African American males (3.0 cases per 100,000), Caucasian females (2.6 cases per 100,000), African American females (2.1 cases per 100,000), Asian American males (1.4 cases per 100,000), and Asian American females (1 case per 100,000). About 10 percent of cases of Hodgkin are diagnosed in children below the age of fourteen; 85 percent of these are boys.

Although the cause of Hodgkin disease is still unknown, researchers have identified several factors that increase a person's risk of developing this form of cancer:

- Age between fifteen and thirty-five or over fifty-five
- Male sex
- Infection with Epstein-Barr virus or infectious mononucleosis
- Family history of Hodgkin disease
- HIV infection
- Organ transplantation or other reasons for therapy that suppresses the immune system

Causes and Symptoms

Although researchers know that Hodgkin disease begins with the formation and multiplication of abnormal cells, they do not yet know what triggers this formation. Some scientists think that certain types of viral infections, genetic factors, or environmental toxins might be involved.

The symptoms of Hodgkin disease include:

- Swelling of the lymph nodes in the neck, armpits, or groin. These are usually painless.
- Tiredness that does not go away.
- Fever and chills.

- Night sweats.
- Unexplained weight loss of 10 percent or more of body weight.
- Itchy skin.
- Loss of appetite.

Some patients also experience heavy sweating, coughing or chest pain, difficulty breathing, enlargement of the spleen, hair loss, or neck pain.

Diagnosis

The doctor usually begins by taking a medical history, because there are many causes other than Hodgkin for swollen lymph nodes, fever, and some of the other early symptoms of the disease. In some cases, a patient with classic Hodgkin has no early symptoms, and the disease is discovered during a routine chest x ray.

In most cases the disease is diagnosed by a tissue biopsy. The doctor removes a small piece of tissue from a swollen lymph node either by cutting directly into the swollen node or by withdrawing a tissue sample through a fine needle. In addition to looking for abnormal cells in the tissue sample, the doctor may use certain types of chemical tests to look for proteins attached to the surface of the abnormal cells.

In addition to a tissue biopsy, the doctor may order blood tests or a bone marrow biopsy. Blood tests are useful in evaluating the type of chemotherapy that would be best for the patient. In addition, imaging tests can be used to determine the location and extent of the disease. These tests may include x-ray studies, magnetic resonance imaging (MRI), computed tomography (CT) scans, positron emission tomography (PET) scans, and a gallium scan. This last type of test uses a radioactive element given intravenously to identify affected lymph nodes.

Treatment

The first step in treating any kind of cancer is called staging. Staging is a description of the location of the cancer, its size, how far it has penetrated into healthy tissue, and whether it has spread to other parts of the body. Hodgkin disease is classified into four stages:

- Stage I: The disease is limited to one lymph node.
- Stage II. The disease involves two or more lymph nodes on the same side of the diaphragm.

- Stage III. The disease has spread to lymph nodes on both sides of the diaphragm and may involve the spleen.
- Stage IV. The disease has spread to one or more organs outside the lymphatic system, such as the lungs or liver.

The next steps in treatment depend on the stage of the disease.

- Stage I and Stage II Hodgkin disease can be treated with radiation therapy, chemotherapy, or a combination of both. Only low-dose radiation therapy is used in girls and women, because standard doses of radiation will increase their risk of breast cancer in later life.
- Stages III and IV. Chemotherapy may be used by itself to treat advanced-stage Hodgkin as well as being combined with radiation therapy. There are five different combinations of drugs that are currently used; some of these are quite toxic and have severe side effects. The drug combination preferred by most doctors in the United States is called ABVD, the initials of the four drugs that are administered.

Patients who are not cured by radiation therapy and chemotherapy, or whose disease recurs after chemotherapy, may be treated with a combination of high-dose chemotherapy and bone marrow transplantation. The bone marrow transplantation is needed because the high doses of anti-cancer chemicals will damage the patient's own bone marrow and lead to a life-threatening shortage of the red and white blood cells produced in the bone marrow.

Prognosis

Hodgkin disease is potentially curable, although the treatments that are currently used increase the patient's risk of developing a second type of cancer later in life. As of 2008, 90 percent of patients with Stage I or II disease lived for five years after treatment. The five-year survival rates for Stages III and IV are 84 percent and 65 percent respectively. Between 20 and 25 percent of all patients diagnosed with Hodgkin will die of the disease. In the first fifteen years after treatment, recurrent Hodgkin is the major cause of death among patients; after fifteen years, death from other causes is more common.

Prevention

There is no way to prevent Hodgkin disease, because its causes are still unknown.

WORDS TO KNOW

Diaphragm: A sheet of muscle extending across the bottom of the rib cage that separates the chest from the abdomen.

Lymph nodes: Small rounded masses of lymphoid tissue found at various points along the lymphatic vessels.

Lymphocyte: A type of white blood cell that fights infection. Lymphocytes are divided into two types, T cells (produced in the thymus gland) and B cells (produced in the bone marrow).

Popcorn cell: An abnormal cell found in nodular lymphocyte predominant Hodgkin disease (NLPHD).

Reed-Sternberg cell: An abnormal type of B lymphocyte that is found in classic Hodgkin lymphoma.

Staging: Measuring the severity or spread of a cancer.

Thymus: A small organ located behind the breastbone that is part of the lymphatic system and produces T cells.

The Future

Current research on Hodgkin disease is focused on the possible role of viruses in causing the disease and on exploring newer forms of treatment. Although radiation therapy and chemotherapy are highly effective treatments for this form of cancer, they have a number of long-term as well as short-term side effects. Because Hodgkin disease is a relatively rare form of cancer and because there are still unanswered questions about the best way to treat it, researchers are actively looking for Hodgkin patients to participate in clinical studies.

SEE ALSO Infectious mononucleosis; Lymphoma

For more information

BOOKS

Adler, Elizabeth M. *Living with Lymphoma: A Patient's Guide*. Baltimore, MD: Johns Hopkins University Press, 2005.

Holman, Peter, Jodi Garrett, and William D. Jansen. *100 Questions and Answers about Lymphoma*. Sudbury, MA: Jones and Bartlett, Publishers, 2004.

PERIODICALS

Preidt, Robert. "Young Hodgkin Survivors Face Later Risk of Second Cancers." *HealthDay*, June 2, 2008. Available online at http://www.nlm.nih.gov/medlineplus/news/fullstory_65263.html (accessed June 17, 2008).

WEB SITES

American Cancer Society (ACS). *Hodgkin Disease.* Available online in PDF format at http://documents.cancer.org/113.00/113.00.pdf (updated March 22, 2008; accessed June 16, 2008).

Lymphoma Research Foundation. *Hodgkin Lymphoma.* Available online at http://www.lymphoma.org/site/pp.asp?c=chKOI6PEImE&b=1574105 (accessed June 17, 2008).

Mayo Clinic. *Hodgkin Disease.* Available online at http://www.mayoclinic.com/health/hodgkins-disease/DS00186 (updated March 26, 2008; accessed June 17, 2008).

National Cancer Institute (NCI). *What You Need to Know about Hodgkin Lymphoma.* Available online at http://www.cancer.gov/cancertopics/wyntk/hodgkin/allpages (updated February 5, 2008; accessed June 16, 2008).

TeensHealth. *Hodgkin Disease.* Available online at http://kidshealth.org/teen/diseases_conditions/cancer/hodgkins.html (updated June 2007; accessed June 17, 2008).

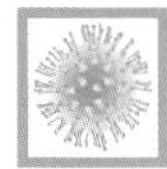

HPV Infection

Definition

HPV infection is a sexually transmitted disease (STD) caused by thirty to forty of the 130 or so known strains of human papillomavirus, the name of a group of viruses that infect the skin and mucous membranes of humans and some animals. In humans these sexually transmitted strains can cause genital warts, precancerous changes in the tissues of the female vagina, or cervical cancer. Other strains of HPV are responsible for warts on the soles of the feet (plantar warts), common warts on the hands, and flat warts on the face or legs.

Also Known As
Human papillomavirus infection, genital warts

Cause
Human papillomavirus

Symptoms
None in most people; genital warts, precancerous tissue changes, cervical cancer

Duration
Months or years after infection

Description

HPV infection is one of the most common sexually transmitted diseases in the United States. Most people who are infected with one of the sexually transmitted strains of the virus, however, do not know that they have it because they have no symptoms. They can easily transmit the infection to a partner.

The various strains of HPV are classified as either low-risk or high-risk according to their potential for causing cancer or other serious health

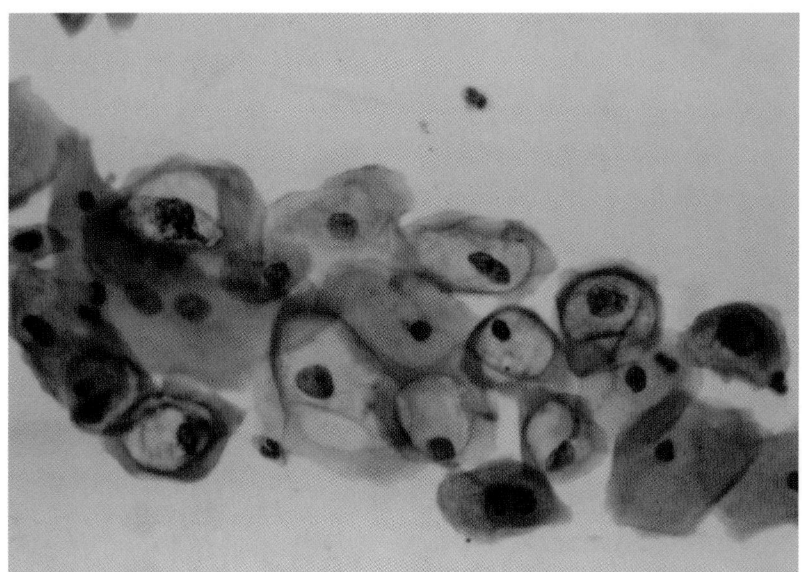

Image of cervical cells infected with HPV. The nucleus of the cell is the black dot; in HPV infection, some cells have more than one nucleus.
DR. E. WALKER / PHOTO RESEARCHERS, INC.

problems. Low-risk strains of HPV may produce genital warts but do not cause cancer. Low-risk types 6 and 11 are responsible for 90 percent of cases of genital warts. High-risk strains of the virus, which include types 16, 18, 31, and 45, may cause cervical cancer in women as well as cancers of the anus and penis in men. These high-risk strains can also cause cancer of the mouth and throat in people who have oral sex. HPV types 16 and 18 are found in more than 70 percent of cervical cancers in women.

Demographics

In recent years HPV infection has become one of the most common STDs in the United States. Approximately 20 million Americans were infected with HPV as of 2008, and another 6.2 million people become newly infected each year. According to one study, 27 percent of women between the ages of fourteen and fifty-nine are infected with one or more types of HPV. The Centers for Disease Control and Prevention (CDC) estimates that more than 80 percent of American women will contract at least one strain of genital HPV by age fifty. About 75–80 percent of sexually active Americans of either sex will be infected with HPV at some point in their lifetime.

As far as is known, men and women are at equal risk of being infected with HPV, as are members of all races and ethnic groups.

Some people are at greater risk of sexually transmitted HPV than others:

- Gay and bisexual men.
- People with HIV or other diseases that weaken the immune system.
- Males or females below age twenty-five. Younger people appear to be more biologically vulnerable to the HPV virus.
- People who have large numbers of sexual partners.
- People in relationships with partners who have sex with many other people.

In terms of specific illnesses associated with HPV, 11,000 women are diagnosed with cervical cancer each year in the United States and 3,900 women die annually of the disease. Another 5,800 women are diagnosed with cancers of the vagina and the external female genitals, while 3,300 men are diagnosed with cancer of the penis or the anal area. The risk of anal cancer is seventeen to thirty-one times higher among gay and bisexual men than among heterosexual men.

Causes and Symptoms

The cause of sexually transmitted HPV infection is one or more strains of the human papillomavirus. The virus enters the body through small breaks in the skin surface or in the mucous membranes lining the genitals. In most cases the body fights off the virus within a few weeks. In some people, however, HPV remains dormant for a period ranging from a few weeks to several years in one of the lower layers of skin cells. The virus then begins to replicate (copy itself) when these cells mature and move upward to the surface of the skin. The virus affects the shape of the cells, leading to the formation of noticeable warts, precancerous changes in skin cells, or cervical cancer. About 1 percent of sexually active adults in the United States have genital warts at any one time; about 10 percent of women with high-risk HPV in the tissues of their cervix will develop long-lasting HPV infections that put them at risk for cervical cancer.

Symptoms of sexually transmitted HPV infection may include:

- Genital warts. These appear as bumps or clusters of fleshy outgrowths around the anus or on the genitals. Some may grow into larger cauliflower-shaped masses. Genital warts usually appear within weeks or months after sexual contact with an infected person. If left untreated, genital warts may go away, remain unchanged, or increase in size or number but will not turn into cancers. It is possible, however, for a person to be infected with a high-risk strain of HPV as well as one of the strains that cause genital warts; therefore the appearance of genital warts does not necessarily mean that the person is not at risk of cancer.

- Precancerous changes in the tissues of the female cervix. These are flat growths on the cervix that cannot be seen or felt by the infected woman.
- Cancer. High-risk strains of HPV can cause cancers of the mouth and throat as well as cancers of the anal area and the male and female genitals. These typically take years to develop after infection. In men, symptoms of anal cancer may include bleeding, pain, or a discharge from the anus, or changes in bowel habits. Early signs of cancer of the penis may include thickening of the skin, tissue growths, or sores.

Diagnosis

There is no general blood, urine, or imaging test for HPV infection. The diagnosis of genital warts is obvious based on their location and appearance. The doctor may, however, use a vinegar solution to identify HPV-infected areas on the skin of the genitals. The vinegar solution may turn white if HPV is present. Since genital warts are caused by low-risk strains of HPV, the doctor does not need to identify the specific strain of the virus that is present.

Sexually active women should be screened periodically for the presence of changes in the tissues of the cervix. The most common test is the Papanikolaou test or Pap smear, invented by a Greek physician in the 1940s. To perform a Pap smear, the doctor takes a small spatula to obtain cells from the outer surface of the cervix and smears the collected cells on a slide that is then examined in a laboratory for signs of any abnormal cells. If abnormal or questionable cells are found, the doctor may order an HPV DNA test, which can identify the DNA of 13 high-risk types of HPV in cells taken from the cervix.

There are no HPV screening tests for men.

Treatment

Patients with genital warts should *never* use over-the counter-preparations designed to remove common or flat warts from the hands or face.

WORDS TO KNOW

Cervix: The narrow neck or outlet of a woman's uterus.

Cryotherapy: The use of liquid nitrogen or other forms of extreme cold to treat a skin disorder.

Mucous membrane: Soft tissues that line the nose, throat, stomach, and intestines.

Pap test: A screening test for cervical cancer devised by Giorgios Papanikolaou (1883–1962) in the 1940s.

Topical: Referring to a type of medication applied directly to the skin or outside of the body.

Doctors can treat genital warts with various medical or surgical techniques:

- Cryotherapy. Cryotherapy uses liquid nitrogen to freeze the warts. The dead tissue in the wart falls away from the skin beneath in about a week.
- Imiquimod. Imiquimod is a topical cream that gets rid of genital warts by stimulating the body's immune system to fight the virus that causes the warts.
- Podofilox. This is a topical medication available in liquid or gel form that destroys the wart tissue.
- Surgery. The doctor can remove the wart by drying it out with an electric needle and then scraping the tissue with a sharp instrument called a curette. Lasers can also be used to remove genital warts.

Low-grade precancerous changes in the tissue of the female cervix are not usually treated directly, because most of them will eventually go away on their own without developing into cancer. The patient should, however, see the doctor for follow-up Pap smears to make sure that the tissues are returning to normal. High-risk precancerous lesions are removed, usually by surgery, cryotherapy, or laser surgery.

Prognosis

The prognosis of sexually transmitted HPV infections depends on the patient's age, number of sexual partners, gender, and the condition of their immune system. Women are significantly more likely than men to develop cancers following HPV infection. However, most people of either sex with normally functioning immune systems who are infected with HPV will clear the infection from their bodies within two years.

Prevention

Preventive measures that people can take to lower their risk of HPV infection include:

- Abstaining from sex, or having sex only with an uninfected partner who is faithful.
- Reducing the number of sexual partners.
- Using condoms regularly during sexual intercourse.
- For women, using a new vaccine called Gardasil. Approved by the Food and Drug Administration in 2006, Gardasil is a vaccine that protects against the four types of HPV that cause most cervical cancers and genital warts. The vaccine is recommended for eleven- and twelve-year-old girls. It is also recommended for girls and women age thirteen through twenty-six who have not yet been vaccinated or completed the vaccine series. Gardasil works best in girls who have not yet been sexually active. It is given as a series of three shots over a six-month period.

The Future

Researchers are working on developing vaccines that protect against additional types of the HPV virus. Other scientists are studying the possibility that the transmission of HPV could be prevented by applying substances that would kill bacteria or viruses directly to the skin of the genitals or to condoms. Several different gels and creams were in clinical trials as of 2008.

SEE ALSO Warts

For more information

BOOKS

Gonzales, Lissette. *Frequently Asked Questions about Human Papillomavirus.* New York: Rosen, 2007.

Marr, Lisa. *Sexually Transmitted Diseases: A Physician Tells You What You Need to Know,* 2nd ed. Baltimore, MD: Johns Hopkins University Press, 2007.

Nardo, Don. *Human Papillomavirus (HPV).* Detroit, MI: Lucent Books, 2007.

PERIODICALS

Brody, Jane. "Personal Health: HPV Vaccine; Few Risks, Many Benefits." *New York Times,* May 15, 2007. Available online at http://query.nytimes.com/gst/

fullpage.html?res=9805E1DE1331F936A25756C0A9619C8B63&sec=&spon=&pagewanted=all (accessed July 8, 2008).

WEB SITES

Centers for Disease Control and Prevention (CDC). *Human Papillomavirus (HPV) Infection*. Available online at http://www.cdc.gov/std/hpv/default.htm (updated June 30, 2008; accessed July 8, 2008).

Centers for Disease Control and Prevention (CDC) Fact Sheet. *HPV and Men*. Available online at http://www.cdc.gov/std/hpv/STDFact-HPV-and-men.htm (updated August 14, 2007; accessed July 8, 2008).

Mayo Clinic. *HPV Infection*. Available online at http://www.mayoclinic.com/health/hpv-infection/DS00906 (updated March 13, 2007; accessed July 8, 2008).

National Cancer Institute (NCI). *Human Papillomaviruses and Cancer: Questions and Answers*. Available online at http://www.cancer.gov/cancertopics/factsheet/Risk/HPV (updated February 14, 2008; accessed July 8, 2008).

National Institute of Allergy and Infectious Diseases (NIAID). *Human Papillomavirus and Genital Warts*. Available online at http://www3.niaid.nih.gov/healthscience/healthtopics/human_papillomavirus/overview.htm (updated February 8, 2007; accessed July 8, 2008).

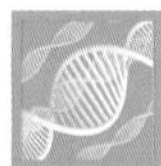

Huntington Disease

Also Known As
Huntington's chorea, HD, St. Vitus' dance

Cause
Defective gene on chromosome 4

Symptoms
Jerky, random physical movements followed by mental decline and eventual death

Duration
Ten to twenty-five years after symptoms appear

Definition

Huntington disease, or HD, is a rare and incurable genetic disorder caused by a defective gene on chromosome 4.

Description

HD is a rare but invariably fatal disease caused by an abnormal stretch of DNA in a single gene on chromosome 4. It has been known for centuries; in the Middle Ages it was grouped together with other movement disorders under the name of St. Vitus' dance. Huntington disease got its present name from Dr. George Huntington (1850–1916), an American doctor who published the first medical description of the disease in 1872, one year after completing medical school. Dr. Huntington was the first writer to prove that the disease is inherited; his grandfather and father had both practiced medicine on Long Island and had kept records of a single family with four generations of members with HD.

It was not until 1983, however, that geneticists were able to find out which of the twenty-three pairs of human chromosomes carries the gene that causes HD. In that year it was discovered that the gene was located somewhere on chromosome 4, although the gene itself was not pinpointed until 1993. In the meantime researchers were studying families living in poor fishing villages along the shores of Lake Maracaibo in Venezuela. This group of families has the highest rate of HD in the world—700 per 100,000 people. Tissue samples from these families helped to locate the gene that causes HD.

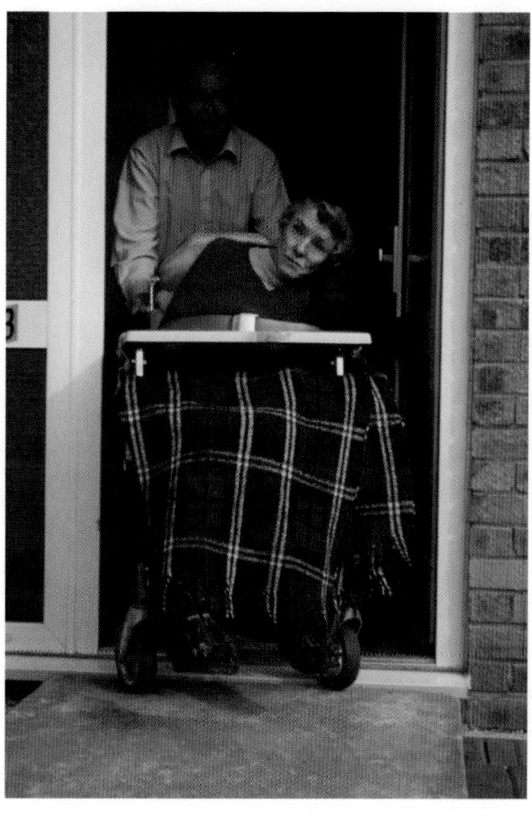

Elderly woman suffering from Huntington's disease. CONOR CAFFREY / PHOTO RESEARCHERS, INC.

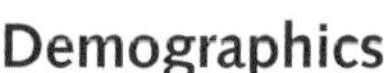

Demographics

Huntington disease is uncommon, affecting between four and eight people per 100,000 in the United States and between two and ten per 100,000 in Europe. There are a few countries other than Venezuela with higher than average rates of HD, including Mauritius (forty-six per 100,000 people) and Tasmania (eighteen per 100,000 people). The disease appears to be somewhat more common among people of European ancestry than among Africans or Asians.

Men and women are equally likely to inherit the defective gene, develop the disease, and pass it on to their children. Huntington disease is one of only a few genetic disorders occurring as a dominant trait, that is, to develop the disease a person only requires one abnormal gene (whereas with recessive traits, to cause overt disease, one must have abnormal genes on both pairs of the chromosome). In many cases the first symptoms appear when patients are in their late 30s or early 40s; however, 10 percent of all cases appear in people younger than twenty. This form of the disease is called juvenile HD. The disease has been known to appear in children as young as two years and in adults over eighty years of age. Most patients die between ten and twenty-five years after the first symptoms appear.

The House of Love and Faith

The House of Love and Faith, or *Casa Hogar Amor y Fe* in Spanish, is a clinic in Venezuela run by Dr. Margot de Young for the families near Lake Maracaibo affected by Huntington disease. There are 14,000 descendants of the first known family member who developed the disease in the 1800s living in this area. Many are at risk of developing HD themselves. The fishing villages around the lake have been impoverished by the disease; children often quit school at age seven or eight in order to care for older relatives dying of HD. By the time they are teenagers, many have had children, thus passing on the gene for the disease to the next generation. Because many families in the villages have ten to twelve children, it is not unusual for such families to have five or more children with juvenile HD.

Dr. de Young's clinic, located in a building that was once a bar, has thirty-four beds for patients in the last stages of Huntington disease. The doctor also provides food, medicines, and basic information about health care and nutrition to the patients' family members. The clinic selectively hires its health care workers from among the HD families; they are proud of their work in the small clinic and do their best to keep it a clean and welcoming place.

Causes and Symptoms

Huntington disease is caused by a defective gene on chromosome 4 that produces an abnormal protein. This protein causes the death of nerve cells in various parts of the brain that control movement, cognition (thinking), and behavior. The defect in the gene is a DNA repeat that occurs from thirty-six to 120 times, whereas there are only seven to thirty-five repeats in a normal gene. The larger the number of repeats, the earlier the symptoms of HD are likely to appear; people with more than sixty repeats are likely to develop juvenile HD. Moreover, the number of repeats increases in each successive generation of people with the defective gene; this characteristic of the disease is known as anticipation.

People can inherit the faulty gene from either parent; however, inheriting it from the father appears to speed up the onset of the disease. Most people who develop juvenile HD inherited the defective gene from the father, whereas people who first develop symptoms after age thirty-five are more likely to have inherited the defective gene from their mother.

The symptoms of Huntington disease include physical, mental, and emotional symptoms. In most cases the physical indications of the disease are the first to appear, although some patients have memory problems or emotional disturbances as the earliest symptoms.

- Physical symptoms: uncontrollable fidgeting or sudden jerky movements (chorea); loss of coordination and balance; difficulty changing the direction of the eyes without moving the entire head; uncontrollable facial grimaces; difficulties with speech and swallowing.
- Cognitive symptoms: dementia (loss of memory and ability to make plans or solve problems); disorientation and confusion.

- Emotional changes: depression; personality changes; antisocial behavior; hallucinations; psychosis (complete loss of contact with reality).

Younger patients with juvenile HD may have symptoms resembling those of Parkinson's disease, such as rigid muscles, slow movement, drooling, and frequent falls. Between 30 and 50 percent of these patients also develop seizures.

As the disease progresses, patients gradually lose their ability to walk or stand and may be confined to a wheelchair or completely bedridden. They may become completely stiff or unable to eat; most patients eventually have to be institutionalized.

Diagnosis

The doctor may order various imaging studies of the brain, such as a computed tomography (CT) scan or magnetic resonance imaging (MRI). Patients with HD will typically show some loss of brain tissue in a specific area of the brain called the caudate nucleus. This part of the brain primarily controls movement but is also involved in learning and memory. It is one of the first parts of the brain to be damaged by the disease.

Genetic testing can be done to confirm the diagnosis of Huntington disease. It involves a blood sample that counts the number of DNA repetitions in the HD gene. People who are at risk for HD can request the test before they develop symptoms. They must undergo several counseling sessions before the test, however, to make sure that they can cope with the results because there is no way to cure HD or slow its appearance.

Treatment

Treatments for Huntington disease are primarily intended to help patients manage their symptoms, since there is no cure for the disease. Most patients are given several medications, which may include antiseizure drugs, antidepressants, tranquilizers, drugs to control hallucinations and other symptoms of psychosis, and drugs to control involuntary body movements.

Other treatments include physical therapy to help keep the patient's muscles strong and flexible, speech therapy to help with difficulties in talking clearly, and occupational therapy to help the patient take care of dressing, bathing, and other basic needs as long as possible.

Prognosis

There is no cure for HD. Patients die about nineteen years on average after the first symptoms appear, most commonly of pneumonia or another infection, malnutrition from inability to eat, or suicide.

Prevention

One reason why Huntington disease has not died out among humans is that the earliest symptoms often do not appear until after the affected person has had children and thus conveyed the defective gene into the next generation. People with a parent who has the defective gene should receive genetic counseling before starting a family. Some younger people choose to be tested for the gene before marrying in order to tell whether they will develop HD themselves as well as risk passing on the defective gene to children. People at risk for HD can consider adoption if they wish to start a family, or they can use a form of assisted reproduction in which embryos are screened for the Huntington gene mutation before being implanted in the woman's uterus.

The Future

It is not likely that HD will ever be completely wiped out even if everyone who presently might have the defective gene agreed to be tested and further agreed not to have children if they turned out to have the gene. The reason why HD would reappear at some point is that some people can develop the disease even without a family history of HD because of a spontaneous mutation (change in their genetic material).

Researchers are looking in several different directions for a possible cure for Huntington disease. One possibility is gene silencing, a technique that would involve using a short sequence of DNA to block the expression of the DNA repeats on the Huntington gene. Another possibility is a combination of certain drugs used to treat cancer with other drugs used to treat AIDS. This type of drug therapy has not yet been tested in humans, however. Still a third possibility is implanting stem cells in the damaged parts of the brain to replace the nerve cells that have already been destroyed.

WORDS TO KNOW

Anticipation: A condition in which the symptoms of a genetic disorder appear earlier and earlier in each successive generation.

Chorea: A general term for movement disorders marked by loss of coordination and involuntary motions of the head and limbs.

Dementia: Loss of memory and other mental functions related to thinking or problem-solving.

Mutation: A change in the genetic material of an organism.

Psychosis: A severe form of mental illness involving loss of contact with reality.

Stem cell: An unspecialized human cell that has the capacity to form itself into a nerve cell or other type of specialized cell.

SEE ALSO Parkinson disease

For more information

BOOKS

Huntington's Disease Society of America (HDSA). *Huntington's Disease.* New York: HDSA, 2007. Available online in PDF format at http://www.hdsa.org/images/content/1/1/11287.pdf (accessed November 4, 2008).

Knowles, Johanna. *Huntington's Disease.* New York: Rosen Publishing Group, 2007.

Quarrell, Oliver. *Huntington's Disease.* New York: Oxford University Press, 2008.

PERIODICALS

Goldberg, Carey. "Huntington's Gene Has Led to Clues, But Not Yet Cures." *Boston Globe*, October 23, 2006. Available online at http://www.boston.com/news/globe/health_science/articles/2006/10/23/huntingtons_gene_has_led_to_clues_but_not_yet_cures/?page=full (accessed April 23, 2008).

Harmon, Amy. "Facing Life with a Lethal Gene." *New York Times*, March 18, 2007. Available online at http://query.nytimes.com/gst/fullpage.html?res=9501E4DD1630F93BA25750C0A9619C8B63&sec=&spon=&pagewanted=all# (accessed April 23, 2008). Article about a young woman who chose to be tested for the Huntington's gene and is coping with the test results. A video about the article is available on the newspaper's website at http://video.on.nytimes.com/index.jsp?fr_story=d962010d883be3d1278974769d1226cf0ed34933 (accessed April 23, 2008). The video shows some patients with HD and is about 3 minutes in length.

Hoag, Christina. "A Tale of Pain and Hope on Lake Maracaibo." *Business Week*, May 29, 2000. Available online at http://www.businessweek.com/2000/00_22/c3683206.htm (accessed April 23, 2008). This is an article about the village in Venezuela with the highest rate of HD in the world.

WEB SITES

Conomy, John P. "Dr. George Huntington and the Disease Bearing His Name." *Huntington's Disease Society of America, Northeast Ohio Chapter.* Available online at http://www.lkwdpl.org/hdsa/conomy.htm (accessed April 23, 2008). This is a short biography of the doctor who first described HD.

Genetics Home Reference. *Huntington Disease.* Available online at http://ghr.nlm.nih.gov/condition=huntingtondisease (updated July 2006; accessed April 23, 2008).

Mayo Clinic. *Huntington's Disease.* Available online at http://www.mayoclinic.com/health/huntingtons-disease/DS00401 (updated May 9, 2007; accessed April 23, 2008).

Understanding Evolution. *Huntington's Chorea: Evolution and Genetic Disease.* Available online at http://evolution.berkeley.edu/evolibrary/article/0_0_0/medicine_05 (accessed April 23, 2008).

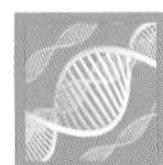

Hutchinson-Gilford Syndrome

Definition

Hutchinson-Gilford progeria syndrome, or HGPS, is a genetic disorder characterized by premature aging and early death.

Also Known As
Hutchinson-Gilford progeria syndrome, HGPS

Cause
Mutations of the LMNA gene

Symptoms
Premature aging, hair loss, wrinkled skin, hardening of the arteries, early death

Duration
Lifelong; average life expectancy is thirteen years

Description

HGPS is a sporadic genetic disorder, which means that it usually occurs at random and occurs in families only rarely. It was first described in 1886 by Jonathan Hutchinson (1828–1913), a British surgeon, and independently reported in 1897 by Hastings Gilford (1861–1941), also a British surgeon.

Children with HGPS look normal at birth but begin to show signs of the disorder during the first two years of life. Their growth slows down; this condition is called failure to thrive or FTT. The child is short and small for his or her age, develops wrinkled skin like that of an elderly person, loses the body fat beneath the skin, and has a fragile-looking body with joints that stick out and easily dislocated hips. The child's facial features are also distinctive, with large eyes, loss of scalp hair, a beaklike nose, thin lips, a small chin, and large ears. Some children have missing teeth or teeth that are late to come in. The child's body ages six to eight times faster than normal aging; however, these children do not develop certain age-related problems like cataracts or an increased risk of cancer.

The disorder does not interfere with intellectual development or with sitting, standing, and walking. Children with HGPS can go to school with other children and participate in activities with them.

The disease leads to death at an early age from heart attack or stroke caused by premature hardening of the arteries. Children with HGPS frequently experience angina—chest pain caused by an inadequate supply of oxygen to the heart muscle. They also suffer from high blood pressure and enlargement of the heart.

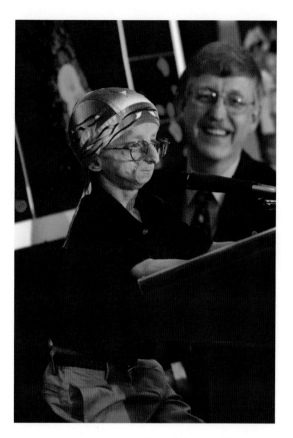

John Tacket, age fifteen, has Hutchinson-Gilford syndrome, or progeria, a rare disease of accelerated aging. AP IMAGES.

Demographics

HGPS is a very rare disorder, thought to affect between one in 8 million and one in 4 million children. About 130 cases have been reported in medical journals since the disease was first described in 1886. There were seven children in the United States with progeria in 2005.

As of 2008, 97 percent of reported cases of HGPS had been found in Caucasians. The reason for this racial disparity is not yet known; since some researchers think that the disorder is misdiagnosed in some cases, it is possible that the racial difference is at least partly a matter of reporting.

HGPS affects boys slightly more often than girls; the gender ratio is about 1.5 boys for every girl.

For many years it was thought that HGPS does not run in families. Since the early 2000s, however, two families have been identified with more than one child affected by the disorder. The first is a family in India with five children with HGPS, first described by a pediatrician in Calcutta in 2005. The other is a family in Belgium with two children with HGPS that was diagnosed in 2006.

Causes and Symptoms

Hutchinson-Gilford progeria syndrome is caused by a mutation in a gene on chromosome 1 called the LMNA gene. This gene tells cells how to make a protein called lamin A, which helps to shape the cell nucleus inside the cell. The defective gene involved in HGPS cannot give the cell proper instructions for making lamin A. As a result, the cell nucleus develops into a strange and twisted shape rather than the normal round shape. It is not known, however, just how the unstable shape of the cell nucleus is related to the characteristic symptoms of HGPS.

Coping with Unfair Suffering

Although Hutchinson-Gilford syndrome is an extremely rare disorder, it played a role in the writing of a well-known book on the meaning of human suffering. *When Bad Things Happen to Good People* was first published in 1981 and reissued in 2001 with a new preface. The author, Harold S. Kushner, was moved to write the book following the death of his son Aaron in 1977 at the age of fourteen. Rabbi Kushner had been the spiritual leader of Temple Israel in Natick, Massachusetts, when his son was diagnosed with progeria at the age of three in 1966. He promised his dying son that he would tell his story so that Aaron would not be forgotten. Four years after Aaron's death, the book was finally ready for publication.

Written in a warm, accessible tone, *When Bad Things Happen to Good People* quickly became a best seller, bringing comfort to literally millions of people struggling with sorrow and loss. The book was eventually translated into fourteen languages and still prompts readers to send thank-you notes to its author. Rabbi Kushner is not, however, concerned with being remembered as an author. He told an interviewer in 2003, "I want to be remembered that, when my son was dying and in pain, I could make him laugh."

Diagnosis

Children with HGPS are usually diagnosed around two years of age, when the changes in their skin, their distinctive facial features, and their failure to grow normally become apparent. The diagnosis can be confirmed by a blood test that was developed in 2003 after the gene that causes the disorder was first identified.

The doctor may also take a small sample of skin to examine it under the microscope for the changes that indicate HGPS, but this test is not necessary to diagnose the disorder.

Treatment

There is no treatment that can cure HGPS. Therapy is intended to give the child as normal a life as possible. Some children are given a daily aspirin to counteract the risk of heart attack or stroke, and doctors commonly recommend a high-calorie diet to help them gain weight. Children with HGPS may also benefit from physical therapy to keep their muscles and joints from weakening.

Children with HGPS must see the doctor periodically to have the condition of their heart and major blood vessels checked and to have their food intake adjusted when necessary.

Prognosis

HGPS is invariably fatal; 90 percent of children with the disorder die of heart attacks or stroke. The average life expectancy is thirteen years,

WORDS TO KNOW

Angina: Chest pain caused by an inadequate supply of blood to the heart muscle.

Failure to thrive: A term used to describe children whose present weight or rate of weight gain is markedly lower than that of other children of their age and sex.

Progeria: A disease characterized by abnormally rapid aging. The term can be used to refer specifically to Hutchinson-Gilford syndrome or to a group of diseases characterized by accelerated aging.

Werner syndrome: Another genetic disease characterized by accelerated aging.

although some children die as young as six or seven. The longest-lived person with HGPS died at twenty-nine.

Prevention

Since HGPS is a genetic disorder, there is no known way to prevent it.

The Future

HGPS is of interest to researchers, along with such other disorders of accelerated aging as Werner syndrome, because they think these diseases may hold clues to the normal process of human aging. In regard to a possible cure for HGPS, a clinical trial of a drug called lonafarnib, originally developed to treat cancer, began in May 2007. Some researchers are experimenting with growth hormone as a possible treatment for HGPS, but the results have not been encouraging.

SEE ALSO Heart attack; Stroke

For more information

BOOKS

Bellenir, Karen, ed. *Genetic Disorders Sourcebook: Basic Consumer Health Information*, 3rd ed. Detroit, MI: Omnigraphics, 2004.

PERIODICALS

Grant, Matthew. "Family Tormented by Ageing Disease." *BBC News*, February 22, 2005. Available online at http://news.bbc.co.uk/2/hi/south_asia/4286347.stm (accessed April 5, 2008).

Smith, Carol. "Seth Cook, 1993–2007: Darrington Teen with Rare Disorder Dies." *Seattle Post-Intelligencer*, June 27, 2007. Available online at http://seattlepi.nwsource.com/local/321200_seth26.html (accessed April 5, 2008). Page includes a video of Seth about 90 seconds in length.

Smith, Carol. "A Time to Live: A Boy Embraces Life as a Rare Disease Hastens His Aging." *Seattle Post-Intelligencer*, September 16, 2004. Available online at http://seattlepi.nwsource.com/specials/seth/190908_progeriamain.asp (accessed April 5, 2008). This is a six-part series on the daily life of Seth Cook, a boy with HGPS who was 10 at the time the series was printed.

WEB SITES

Genetics Home Reference. *Hutchinson-Gilford Progeria Syndrome.* http://ghr.nlm.nih.gov/condition=hutchinsongilfordprogeriasyndrome (accessed April 5, 2008).

Madisons Foundation. *Progeria.* http://www.madisonsfoundation.org/index.php/component/option,com_mpower/diseaseID,641/ (posted October 2005; accessed April 5, 2008).

MayoClinic.com. *Children's Health: Progeria.* http://www.mayoclinic.com/health/progeria/DS00936/DSECTION=1 (accessed April 5, 2008).

Progeria Research Foundation. *Progeria 101/FAQs.* http://www.progeriaresearch.org/progeria_101.html (accessed April 5, 2008).

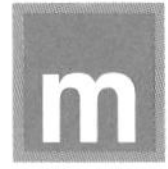

Hydrocephalus

Also Known As
Water on the brain

Cause
Birth defects, head injuries, brain tumors, stroke, infections, bleeding in the brain

Symptoms
Swollen head (infants); headache, nausea and vomiting, loss of balance, problems with memory

Duration
Months to years unless corrected

Definition

Hydrocephalus is a condition in which the flow of cerebrospinal fluid (CSF) in the central nervous system is interrupted or blocked. CSF is the liquid that circulates between the layers of tissue that cover the brain, within the ventricles (hollow cavities) of the brain, and around the spinal cord. It serves to cushion the structures of the central nervous system, deliver nutrients to the brain, and regulate the amount of blood within the brain. In normal circumstances, the CSF moves within the ventricles in the brain, exits through closed spaces at the base of the brain, flows over the surface of the brain and spinal cord, and is then reabsorbed into the bloodstream.

Hydrocephalus develops when there is an imbalance between the production of CSF and its reabsorption or when its flow is blocked. The cerebrospinal fluid builds up inside the brain, putting pressure on the tissues of the central nervous system and causing symptoms ranging from visual disturbances and headache to mental disturbances and difficulty walking.

Doctors classify hydrocephalus into several different categories:

- Congenital. This type of hydrocephalus is present at birth and may be caused by genetic disorders or problems that occur during the baby's development before birth.
- Acquired. Acquired hydrocephalus develops later in life as the result of brain tumors, head injuries, infections of the brain, or other brain disorders.
- Communicating. This type of hydrocephalus is one in which the CSF can flow between the ventricles of the brain but is blocked from leaving the brain.
- Noncommunicating or obstructive. In this type of hydrocephalus, the CSF cannot flow freely among the ventricles inside the brain.
- Normal pressure hydrocephalus (NPH). This is a form of communicating hydrocephalus most commonly found in the elderly. It is a condition in which CSF builds up within the ventricles of the brain.

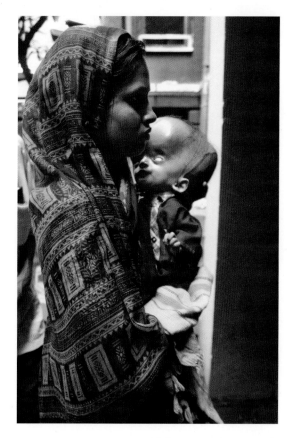

Mother carrying her six-month-old son, who has hydrocephalus, in Calcutta, India. AP IMAGES.

Description

The symptoms and course of hydrocephalus vary widely depending on the person's age, the cause of the condition, and its severity. In infants, the bony plates that form the skull have not yet completed their joining together. This incomplete development of the skull allows the infant's head to expand from the pressure of the CSF, sometimes very rapidly. The baby may vomit, sleep a lot, be irritable, or have seizures. In older children and adults, the skull has already completed its development and the buildup of CSF results in increased pressure on the tissues of the brain and spinal cord. Hydrocephalus in these age groups is more likely to produce such symptoms as headaches, double vision, vomiting, problems with balance or coordination, drowsiness, personality changes, or other signs of damage to the central nervous system.

An Unusual Case of Hydrocephalus

In July 2007, the British medical journal *The Lancet* published a report by three French surgeons who had treated a forty-four-year-old man in a Marseille hospital for weakness in his left leg. When the doctors performed some imaging studies of the man's brain, they were amazed to find that the ventricles in his brain had filled with cerebrospinal fluid (CSF) to the point that his brain had been crushed against the sides of his skull. There was very little brain tissue left. The chief surgeon was quoted as saying, "The images [from the scans] were most unusual...the brain was virtually absent."

The surgeons thought that the man's condition was the result of an operation he had had at the age of six months to treat hydrocephalus. Although the man had an IQ of 75, somewhat below normal, he had led a normal life without any unusual medical symptoms until his leg disorder. He was married and the father of two children and was employed as a civil servant. The surgeons treated the man by inserting a new shunt to drain the excess CSF, which relieved his leg symptoms and allowed him to return to work.

Elderly adults with normal-pressure hydrocephalus often have difficulties with bladder control and movement as well as dementia. Because these symptoms are also found in such disorders as Parkinson disease or Alzheimer disease, many older adults with NPH are never properly diagnosed or treated.

Demographics

The exact number of people with hydrocephalus in the United States is not known because the disorder has so many possible causes—particularly acquired hydrocephalus—and because the diagnosis is often missed in elderly patients. The National Institutes of Health (NIH) estimates that there are 700,000 children and adults living with hydrocephalus in the United States. It is the leading cause of brain surgery for American children and costs the nation about $1 billion every year in health care expenses. The disorder is most common in the very young and the very old. About three babies in every 1,000 are diagnosed with congenital hydrocephalus. About 60 percent of cases of acquired hydrocephalus occur in children, with the remaining 40 percent in adults.

As far as is known, hydrocephalus is equally common in both sexes and in all races and ethnic groups.

Risk factors for hydrocephalus in infants and young children include:

- Premature birth. Prematurity increases the risk of bleeding into the brain.
- Spina bifida. This is a condition in which the spinal column fails to close completely over the spinal cord.
- An infection within the mother's uterus.

Causes and Symptoms

The causes of hydrocephalus range from genetic disorders and incomplete development before birth to brain tumors, head injuries, infectious diseases that affect the brain, and bleeding in the brain.

The symptoms of hydrocephalus depend partly on the patient's age:

- Infants: Enlargement of the skull; bulging of the soft spot at the top of the skull; veins in the scalp are enlarged; baby feeds poorly, vomits, has seizures, sleeps a great deal, or has eyes that look downward much of the time ("sunsetting").
- Children: Headache; nausea; vomiting; fever; blurred or double vision; unstable balance; irritability; sleepiness; delayed progress in walking or talking; poor coordination; change in personality; difficulty staying awake or waking from sleep.
- Adults: Headache; constant drowsiness; loss of ability to think clearly or concentrate; difficulty walking; personality changes and loss of social skills. Job performance is often affected.
- Elderly adults: Loss of coordination or balance; shuffling gait, memory loss; headache; or bladder control problems.

Diagnosis

The specific diagnostic techniques that the doctor will use depend on the person's age and recent medical history. The doctor will note the specific symptoms and when they first appeared. If the patient is an infant, his or her head will be measured and compared to the normal range for babies of the same sex and age. A head larger than 97 percent of the heads of normal children usually indicates hydrocephalus.

Older children and adult patients will usually be referred to a neurologist (a doctor who specializes in treating disorders of the central nervous system) for a complete evaluation of his or her vision, memory, coordination, and other functions that may be affected by hydrocephalus.

The neurologist will order one or more imaging studies of the brain in order to determine whether the hydrocephalus is communicating or noncommunicating and whether other abnormalities of the brain are present. Ultrasound is often used to evaluate hydrocephalus in infants, and computed tomography (CT) scans or magnetic resonance imaging (MRI) is used for older children and adults.

Normal-pressure hydrocephalus is diagnosed by lumbar puncture (spinal tap) followed by withdrawal of some of the cerebrospinal fluid. If the patient has NPH, their symptoms will usually improve after the fluid is removed. This test is known as the Fisher test.

Treatment

The usual treatment of hydrocephalus, whatever its cause, is the surgical insertion of a shunt system. A shunt is a flexible plastic tube that carries extra CSF away from the brain. The shunt system consists of the shunt itself, a valve that keeps the CSF flowing in the correct direction, and a long thin tube called a catheter. The shunt is inserted into one of the brain's ventricles. The catheter and valve are attached to it, and the catheter tubing is threaded underneath the skin to another part of the body (usually the heart or the abdomen) where the excess CSF can be absorbed. The shunt system needs periodic replacement in children as they grow or in adults if the tubing becomes blocked or infected.

A few people with noncommunicating hydrocephalus can be treated by surgery on the third of the brain's four ventricles. In this procedure, the surgeon uses a miniature camera and instrument to locate the third ventricle and cut a small hole in its floor. This hole allows the CSF to bypass the blockage between the ventricles and flow toward its normal outlet from the brain.

Prognosis

Hydrocephalus cannot be cured. The outcome for a given patient is difficult to predict, as the condition has so many different possible causes. The insertion of a shunt system carries some risk of further brain damage. An estimated 50 percent of all shunts fail within two years, requiring further surgery to replace them. Since 1980, however, death rates associated with hydrocephalus have decreased from 54 percent to 5 percent; and intellectual disability in children with hydrocephalus has decreased from 62 percent to 30 percent.

Prevention

The best way to prevent hydrocephalus in newborns is to take steps to reduce the risk of premature birth and to protect infants and small children against head injuries. In addition, vaccinating children against meningitis—a type of infection that can cause hydrocephalus—offers further protection.

The Future

Some possible new treatments for hydrocephalus as well as various improvements in shunt systems are currently being studied in clinical

WORDS TO KNOW

Dementia: Loss of memory and other mental functions related to thinking or problem-solving.

Shunt: A flexible plastic tube inserted by a surgeon to drain cerebrospinal fluid from the brain and redirect it to another part of the body.

Sunsetting: A term used to describe a downward focusing of the eyes.

Ventricle: One of four hollow spaces or cavities in the brain that hold cerebrospinal fluid.

trials. As of 2008 the NIH was sponsoring thirty-two separate trials for these treatments.

SEE ALSO Alzheimer disease; Brain tumors; Meningitis; Prematurity; Spina bifida; Stroke

For more information

BOOKS

Judd, Sandra J., ed. *Brain Disorders Sourcebook*, 2nd ed. Detroit, MI: Omnigraphics, 2005.

Judd, Sandra J., ed. *Congenital Disorders Sourcebook*, 2nd ed. Detroit, MI: Omnigraphics, 2007.

PERIODICALS

Jablons, Beverly. "Cases: A Mind Emerges after Years Lost in a Cloud." *New York Times*, February 10, 2004. Available online at http://query.nytimes.com/gst/fullpage.html?res=9907E7DC173AF933A25751-C0A9629C8B63&sec=&spon=&pagewanted=all (accessed July 19, 2008). This is an article about the effects of undiagnosed hydrocephalus on a writer and her recovery following surgical treatment.

"Report: Man with Almost No Brain Has Led Normal Life." *Fox News*, July 25, 2007. Available online at http://www.foxnews.com/story/0,2933,290610,00.html (accessed July 21, 2008). This is a news item about the patient in the *Lancet* article described in the sidebar. It includes a photo of the patient's brain scan.

WEB SITES

American Association of Neurological Surgeons. *Hydrocephalus*. Available online at http://www.neurosurgerytoday.org/what/patient_e/hydrocephalus.asp (updated September 2005; accessed November 5, 2008).

Hydrocephalus Association. *FAQs: What Is Hydrocephalus?* Available online at http://www.hydroassoc.org/education_support/faq#22 (updated December 2007; accessed July 20, 2008).

National Institute of Neurological Disorders and Stroke (NINDS). *Hydrocephalus Fact Sheet*. Available online at http://www.ninds.nih.gov/disorders/

hydrocephalus/detail_hydrocephalus.htm (updated June 23, 2008; accessed July 20, 2008).

National Institute of Neurological Disorders and Stroke (NINDS). *Normal Pressure Hydrocephalus Information Page*. Available online at http://www.ninds.nih.gov/disorders/normal_pressure_hydrocephalus/normal_pressure_hydrocephalus.htm (updated June 23, 2008; accessed July 20, 2008).

Neuroanimations. *What Is Hydrocephalus?* Available online at http://www.neuroanimations.com/Defn_Obst_Com/Definition.html (accessed July 20, 2008). There are other animations and text explanations of hydrocephalus on this website listed on the home page.

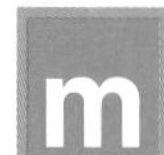

Hypercholesterolemia

Definition

Hypercholesterolemia is the medical term for high blood cholesterol levels. It is not a disease as such but a condition that raises a person's risk of coronary heart disease, stroke, and other disorders of the circulatory system.

Description

Cholesterol is a waxy or fatty substance that the human body produces normally. About 75 percent of the cholesterol in the body is made by the liver and other cells; the remaining 25 percent comes from food. A certain amount of cholesterol is necessary to maintain the function of cell membranes; thus cholesterol is present in the walls of all body cells, including those in the skin, muscle tissue, nervous system, digestive tract, and other parts of the body.

The body also needs cholesterol to make bile (a substance produced in the liver that helps to digest fat), hormones, and vitamin D. This cholesterol is carried in the bloodstream attached to protein molecules. These combinations of cholesterol and protein molecules are called lipoproteins. If more cholesterol is made than is needed for the body's functions, the waxy cholesterol may form deposits on the inner walls of arteries known as plaques.

Fatty plaque deposits are particularly likely to build up in the arteries that supply the heart with blood. These blood vessels are known as the

Also Known As
High blood cholesterol

Cause
Genetic factors, obesity, high-fat diet

Symptoms
None; requires a blood test to detect

Duration
Years

coronary arteries. Plaque deposits can become thick enough to partially block the coronary arteries. If the deposits remain in place, they eventually cause the arteries to stiffen or harden—a condition known as atherosclerosis. If the arteries become too narrow because of the plaques, they cannot carry enough blood to the heart to meet the needs of the heart muscle for oxygen. The oxygen-starved muscle may then produce a kind of chest pain known as angina. The fatty plaques can also come loose from the walls of the artery, resulting in the formation of a clot, a complete blockage of the coronary artery, and a heart attack.

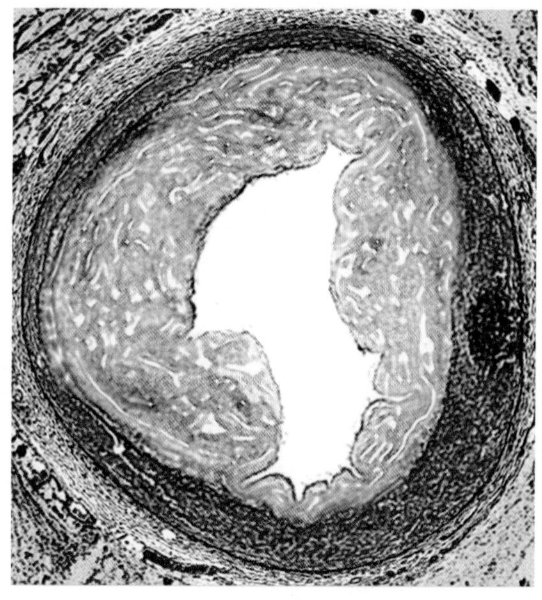

Cross section of an artery around the heart. The inside is coated with plaque, making the opening smaller. © PHOTOTAKE INC. / ALAMY.

It is important to understand that there are three different types of cholesterol and lipoproteins in the human body:

- Low-density lipoprotein (LDL). Often called "bad" cholesterol, LDL is the type of cholesterol that forms plaques on the walls of the coronary arteries.
- High-density lipoprotein (HDL). The "good" cholesterol, HDL picks up LDL and takes it back to the liver. Between 25 and 32 percent of the body's cholesterol is HDL.
- Very low-density lipoprotein (VLDL). This type of cholesterol contains the highest levels of triglycerides (a type of fat) attached to its protein molecules. VLDL is converted in the bloodstream to LDL and can increase the size of LDL particles, thus speeding up the formation of plaques and atherosclerosis.

Demographics

High blood cholesterol levels are largely an adult health problem. Women in the United States before menopause usually have lower blood cholesterol levels than men of the same age. As women and men age, however, their blood cholesterol levels rise until about sixty to sixty-five years of age. After about age fifty, women often have higher total cholesterol levels than men of the same age.

Race and ethnicity appear to affect the rates of hypercholesterolemia in the United States. According to a government health survey carried out in the 1990s, Caucasian adults are more likely (19 percent) to have high blood cholesterol levels than Hispanics (15 percent) or African Americans (16 percent).

Other risk factors for high blood cholesterol include:

- Smoking. Smoking damages the walls of the coronary arteries, making it easier for plaques to form. It also lowers the level of HDL cholesterol.
- Obesity.
- A high-fat diet. Such high-fat foods as red meat, eggs, and full-fat milk and cheese raise blood cholesterol levels.
- Lack of exercise. Exercise helps to raise HDL levels and lower LDL levels.
- High blood pressure. Like smoking, high blood pressure damages the walls of the coronary arteries.
- Diabetes. High levels of blood sugar raise LDL levels and lower HDL levels.
- Family history of heart disease. A parent or sibling who developed heart disease before age fifty-five places a person with high cholesterol levels at a greater than average risk of developing heart disease.
- Emotional stress. Several studies have shown that high stress levels for long periods of time raise blood cholesterol levels.

Causes and Symptoms

The basic cause of high blood cholesterol levels is a combination of genetic factors and lifestyle factors, particularly diet. There is one specific form of hypercholesterolemia called familial hypercholesterolemia that affects about one person in every 500 in the United States. Familial hypercholesterolemia is caused by a mutation in one specific gene known as the LDLR gene.

Genetic factors, however, also affect other people's risk of hypercholesterolemia. As of 2008 no other specific genes had been associated with high blood cholesterol levels in the general population; researchers think that there are probably several such genes rather than only one. These genetic factors contribute to high cholesterol levels either by interfering with the body's ability to remove LDL cholesterol from the bloodstream or by allowing the liver to produce too much cholesterol.

A person can have high blood cholesterol levels without any noticeable symptoms. Because of this fact, the National Cholesterol Education Program (NCEP) guidelines suggest that everyone aged twenty years and older should have their blood cholesterol level measured at least once every five years.

Diagnosis

Blood cholesterol levels are measured by a blood test taken early in the morning after nine to twelve hours of fasting. The doctor will ask the patient about a family history of high cholesterol or heart disease as well as drawing the blood, since high cholesterol levels can be hereditary.

The blood cholesterol test measures total blood cholesterol, LDL, HDL, and triglyceride levels using units called milligrams per deciliter (mg/dL).

- Total cholesterol: Less than 200 mg/dL is a desirable level that lowers a person's risk for heart disease. A cholesterol level of 200 mg/dL or greater increases the risk. A level of 240 mg/dL and above is considered high blood cholesterol. The risk of heart disease at this level is twice that of a person whose total cholesterol level is 200 mg/dL.
- LDL: Less than 100 mg/dL is considered the best level; a level of 100–129 mg/dL is good; a level of 130–159 mg/dL is borderline high; a level of 160–189 mg/dL is high; and a level of 190 mg/dL and above is very high.
- HDL: A level below 40 mg/dL is considered a major risk factor for heart disease; a level between 40 and 59 mg/dL is better; and a level above 60 mg/dL is considered protective against heart disease.
- Triglycerides: Less than 150 mg/dL is normal; a level of 150–199 mg/dL is borderline high; a level of 200–499 mg/dL is high; and a level of 500 mg/dL or above is very high.

Treatment

Treatment for hypercholesterolemia begins with lifestyle changes, including following strict dietary guidelines and increasing one's amount of daily exercise. There is some evidence that a vegetarian diet is beneficial.

In addition to lifestyle changes, the patient's doctor may recommend one or more medications to lower LDL and/or triglyceride levels.

The most common types of drugs used to control hypercholesterolemia are:

- Statins. These are drugs that block the liver from using a substance it needs to make cholesterol. As the level of cholesterol in the liver drops, the liver begins to remove excess cholesterol from the bloodstream.
- Bile acid-binding resins. These are drugs that work by prompting the liver to make more bile acid; to do this, the liver needs to draw cholesterol from the blood.
- Cholesterol absorption inhibitors. These medications work by limiting the amount of cholesterol that the small intestine can absorb from food.
- Fibrates. These are drugs that speed up the removal of triglycerides from the bloodstream.
- Niaspan. Niaspan is a prescription form of niacin (a B vitamin) that works by limiting the liver's ability to produce VLDL and LDL cholesterol.

Prognosis

The prognosis of hypercholesterolemia depends on the person's age, sex, family history, and willingness to follow a treatment program. The statins in particular have greatly improved a person's ability to lower his or her risk of coronary heart disease. The United States Preventive Services Task Force (USPSTF) has estimated that five to seven years of treatment with statins can lower the risk of heart disease by 30 percent.

Prevention

People cannot change their age, sex, genetic factors, or family history that may increase their risk of high cholesterol levels, but they can manage their risk by getting plenty of exercise, keeping their weight at a healthy level, quitting smoking, and eating foods that help to lower LDL levels.

Specific dietary recommendations include:

- Eating foods that are low in saturated fats.
- Keeping cholesterol intake from foods below 200 milligrams per day. One egg, for example, contains about 210 milligrams of cholesterol. Eating lean meats, drinking skim instead of whole milk, and using egg substitutes are good ways to lower one's intake of cholesterol from foods.

WORDS TO KNOW

Angina: Chest pain caused by inadequate supply of oxygen to the heart muscles.

Atherosclerosis: Stiffening or hardening of the arteries caused by the formation of plaques within the arteries.

Cholesterol: A fatty substance produced naturally by the body that is found in the membranes of all body cells and is carried by the blood.

Plaque: A deposit of cholesterol along the inside wall of an artery.

Triglyceride: A type of fat made in the body.

- Eating whole-grain breads.
- Adding more servings of fruits and vegetables to the diet. These foods are rich in fiber, which can lower blood cholesterol levels.
- Eating more fish. Some types of fish, such as cod, halibut, and tuna, are lower in fat and cholesterol than poultry or red meat.
- Keeping one's alcohol intake moderate.

The Future

Researchers are presently focusing on the genetic factors involved in hypercholesterolemia as well as potential new treatments for it. As of 2008, the National Institutes of Health (NIH) was conducting almost 400 separate studies on high blood cholesterol, ranging from clinical trials of new statins to studies of statins in combination with other drugs, and several experimental drugs.

SEE ALSO Coronary artery disease; Heart attack; Stroke

For more information

BOOKS

American Heart Association. *To Your Health! A Guide to Heart-Smart Living.* New York: Clarkson Potter, 2001.

Durstine, J. Larry. *Action Plan for High Cholesterol.* Champaign, IL: Human Kinetics, 2006.

WEB SITES

American Academy of Family Physicians (AAFP). *Cholesterol: What Your Level Means.* Available online at http://familydoctor.org/online/famdocen/home/

common/heartdisease/risk/029.html (updated October 2007; accessed on August 4, 2008).

American Heart Association (AHA). *About Cholesterol.* Available online at http://www.americanheart.org/presenter.jhtml?identifier=512 (updated April 3, 2008; accessed on August 4, 2009).

National Heart, Lung, and Blood Institute (NHLBI). *High Blood Cholesterol.* Available online at http://www.nhlbi.nih.gov/health/dci/Diseases/Hbc/HBC_WhatIs.html (updated February 2006; accessed on August 4, 2008).

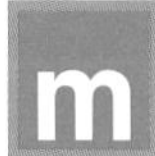

Hyperopia

Definition

Hyperopia is one of several eye conditions called refractive errors, which means that light entering the eye is not properly focused on the retina (the light-sensitive layer of tissue at the back of the eyeball). It is not a disease of the eye in the strict sense.

Description

Hyperopia, or farsightedness, is a condition that develops when a person's eyeball is abnormally short from front to back, or when the cornea (the clear front portion of the eyeball) is abnormally flat. In a normal eye, light entering the eye through the cornea is focused by the lens of the eye on the retina. In hyperopia, the abnormal shortness of the eye or the flatness of the cornea causes the lens to focus images behind the retina. This incorrect focus means that objects at a distance can be seen more clearly than those that are close to the viewer. If the hyperopia is severe, the person may be able to see clearly only objects that are quite far away.

Also Known As
Farsightedness

Cause
Short eyeball or overly flat cornea

Symptoms
Blurry near vision; sometimes blurry far vision as well

Duration
May be lifelong

Demographics

Hyperopia is a common refractive error in the general population, affecting about 25 percent of the general population. In addition, the condition tends to run in families. Hyperopia is often combined with astigmatism, another type of refractive error caused by irregularities in the curvature of the cornea or the lens of the eye.

Most babies are mildly hyperopic at birth. Hyperopia in children is usually less severe than hyperopia in adults, partly because the eyeball in many children lengthens as they grow older and allows the eye to focus

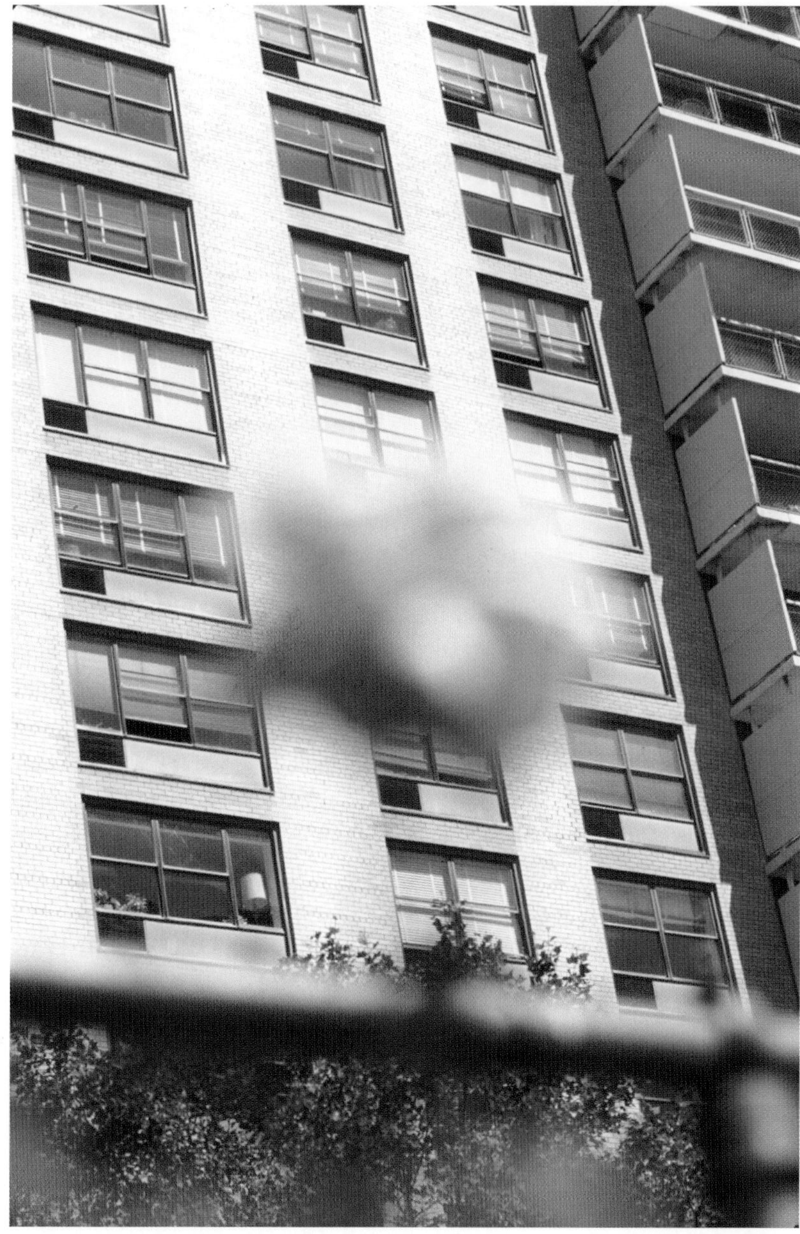

A person with hyperopia can see objects that are far away, like this building, more clearly than objects that are near, like the flower and railing. LEONARD LESSIN / PETER ARNOLD INC.

normally. It is thought that between 6 and 9 percent of children in the United States may have mild hyperopia. Boys and girls are equally affected. There are, however, racial and ethnic differences, with Native Americans, African Americans, and Pacific Islanders having higher than average rates of hyperopia.

Preventive Eye Care

Protection of one's vision is an important part of preventive health care. Eye doctors recommend the following schedule of eye examinations for children and adults:

- Children: should have their eyes tested by their pediatrician or an ophthalmologist between birth and three months; between six months and one year; at three years; and at five years.
- Older children and adolescents: should be seen yearly if they wear corrective lenses, have other eye problems, or have diseases like diabetes that affect the eyes.
- Adults between twenty and thirty-nine: should have the eyes checked every three to five years.
- Adults over thirty-nine who do not wear glasses and are at low risk of eye disease: should be checked every two years between forty and sixty-four, and every year after age sixty-five.
- Adults over thirty-nine who do wear eyeglasses or contact lenses: should have an eye checkup every year.

People who notice blurriness, pain, or any other visual problem should make an appointment with their eye doctor as soon as possible even if they recently had an eye checkup.

There is a condition similar to hyperopia called presbyopia that appears in middle-aged adults. Presbyopia is a type of farsightedness that develops because the lens of the eye becomes less flexible with age and cannot change its shape as easily when the person is trying to focus on near objects (usually reading materials). Most people over forty will develop some degree of presbyopia. Hyperopia that went unnoticed during a person's younger years may become apparent in middle age, when the person begins to develop presbyopia as well.

Causes and Symptoms

In addition to a short eyeball or flatter cornea, hyperopia can be caused in some people by abnormal development of the eye or by trauma to the eye. In a very few cases, hyperopia may be related to disorders of the nervous system or to medications that affect the eye's ability to focus. In general, genetic factors are thought to play a more important role in hyperopia than environmental factors or personal history.

Hyperopia in younger children may not cause noticeable symptoms. Older children and adults, however, will often develop the following symptoms:

- Having to squint while reading.
- Frequent blinking and difficulty focusing on close objects.
- Red or teary eyes, or burning or aching in the eyes.
- Blurry vision.
- Headaches or general discomfort in the eye after a long period of reading, writing, or doing other close work.

People who have these symptoms should make an appointment with an optometrist (an eye care professional who is trained to diagnose refractive errors) or an ophthalmologist (a doctor who specializes in diagnosing diseases of the eye) to find out whether they need corrective lenses.

Diagnosis

Hyperopia and other refractive errors are evaluated by a series of vision tests. After the examiner takes a history of the patient's symptoms (including a family history of eye problems), the patient is usually asked to read the letters on an eye chart. The examiner may also shine lights into the eyes or administer eye drops that allow him or her to see all the structures inside the eye clearly.

To measure the strength of the lens needed to correct the patient's hyperopia, the examiner uses a device called a photopter (or refractor). The photopter is placed in front of the patient's eyes, and the examiner moves various lenses in and out of the device while the patient reads letters on an eye chart located 20 feet (6 meters) away.

Treatment

Screening for and treatment of hyperopia in school-age children is important because significant hyperopia can lead to strabismus (inability of the eyes to work together) or amblyopia, a condition in which there is poor vision in one eye that is not caused by disease. In addition, uncorrected hyperopia can lead to problems in school, including learning disorders and loss of interest in reading.

Hyperopia can be treated nonsurgically by prescription eyeglasses or contact lenses, which are prescribed by the optometrist or ophthalmologist but made and fitted by an optician. There are also surgical options for people who dislike glasses or contact lenses. The two most common surgical procedures for hyperopia involve reshaping the cornea with a laser or implanting an artificial lens in the front of the eye. Reshaping the cornea works better if the refractive error is only low to moderate. Patients with a high degree of refractive error generally do better with lens implantation.

There are drawbacks to surgical correction for refractive errors, however. These include the risks of infection, development of haze in the cornea, or dry eyes. In some cases the surgeon may need to perform a second operation if the first one either overcorrected or undercorrected the shape of the patient's cornea.

It is important for a patient diagnosed with hyperopia to discuss all the treatment options with the optometrist or ophthalmologist, as no

WORDS TO KNOW

Amblyopia: Dimness of sight in one eye without any change in the structure of the eye.

Astigmatism: A refractive error caused by irregularities in the shape of the cornea or the lens of the eye.

Cornea: The transparent front part of the eye where light enters the eye.

Ophthalmologist: A doctor who specializes in diagnosing and treating eye disorders and can perform eye surgery.

Optician: An eye care professional who fills prescriptions for eyeglasses and corrective lenses.

Optometrist: An eye care professional who diagnoses refractive errors and other eye problems and prescribes corrective lenses.

Photopter: A device positioned in front of a patient's eyes during an eye examination that allows the examiner to place various lenses in front of the eyes to determine the strength of corrective lenses required.

Presbyopia: Age-related farsightedness caused by loss of flexibility in the lens of the eye.

Refractive error: A general term for vision problems caused by the eye's inability to focus light correctly.

Strabismus: A condition in which the eyes are not properly aligned with each other.

two people will have exactly the same degree of farsightedness or the same lifestyle.

Prognosis

Most patients with hyperopia do well after being fitted with corrective lenses or having eye surgery. Hyperopia caused by the shape of the eyeball or the cornea does not get worse with age and is unlikely to lead to vision loss.

Prevention

Hyperopia is largely a matter of heredity and cannot be prevented. People can, however, prevent strabismus or other complications of hyperopia by visual screening in childhood and regular eye checkups at all ages.

The Future

It is possible that laser treatment and other types of vision surgery will be further refined in the future and have fewer risks or side effects.

SEE ALSO Astigmatism; Myopia; Strabismus

For more information

BOOKS

Viegas, Jennifer. *The Eye: Learning How We See.* New York: Rosen Publishing Group, 2002.

PERIODICALS

Freudenheim, Milt. "To Read the Menu, Baby Boomers Turn to Eye Treatments." *New York Times*, April 11, 2004. Available online at http://query.nytimes.com/gst/fullpage.html?res=9A0CE3DF1138F932A25757C0A9629C8B63&sec=&spon=&pagewanted=all (accessed April 29, 2008). This is an article about the application of radio waves to the cornea of the eye to treat hyperopia.

WEB SITES

American Optometric Association (AOA). *Hyperopia.* Available online at http://www.aoa.org/hyperopia.xml (accessed April 29, 2008). The page includes two animations about hyperopia that have a total playing time of about 1 minute.

EyeCareAmerica. *Refractive Errors.* Available online at http://www.eyecareamerica.org/eyecare/conditions/refractive-errors/index.cfm (updated May 2007; accessed April 29, 2008).

Mayo Clinic. *Farsightedness.* Available online at http://www.mayoclinic.com/health/farsightedness/DS00527 (updated February 8, 2008; accessed April 29, 2008).

Montreal Vision Clinic. *EyeMotion: Myopia and Hyperopia.* Available online at http://www.eyemotion.com/eyemotion/library/_montrealeyefr.php?src=8 (accessed April 29, 2008). This is a one-minute animation of the refractive errors involved in nearsightedness and farsightedness.

National Eye Institute (NEI). *Questions and Answers about Refractive Errors.* Available online at http://www.nei.nih.gov/CanWeSee/qa_refractive.asp (updated December 2006; accessed April 29, 2008).

TeensHealth. *Taking Care of Your Vision.* Available online at http://www.kidshealth.org/teen/your_body/take_care/vision_care.html (updated January 2008; accessed April 29, 2008).

Hypertension

Definition

Hypertension, or high blood pressure (HBP), is a condition in which a person's blood pressure is higher than is healthy over a period of time. Blood pressure normally rises and falls over the course of a day; it also rises when a person is anxious or is exercising. Doctors usually take blood pressure readings during two different office visits before diagnosing hypertension.

Blood pressure is measured in millimeters of mercury (mm Hg) because the sphygmomanometer—the device most commonly used to measure blood pressure—contains a column of mercury that rises and falls as the doctor inflates and deflates a cuff around the patient's arm. The first of two numbers in a blood pressure measurement is the systolic blood pressure. It is the peak blood pressure in the patient's arteries. The second measurement is the diastolic blood pressure and represents the lowest blood pressure, which occurs when the heart is resting between beats.

Doctors use the following values, measured in millimeters of mercury (mm Hg), when evaluating a patient for hypertension:

- Normal blood pressure: systolic below 120 mm Hg, diastolic below 80.
- Pre-hypertension: systolic between 120 and 139 mm Hg, diastolic between 80 and 99.
- Stage 1 hypertension: systolic between 140 and 159 mm Hg, diastolic between 90 and 99.
- Stage 2 hypertension: systolic 160 mm Hg or higher, diastolic 100 or higher.

Doctors also distinguish between primary (or essential) hypertension and secondary hypertension. Essential hypertension, which accounts for about 95 percent of cases in American adults, is high blood pressure that develops without any apparent cause. Secondary hypertension, which accounts for the remaining 5 percent, is caused by other diseases or conditions, including pregnancy, abnormalities in the shape of the aorta, kidney disease, alcoholism, thyroid disease, the use of birth control pills, and tumors of the adrenal gland.

Also Known As
High blood pressure, HBP

Cause
Unknown (essential hypertension); medications, eating habits, pregnancy, diseases (secondary)

Symptoms
Often none at all; chest pain, tiredness, ringing in the ears, vision changes

Duration
Years

Description

Hypertension is considered a silent disease because a person can have it for years without any noticeable symptoms. Although some people develop nosebleeds, headaches, dizziness, nausea, or changes in their vision as a result of hypertension, the majority of those diagnosed with high blood pressure do not know they have a problem until their doctor checks their blood pressure during a routine physical exam. Sadly, some

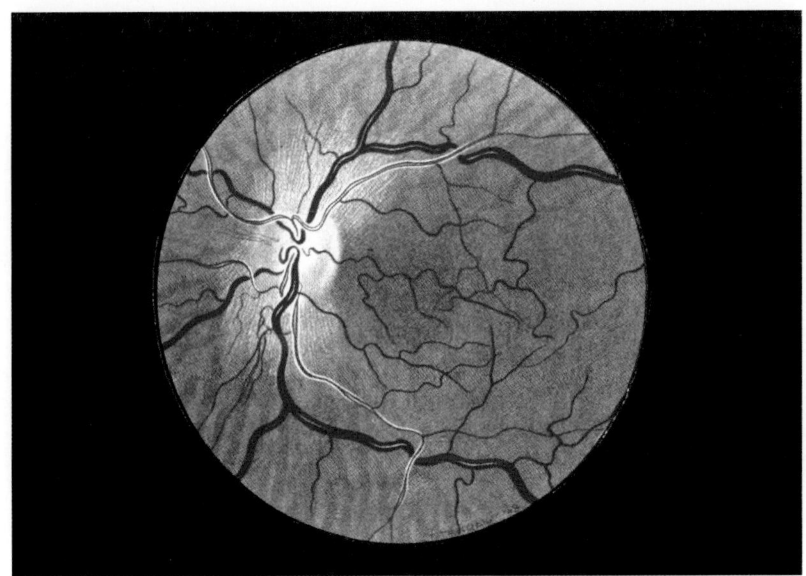

Image of the retina, the lining of the back of eye. In hypertension, the small arteries that are visible get thicker, and push on the veins so they appear nipped as they cross the arteries. © MEDICAL-ON-LINE / ALAMY.

people do not know they have high blood pressure until they have a stroke or heart attack.

Untreated hypertension can damage the heart and other organs:

- High blood pressure can lead to heart failure by causing the heart to enlarge or grow weaker.
- Hypertension can lead to stroke by causing a bulge or weak spot along the wall of an artery known as an aneurysm.
- Blood vessels in the eye can burst or bleed as a result of high blood pressure, leading to loss of vision.
- High blood pressure can cause the blood vessels in the kidneys to become too narrow, leading eventually to kidney failure. Narrowing of the blood vessels in the heart may eventually cause a heart attack.

Demographics

Hypertension is almost entirely a disorder of adults; it affects only 1–3 percent of children and teenagers. About 35 percent of adults in the United States have high blood pressure. Worldwide, hypertension is a leading cause of illness and death; it is the most important factor that people can control in regard to their risk of heart failure, heart disease, stroke, and kidney failure.

Risk factors for hypertension include:

- Age: As people get older, their arteries tend to stiffen, thus contributing to high blood pressure.
- Race: African Americans develop hypertension at higher rates than members of other races in the United States. They also develop high blood pressure at younger ages.
- Sex: Men are more likely to develop hypertension than women.
- Obesity: People with a body mass index (BMI) over thirty are at increased risk of high blood pressure.
- Family history: Hypertension is known to run in families.
- Lack of exercise.
- Drugs of abuse: Cocaine, amphetamines, and heavy alcohol use all increase a person's risk of hypertension.

Causes and Symptoms

The causes of essential hypertension are not known.

Causes of secondary hypertension include:

- Chronic kidney disease
- Tumors or other diseases affecting the adrenal gland
- An unusually narrow aorta (Some people are born with this condition.)
- Pregnancy
- Use of birth control pills
- Thyroid disorders

Diagnosis

Hypertension is diagnosed in the doctor's office by the use of a sphygmomanometer. The doctor places a cuff around the patient's upper arm and inflates it while listening through a stethoscope. The cuff is inflated until the air pressure squeezes the large artery in the upper arm shut. The doctor then releases pressure in the cuff until he or she can start to hear the sounds of the patient's pulse. This is the systolic pressure. The doctor then continues to release pressure until the sounds disappear. This second reading is the diastolic pressure.

In addition to measuring the patient's blood pressure, the doctor may order additional tests to look for possible causes of the hypertension or signs of damage to other organs:

- Blood and urine tests. These can be done to look for evidence of kidney or thyroid disease or to measure the levels of cholesterol in the patient's blood.
- X-ray studies of the chest or the kidneys.
- Electrocardiogram (ECG or EKG). This test measures the electrical activity of the heart and may be done to evaluate the condition of the patient's heart muscle.

Treatment

There is no cure for hypertension. Treatment for the disorder comprises a combination of lifestyle changes and medications. Some people can lower their blood pressure by losing weight and getting more exercise, but most need to take medications to keep their blood pressure within the normal range.

The doctor may prescribe one or a combination of medications to control the patient's blood pressure. In most cases the patient will be asked to see the doctor every three to four months to see whether the drugs or their dosage levels need to be adjusted. Although these drugs can produce side effects, the patient should not stop taking them without consulting the doctor. The various types of drugs given to control hypertension include:

- Diuretics. Sometimes called water pills, diuretics increase salt and urine output. They are often prescribed in combination with other types of pills.
- ACE inhibitors. These drugs work to lower blood pressure by blocking the production of a chemical that causes blood vessels to tighten.
- Calcium channel blockers. These drugs work by reducing the force of the contraction of the heart muscle.
- Beta blockers. Drugs in this group slow down the heart rate. They are often prescribed for people who have had a heart attack or a history of heart disease.
- Vasodilators. These drugs cause blood vessels to open up, which lowers blood pressure. They may be given intravenously if the patient's blood pressure has risen very high very quickly.

- Alpha blockers. Drugs in this group block nerve impulses that cause blood vessels to tighten up. The blood can then move more freely through the blood vessels, thus lowering blood pressure.

Prognosis

Most patients with hypertension can keep their blood pressure at a healthy level provided they follow their doctor's recommendations about diet and exercise and take their blood pressure medications. They should watch their blood pressure carefully as they age because hypertension tends to get worse as people get older. Even mild hypertension, if untreated, increases a person's risk of heart disease by 30 percent and kidney damage by 50 percent within eight to ten years after it starts.

Prevention

Hypertension is a lifelong disorder that requires long-term commitment to healthy lifestyle changes and regular use of prescribed medications.

Specific lifestyle changes recommended by the National Institutes of Health (NIH) for controlling hypertension include:

- Eating a healthful diet. A good place to start is the Dietary Approaches to Stop Hypertension (DASH) diet, which emphasizes eating more fruits, vegetables, and low-fat dairy products, and cutting back on salt and alcohol.
- Get regular physical exercise, preferably at least thirty minutes a day.
- Stop smoking (or do not start).
- Learn to manage emotional stress effectively; relaxation techniques, biofeedback, meditation, or yoga work well for many people.
- Lose weight if the doctor recommends it.
- Avoid cocaine, heavy drinking, and other recreational drugs that raise blood pressure.
- Have blood pressure checked regularly and take all medications for hypertension on a daily basis even if you feel fine.

The Future

The rates of hypertension in all developed countries are expected to rise over the next several decades as populations get older and the rates of obesity continue to increase. A major difficulty in treating hypertension is that

WORDS TO KNOW

Aneurysm: A weak or thin spot on the wall of an artery.

Aorta: The large artery that carries blood away from the heart to be distributed to the rest of the body.

Diastolic blood pressure: The blood pressure when the heart is resting between beats.

Essential hypertension: High blood pressure that is not caused by medications, pregnancy, or another disease.

Sphygmomanometer: The device used to measure blood pressure. It consists of an inflatable cuff that compresses an artery in the arm. The doctor listens through a stethoscope as the air pressure in the cuff is released in order to measure the blood pressure.

Systolic blood pressure: The blood pressure at the peak of each heartbeat.

many people do not know they have it, and others stop taking their blood pressure medications because they dislike the side effects or do not think their drugs are necessary. As of 2008, only 20 percent of Americans diagnosed with high blood pressure were following their doctors' recommendations and getting adequate treatment. Researchers are looking at patient education programs and behavioral approaches to treatment as much as new drugs and new methods of screening for hypertension.

SEE ALSO Diabetes; Heart attack; Heart failure; Obesity; Stroke

For more information

BOOKS

Rubin, Alan L. *High Blood Pressure for Dummies*, 2nd ed. Indianapolis, IN: Wiley Publishing, 2007.

Sheps, Sheldon G., ed. *Mayo Clinic 5 Steps to Controlling High Blood Pressure.* Rochester, MN: Mayo Clinic, 2008.

Townsend, Raymond R. *100 Questions and Answers about High Blood Pressure (Hypertension).* Sudbury, MA: Jones and Bartlett Publishers, 2008.

PERIODICALS

Sabo, Eric. "Practical Blood Pressure Advice, Too Often Shelved for Convenience." *New York Times*, April 4, 2008. Available online at http://health.nytimes.com/ref/health/healthguide/esn-hypertension-ess.html (accessed on September 22, 2008). This is an article about the DASH diet and limiting salt intake in controlling hypertension.

WEB SITES

American Academy of Family Physicians (AAFP). *High Blood Pressure: Things You Can Do to Lower Yours.* Available online at http://familydoctor.org/

online/famdocen/home/common/heartdisease/risk/092.html (updated November 2006; accessed on September 22, 2008).

American Heart Association. *What Is High Blood Pressure?* Available online at http://www.americanheart.org/presenter.jhtml?identifier=2112 (updated April 18, 2008; accessed on September 22, 2008).

Centers for Disease Control and Prevention (CDC). *About High Blood Pressure.* Available online at http://www.cdc.gov/bloodpressure/about.htm (updated August 2007; accessed on September 22, 2008).

eMedicine Health. *High Blood Pressure.* Available online at http://www.emedicinehealth.com/high_blood_pressure/article_em.htm (accessed on September 22, 2008).

National Heart, Lung, and Blood Institute (NHLBI). *What Is High Blood Pressure?* Available online at http://www.nhlbi.nih.gov/health/dci/Diseases/Hbp/HBP_WhatIs.html (updated August 2008; accessed on September 22, 2008).

National Heart, Lung, and Blood Institute (NHLBI). *In Brief: Your Guide to Lowering Your Blood Pressure with DASH.* Available online in PDF format at http://www.nhlbi.nih.gov/health/public/heart/hbp/dash/dash_brief.pdf (updated December 2006; accessed on September 22, 2008). This is a six-page pamphlet about the DASH diet with sample menus and a calorie guide.

National Library of Medicine (NLM). *Essential Hypertension.* Available online at http://www.nlm.nih.gov/medlineplus/tutorials/hypertension/htm/index.htm (accessed on September 22, 2008). This is an online tutorial with voiceover; viewers have the option of a self-playing version, an interactive version with questions, or a text version.

TeensHealth. *Hypertension (High Blood Pressure).* Available onine at http://kidshealth.org/teen/diseases_conditions/heart/hypertension.html (updated August 2008; accessed on September 22, 2008).

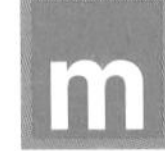

Hypoglycemia

Also Known As
Low blood sugar, glucose disorder

Cause
Difficulty in maintaining a steady level of blood glucose

Symptoms
Hunger, dizziness, shakiness, feeling anxious or weak, sweating, mental confusion

Duration
Minutes to an hour

Definition

Hypoglycemia is a syndrome (group of related symptoms) caused by abnormally low levels of blood sugar. It is not a disease or disorder by itself. Although some doctors disagree about the exact cutoff point for measuring hypoglycemia, the usual standard is 60–70 milligrams per deciliter (mg/dL) of blood.

Description

Hypoglycemia can be understood as the result of the body's difficulty in regulating blood sugar levels. It is normal for people's blood sugar levels

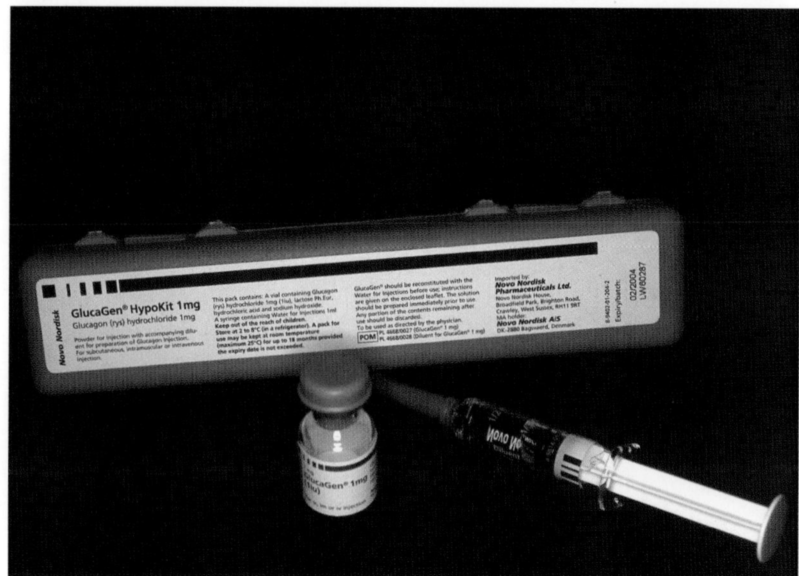

GlucaGen Hypokit, an emergency treatment for low blood sugar, often seen in diabetics. © MEDICAL-ON-LINE / ALAMY.

to rise and fall over the course of a normal day from about 70 mg/dL to 140 mg/dL, depending on whether they has just eaten, if they are digesting their meal, or if they have not eaten for some hours (as when sleeping). The body normally regulates the level of glucose in the blood by means of two hormones secreted by the pancreas, a small organ located near the liver.

When a person eats a meal, the carbohydrates in such foods as rice, potatoes, pasta, sugary foods, and bread are broken down into glucose, which is then absorbed into the bloodstream. As the glucose level in the blood rises, the pancreas secretes insulin, a hormone that helps the body's tissues make use of the glucose. If there is more glucose in the blood than is needed for the body's energy needs at the time, the extra glucose is stored in the liver in a form called glycogen. As the levels of glucose in the blood drop, the pancreas secretes another hormone called glucagon. Glucagon stimulates the liver to convert the stored glycogen back into glucose and release it into the blood. The additional glucose then raises the person's blood sugar level.

What happens in hypoglycemia is that the normal process of blood sugar regulation no longer works smoothly. This problem may develop as a complication of diabetes, a side effect of some medications, or the result of other diseases or tumors. When blood sugar levels drop below about 70 mg/dL, a person with hypoglycemia may begin to experience the mental and physical symptoms of hypoglycemia.

Demographics

It is difficult to tell with certainty how many people in the general American population suffer from hypoglycemia, because some people use the term loosely to refer to irritable feelings or mild anxiety associated with hunger even though they have not had a blood sugar test and may in fact have normal levels of blood glucose. Most doctors think that between 5 and 10 percent of Americans have true hypoglycemia. About 55 percent of patients with diabetes will have mild hypoglycemia at some point during treatment for the disease. Hypoglycemia caused by tumors that secrete insulin is very rare, affecting one or two persons per million.

As far as is known, hypoglycemia affects persons of all races and men and women equally. Reactive or fasting hypoglycemia is more common in adults over thirty-five than in adolescents or young adults. Hypoglycemia related to food allergies or overly low levels of growth hormone occurs mostly in children.

Causes and Symptoms

Hypoglycemia has a number of possible causes: In patients with diabetes, hypoglycemia is usually a side effect of the medications taken to control blood sugar levels. A person's blood sugar level can fall too low if he or she skips meals, exercises too long or too vigorously, takes too large a dose of their diabetes medication, or drinks alcohol.

Patients who do not have diabetes can develop reactive hypoglycemia. This is a condition in which a person's blood sugar drops suddenly between two and five hours after eating sugary foods. Reactive hypoglycemia is not caused by a disease.

Fasting hypoglycemia is a condition that develops in some people as a result of tumors that secrete insulin; certain types of hormone disorders; drinking alcohol; or taking certain medications (particularly sulfa drugs, quinine, and aspirin). It is most noticeable when a person wakes up in the morning.

The symptoms of hypoglycemia are related to the functioning of the central nervous system (CNS) and another part of the nervous system called the sympathetic nervous system. The reason why low blood sugar affects the nervous system before other parts of the body is that the brain and the nerves have higher energy requirements than other tissues. If blood sugar levels drop too low, a hormone called epinephrine is released, which triggers both mental and physical symptoms related to the nervous system.

Mental symptoms that are caused by hypoglycemia include confusion, difficulty thinking clearly, and eventually loss of consciousness or seizures.

Physical symptoms typically include sweating or a clammy feeling, headaches, general weakness or dizziness, speeded-up heartbeat, trembling or shaking, and hunger.

Not everyone with hypoglycemia experiences the same symptoms or experiences them with the same degree of severity. It is possible for a person to have a blood sugar level below 60 mg/dL and have no noticeable symptoms.

Diagnosis

Diagnosis of hypoglycemia is based in part on the patient's history and partly on the results of blood and other tests. If the patient does not have diabetes, the doctor will look for three signs known as Whipple's triad: 1) the patient has the symptoms of hypoglycemia; 2) when tested, the blood sugar level is below 45 mg/dL (in a woman) or 55 mg/dL (in a man); 3) the symptoms are relieved in a few minutes when the patient is given sugar or a sugary drink.

If the patient has diabetes, the doctor will review the patient's treatment history to see whether the dosage or specific drug needs to be adjusted. The doctor may also order laboratory tests to look for breakdown products of insulin in the patient's blood. If the person has an insulin-secreting tumor, their blood insulin levels will be high but the level of insulin breakdown products will be low.

Reactive hypoglycemia is diagnosed by measuring the person's blood glucose in the doctor's office while he or she is having symptoms and then measuring the blood glucose again after the patient eats or drinks. If the patient's blood glucose level was below 70 mg/dL while he or she was having symptoms and the symptoms were relieved by food, the person is diagnosed as having reactive hypoglycemia.

Fasting hypoglycemia is diagnosed by a blood sample that shows a blood glucose level of less than 50 mg/dL after an extended supervised fast (usually seventy-two hours in an adult). A healthy person can usually maintain a blood glucose level above 50 mg/dL for seventy-two hours.

Treatment

Treatment for hypoglycemia depends in part on its cause. Diabetics are usually asked to monitor their lifestyle habits, particularly eating and exercise patterns, as well as paying close attention to the proper use of their medications.

Patients with reactive hypoglycemia are cautioned to avoid sugary foods; have starches, high-protein, and high-fiber foods instead; and eat small meals or snacks every three to four hours rather than three large but widely spaced meals.

Fasting hypoglycemia is usually treated by evaluating the patient's medications and adjusting dosages as necessary; and recommending avoidance of alcohol. Fasting hypoglycemia caused by tumors is treated by surgical removal of the tumor.

Prognosis

Most people recover completely from an episode of hypoglycemia within minutes of taking some form of glucose. In a few cases, people who have fallen into comas before they were treated suffer long-term brain damage. In a very few cases, people may die from hypoglycemia if not treated.

Prevention

Preventive measures vary somewhat for diabetics and for nondiabetics with hypoglycemia. Patients with diabetes should take the following steps to prevent hypoglycemia:

- Take medications exactly as prescribed; measure doses carefully.
- Do not skip meals or eat less than the amount of food prescribed for the insulin dosage.
- Keep alcohol consumption to a minimum.
- Exercise in moderation and check the blood glucose level before exercising.
- Check the blood glucose level with a home meter if early symptoms of hypoglycemia appear. If the level is below 70 mg/dL, take some glucose in the form of five or six pieces of hard candy, 1–2 teaspoons of honey or table sugar, two or three glucose tablets, or one-half cup of fruit juice.
- Measure the blood sugar again in fifteen minutes. If it is still below 70, take another dose of sugar or a sugary food or beverage. Always carry one of these foods or drinks in case of need.

WORDS TO KNOW

Fasting hypoglycemia: A type of hypoglycemia in people without diabetes that is caused by hormone deficiencies, medication side effects, or tumors rather than by reaction to a sugar-rich meal.

Glucagon: A hormone secreted by the pancreas that raises blood sugar levels by signaling the liver to convert glycogen to glucose.

Glycogen: A form of glucose that is stored in the liver as an energy reserve.

Insulin: A hormone secreted by the pancreas that lowers blood sugar levels by allowing body tissues to absorb and make use of the glucose.

Reactive hypoglycemia: A condition in which a person develops hypoglycemia between two and five hours after eating foods containing high levels of glucose.

Whipple triad: A group of three factors used to diagnose hypoglycemia: symptoms; blood sugar measuring below 45 mg/dL for a woman and 55 mg/dL for a man; and rapid recovery following a dose of sugar.

- Wear a medical identification tag or bracelet if you have ever lost consciousness as a result of hypoglycemia.
- Ask the doctor about having a glucagon kit at home or work. People with a history of severe hypoglycemia may need to have a friend or relative inject them with the glucagon if they lose consciousness.
- Never drive a car without checking to see that the blood glucose level is above 70 mg/dL.
- People with reactive hypoglycemia should consult a registered dietitian to help them plan a personalized diet that will lower their risk of hypoglycemic episodes while still allowing them to eat foods they enjoy.
- Follow-up visits to the doctor to evaluate any further symptoms are also an important part of preventive care.

The Future

Research is focusing on a better understanding of the causes of reactive hypoglycemia. Researchers are also studying whether new devices for monitoring blood glucose levels frequently at home will help reduce the risk of hypoglycemic episodes.

SEE ALSO Diabetes

For more information

BOOKS

Chow, Cheryl, and James Chow. *Hypoglycemia for Dummies.* New York: Wiley Publishing, 2003.

Fairview Health Services. *Taking Charge of Your Diabetes.* Minneapolis, MN: Fairview Press, 2006.

PERIODICALS

Kolata, Gina. "Study Undercuts Diabetes Theory." *New York Times,* February 7, 2008. Available online at http://query.nytimes.com/gst/fullpage.html?res=9501E3D8163EF934A35751C0A96E9C8B63&sec=&spon=&pagewanted=all (accessed May 28, 2008). This is a news item about controversial findings from a diabetes study that suggest that trying to lower blood sugar levels to nearly normal in diabetic patients is harmful rather than helpful.

WEB SITES

American Diabetes Association (ADA). "Hypoglycemia." Available online at http://www.diabetes.org/for-parents-and-kids/diabetes-care/hypoglycemia.jsp (accessed May 28, 2008).

National Institute of Diabetes and Digestive and Kidney Diseases (NIDDK). "Hypoglycemia." Available online at http://diabetes.niddk.nih.gov/dm/pubs/hypoglycemia/ (updated March 2003; accessed May 28, 2008).

National Library of Medicine (NLM) online tutorial. "Hypoglycemia." Available online at http://www.nlm.nih.gov/medlineplus/tutorials/hypoglycemia/htm/index.htm (accessed May 28, 2008). This is an online tutorial with voiceover; viewers have the option of a self-playing version or an interactive version with questions.

TeensHealth. "What Is Hypoglycemia?" Available online at http://www.kidshealth.org/teen/question/illness_infection/hypoglycemia.html (updated September 2006; accessed May 28, 2008).

Also Known As
Core temperature drop

Cause
Exposure to cold; surgical procedure; diseases related to aging

Symptoms
Intense shivering; loss of muscle and mental control; heart failure and death

Duration
Depends on length of cold exposure and overall health

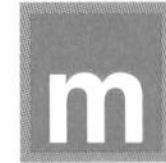

Hypothermia

Definition

Hypothermia is defined as a subnormal body temperature caused by the loss of more body heat than the body can replace. There are several different types of hypothermia. Accidental hypothermia is caused by exposure to cold weather, while intentional or induced hypothermia is a medical technique used to increase a patient's chances of recovery after stroke or cardiac arrest. Primary hypothermia is caused by exposure to a cold or wet environment; secondary hypothermia refers to lowering

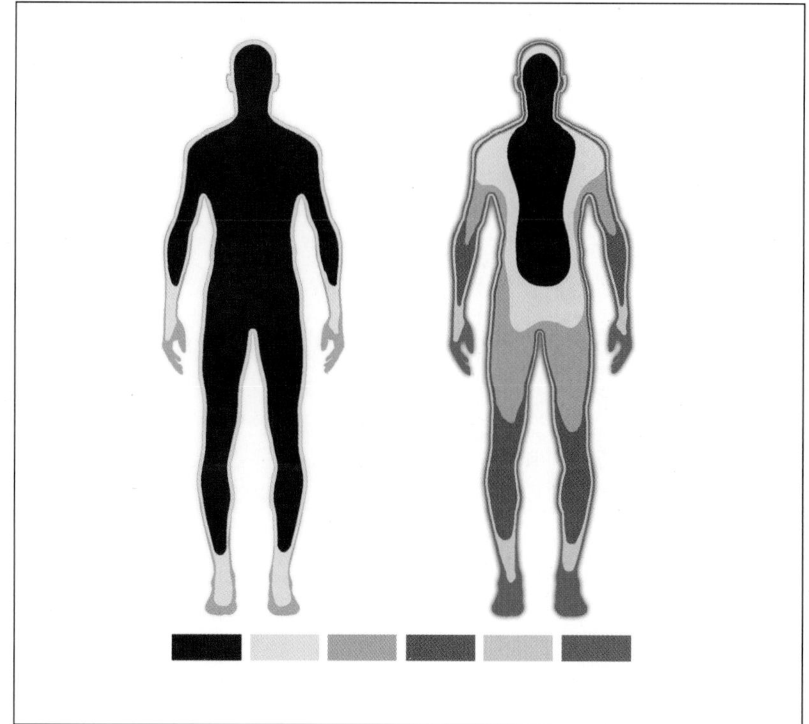

Images of body heat on a warm day (left) and a cold day (right). Red and pink are warmer areas; blue areas are colder. CLAUS LUNAU / BONNIER PUBLICATIONS / PHOTO RESEARCHERS, INC

of body temperature caused by such diseases as Parkinson disease, multiple sclerosis, or brain tumors. Many elderly people with hypothermia have the secondary form.

Description

The normal temperature of the human body is about 97.9°F (36.6°C). Body temperature is regulated by a part of the brain called the hypothalamus. When a person begins to feel cold, the hypothalamus releases chemicals to step up heat production from the body's energy stores. The muscles begin to shiver, which also releases heat. Shivering increases the body's rate of heat production by two to five times.

The hypothalamus also works to control heat loss by slowing down the flow of blood to the arms, hands, legs, and feet. This process is known as vasoconstriction. Vasoconstriction protects the body by helping to keep the heart and other vital organs in the body core functioning as effectively as possible. In most cases, the person will feel uncomfortable enough to go back indoors or put on more clothing. If the person cannot find shelter or otherwise get warm, the person's central nervous system

An Evil Experiment

In the early 1940s Nazi doctors conducted cruel experiments on Russian prisoners of war and concentration camp inmates to see how long it takes people to freeze to death and to try various ways to rewarm people with hypothermia. The reason for these experiments was the high casualty rate suffered by German soldiers during the winter of 1941–1942 following Hitler's invasion of the Soviet Union.

The men used for these experiments were exposed to cold either by being put in vats of icy water or tied naked to stretchers and placed outside in freezing weather. The prisoners put in cold water had probes inserted into their rectums that measured the drop in their body temperature; it was found that they died when their core temperature dropped to 77°F (25°C).

The methods used to warm the men were just as cruel: using sun lamps so hot they burned the skin and forcing scalding-hot water into the stomach, intestines, or bladder. None of the prisoners survived these rewarming treatments.

One of the doctors who conducted these experiments, Sigmund Rascher, was shot on orders of the Nazi leaders in April 1945 before the Allies liberated the concentration camps. Some doctors involved in the experiments were tried for war crimes in 1947 and either executed or sentenced to long prison terms.

(CNS) will eventually be affected and the hypothalamus will no longer be able to regulate the body's temperature. When temperature regulation fails, the heart and other vital organs can no longer function properly.

Hypothermia may come on gradually; the person may not know that his or her body temperature is dropping, though others may notice the person is becoming irritable, slurring their speech, becoming clumsy in their movements, or showing poor judgment. The rate at which a person develops hypothermia depends on basic health, environmental temperature and humidity, and the warmth and dryness of their clothing.

Doctors distinguish three stages of hypothermia according to severity:

- Mild hypothermia: body temperature between 95–90°F (35–32°C).
- Moderate hypothermia: body temperature between 90–82°F (32–28°C).
- Severe hypothermia: body temperature below 82°F (28°C).

Demographics

The true number of people who develop hypothermia in the United States each year is not known; doctors think that those who are taken to hospital emergency rooms are only a small fraction of the actual number of cases. According to the Centers for Disease Control and Prevention, between 650 and 700 people die from hypothermia each year in the United States, or about 0.2 persons per 100,000. Cold-related deaths are twice as common in men as in women. Fifty-two percent of the victims were over the age of sixty-five. The states with the highest rates of deaths from hypothermia are Alaska, New Mexico, North Dakota, Montana, North and South Carolina, and Arizona. Some states have higher-than-average rates because they experience rapid temperature changes at certain times of the year or have mountainous regions with rapid changes in overnight temperatures.

Some people are at greater risk of hypothermia, particularly infants and young children and the elderly. People with diabetes and other illnesses that affect blood circulation are also more likely to develop hypothermia when exposed to cold.

Causes and Symptoms

The most common causes of hypothermia are loss of body heat due to exposure to cold weather or to a combination of cold and dampness. Swimmers or people who fall into a body of water can develop hypothermia even when the water is not icy cold. According to the U.S. Coast Guard, a person who falls into water at 40°F (4°C) will become unconscious in about half an hour and die within another hour; at 32°F (0°C), survival time drops to fifteen minutes.

The symptoms of hypothermia include mental as well as physical symptoms:

- Mild hypothermia: The person shivers vigorously and begins to show confusion and poor judgment. They become moody, may slur their speech, move clumsily, and start breathing heavily.
- Moderate hypothermia: The person's breathing slows down, central nervous activity is lowered and the body loses its ability to generate additional heat by shivering. The heart may develop an abnormal rhythm. A symptom sometimes seen at this stage is paradoxical undressing, in which the person becomes confused, disoriented, and starts to remove their clothing—which speeds up the rate of heat loss. Between 20 and 50 percent of deaths from hypothermia are thought to result from paradoxical undressing.
- Severe hypothermia: The risk of heart failure increases; the person may go into coma and be unresponsive when touched. There may be no pulse and the blood pressure may be abnormally low. The lungs may fill with fluid and breathing may be difficult.

Diagnosis

Diagnosis of hypothermia is usually based on a measurement of body temperature in the emergency room, as many of the physical and mental symptoms of hypothermia can be caused by such other conditions as stroke, alcohol intoxication, medication side effects (common in the elderly), and mental illness. The use of a special low-temperature probe inserted into the rectum or the bladder is thought to give a more accurate reading than a standard thermometer.

Treatment

The first line of emergency treatment for hypothermia includes preventing further heat loss, raising the body core temperature, and preventing heart failure. To lower the risk of the person's developing an abnormal heart rhythm, rescuers are advised to move the person as gently as possible and to begin rewarming the person in the field before taking him or her to the hospital. Wet clothing is removed and replaced with dry clothing and blankets or a dry sleeping bag. Hot water bottles or chemical heat packs are used to warm the body; in extreme emergencies, rescuers can warm the person by skin-to-skin contact.

In the hospital, emergency room doctors will take the person's core temperature to determine the severity of the hypothermia; the lower the body temperature, the more careful the doctors must be in rewarming the patient. Sometimes the person's core temperature continues to drop after rewarming is started; this complication, known as after drop, is thought to result from cooler blood in the patient's extremities being recirculated back into the body's core organs during rewarming.

Various techniques have been used to rewarm people with hypothermia, ranging from wrapping the patient in heated blankets, immersing him or her in warm water in a device known as a Hubbard tank, or giving warmed and humidified oxygen through a face mask or endotracheal tube. Another method that is used is injection of intravenous fluids heated to 113°F (45°C).

Prognosis

The prognosis for recovery from hypothermia depends on its severity. Most people survive mild hypothermia without significant after-effects. The death rate for moderate hypothermia is close to 21 percent; for severe hypothermia, it is close to 40 percent.

Hypothermia can lead to a number of long-term health complications, including frostbite, pneumonia, other infections, disorders of the pancreas and bladder, and lung damage.

Prevention

Accidental hypothermia can be prevented by dressing sensibly for cold-weather activities and by avoiding the use of alcohol and other substances that interfere with good judgment. In the summer, people should be careful not to drink before operating a boat, as falling into water even in summertime temperatures can still cause hypothermia.

In addition, persistent shivering is a sign that the body is losing too much heat; this is an important signal to go back inside as soon as possible. A tip that can help people remember how to dress for winter is the word COLD:

- Cover: Keep head, neck, and face covered with a warm hat, hood, or scarf. Mittens are better than gloves for protecting the hands because they keep the fingers closer together.
- Overexertion: Avoid exercise or other activities that cause heavy sweating, because the combination of moisture on the skin, clothing that becomes damp from sweat, and the cold outside can cause rapid loss of body heat.
- Layer: Loose-fitting layered clothing holds in body heat better than tight-fitting garments. Water-repellent outerwear is a good choice for wet and windy weather.
- Dry: People should stay as dry as possible outdoors, and check mittens and boots from time to time to make sure that snow cannot get inside and melt. It is a good idea to pack an extra pair of dry socks and mittens just in case.

The CDC recommends carrying emergency supplies of food (granola and crackers are good choices), blankets, matches and candles, and extra clothing in the car during the winter in case the car stalls or is stranded in snow. Additional safety precautions include checking the weather forecast before setting out on a trip and letting others know the expected arrival time.

The Future

Hypothermia is thought to be a growing problem in North America because of the increasing numbers of people participating in outdoor sports as well as the increasing numbers of mentally ill and substance-addicted homeless people. Public health doctors and social workers often have trouble convincing homeless people to go into public shelters in the

WORDS TO KNOW

After drop: A term that doctors use to refer to lowering of the body's core temperature that continues while the person is being rewarmed.

Hypothalamus: The part of the brain that controls body temperature, hunger, thirst, and response to stress.

Paradoxical undressing: A symptom sometimes seen in people with moderate or severe hypothermia, thought to be caused by a malfunction of the hypothalamus. The person becomes confused, disoriented, and begins to remove clothing.

Vasoconstriction: A narrowing of the blood vessels in response to cold or certain medications.

cold weather, however, because they claim they are afraid of drug abusers who also use the shelters.

SEE ALSO Frostbite

For more information

BOOKS

Centers for Disease Control and Prevention (CDC). *Extreme Cold: A Prevention Guide to Promote Your Personal Health and Safety*. Atlanta, GA: CDC, 2007. Available online in PDF format at http://emergency.cdc.gov/disasters/winter/pdf/cold_guide.pdf (accessed November 5, 2008).

Giesbrecht, Gordon G. *Hypothermia, Frostbite, and Other Cold Injuries: Prevention, Survival, Rescue and Treatment*, 2nd ed. Seattle, WA: Mountaineers Books, 2006.

PERIODICALS

Fagan, Kevin. "Shame of the City: A Rugged Refuge." *San Francisco Chronicle*, December 2, 2003. Available online at http://www.sfgate.com/cgi-bin/article.cgi?file=/c/a/2003/12/02/MNGB13E11F1.DTL (accessed April 3, 2008). This article is the third of a five-part series on homelessness in San Francisco.

McNeil, Donald G. "Chill Therapy Is Endorsed for Some Heart Attacks." *New York Times*, July 8, 2003. Available online at http://query.nytimes.com/gst/fullpage.html?res=9502E2DF153DF93BA35754C0A9659C8B63 (accessed April 3, 2008). This article describes the use of induced hypothermia in the treatment of people with stroke or cardiac arrest.

WEB SITES

MayoClinic.com. *Hypothermia*, http://www.mayoclinic.com/health/hypothermia/DS00333 (accessed November 5, 2008).

Nova. *Deadly Ascent*. http://www.pbs.org/wgbh/nova/denali/ (accessed November 5, 2008). This is a website with interactive features that explores hypothermia and other health conditions related to mountain climbing.

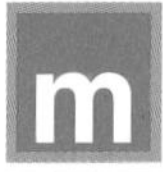

Hypothyroidism

Definition

Hypothyroidism is a condition in which a person's thyroid gland is not producing enough hormone. It may be caused by an autoimmune disorder, a genetic defect in a newborn, certain medications, surgical removal of the thyroid gland, radiation therapy for cancer, and other reasons. Hypothyroidism is sometimes categorized as either primary (caused by a problem in the thyroid gland itself) or secondary (caused by the lack of hormones that ordinarily stimulate the thyroid gland to produce thyroid hormone).

Description

Hypothyroidism is an endocrine disorder. It is caused by underfunctioning of a gland that is part of the endocrine system—a group of small organs located throughout the body that regulate growth, metabolism, tissue function, and emotional mood. The thyroid gland itself is a butterfly-shaped organ that lies at the base of the throat below the Adam's apple.

Hypothyroidism is not easy to diagnose because its symptoms are found in a number of other diseases; it often comes on slowly; and it may produce few or no symptoms in younger adults. In general, hypothyroidism is characterized by a slowing down of both physical and mental activities.

Also Known As
Myxedema, if the hypothyroidism is severe

Cause
Underproduction of the thyroid hormone

Symptoms
Fatigue, weight gain, brittle nails and hair, menstrual problems, sensitivity to cold

Duration
Develops slowly over months to years

Demographics

About 3 percent of the general population in the United States and Canada have some form of hypothyroidism. Apart from cretinism, which affects one child in every 3,000 to 4,000, hypothyroidism is largely a disease of adults. The most common form of primary hypothyroidism in North America is Hashimoto disease, an autoimmune disorder that is diagnosed in about fourteen women out of every 1,000 and one man in every 2,000. Internationally, however, the most common cause of hypothyroidism is a lack of iodine in the diet.

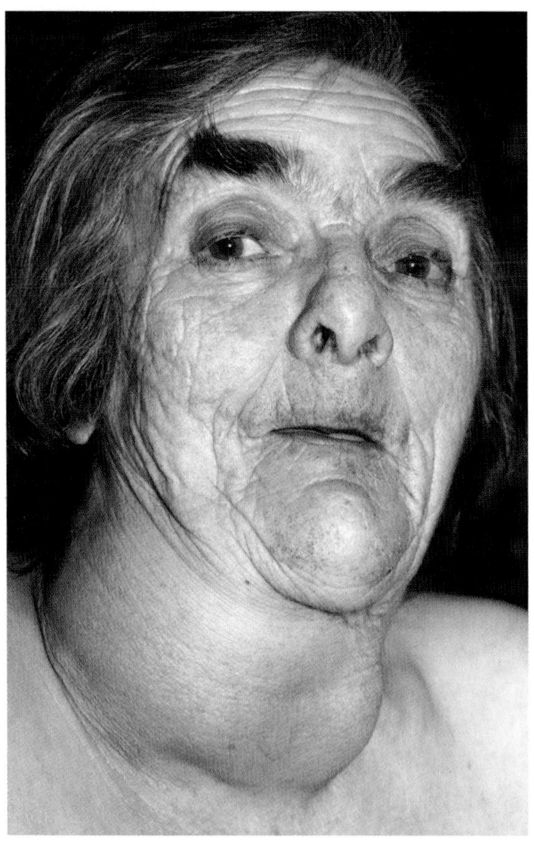

Woman with hypothyroidism, shown by the swelling of her neck, called a goiter. DR. P.

Some people are at increased risk of hypothyroidism:

- Women. Women are two to eight times as likely to have hypothyroidism, depending on the age group being studied.
- Age over fifty. In one Massachusetts study, 6 percent of women over age sixty and 2.5 percent of men over age sixty were found to be hypothyroid.
- Race. According to the National Institutes of Health (NIH), the rates of hypothyroidism in the United States are highest among Caucasians (5.1 percent) and Hispanics (4.1 percent) and lowest among African Americans (1.7 percent).
- Obesity.
- People who have close relatives with an autoimmune disease.

Causes and Symptoms

The most common causes of hypothyroidism are:

- Hashimoto disease. This is an autoimmune disorder in which the patient's immune system attacks the thyroid gland, leading to tissue destruction.
- Treatment for hyperthyroidism. People who have been treated for an oversupply of thyroid hormone with radioactive iodine may lose their ability to produce enough thyroid hormone.
- Surgery on the thyroid gland.
- Radiation therapy for the treatment of head or neck cancer.
- Medications. Lithium, given to treat some psychiatric disorders, and certain heart medications may affect the functioning of the thyroid gland.
- Pregnancy. As many as 10 percent of women may become hypothyroid in the first year after childbirth, particularly if they have diabetes.

An Olympic Champion's Story

Carl Lewis (1961–), a track and field superstar, was the first athlete to equal Jesse Owens's (1913–1980) feat of winning four gold medals in a single Olympic Games in 1936. In 1984 Lewis won his four medals at the Games held in Los Angeles. He continued to dominate track and field events into the 1990s.

Shortly before competing in the 1996 Olympic Games in Atlanta, however, Lewis was diagnosed with hypothyroidism. His early symptoms were easy to miss, such as a weight gain that could be explained as the result of a muscle-building program that was part of his training for the games. He began treatment with synthetic thyroid hormone at once. In July 1996, he won the long jump at the Atlanta Games and became one of only several athletes in the history of the Olympics to win a total of nine gold medals in the course of his career.

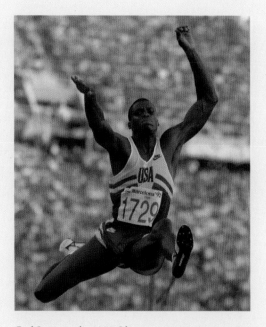

Carl Lewis in the 1992 Olympics. AP IMAGES.

Lewis later published a book about his condition in which he said, "As is the case with most people with thyroid conditions, I had no clue that I had the condition at all. The fact that I was checked was a fortunate accident.... I knew nothing about thyroid problems before discovering that I had one myself. Educate yourself, and follow prescribed treatment. As I showed in the Olympics, you can go back to being 100 percent. I feel even better now than I did in Atlanta, now that my stress level is on a more even keel and my medication levels are just right."

- Viral infections. These can cause a short-term inflammation of the thyroid gland in some people.
- A tumor in the pituitary gland. The pituitary gland produces a hormone called thyroid-stimulating hormone or TSH. Low levels of TSH can lead to secondary hypothyroidism.
- Congenital. About one baby in every 3,000 to 4,000 is born with a defective thyroid gland or no gland at all.
- Too little iodine in the diet. This cause of hypothyroidism is most common in developing countries; it is rare in North America and Europe.

Hypothyroidism can be difficult to diagnose because many of its early symptoms are not unique to it. In addition, the symptoms typically come on gradually. The person may simply feel tired or less energetic than usual, or develop dry, itchy skin and brittle hair that falls out easily. The classic symptoms of hypothyroidism—sensitivity to cold, puffy complexion, decreased sweating, and coarse skin—may occur in only 60 percent of patients. It may take months to years before the person or his or her doctor begins to suspect a problem with the thyroid gland.

Not every patient with an underactive thyroid has the same symptoms or has them with the same severity. Common symptoms of hypothyroidism, however, include the following:

- Increased sensitivity to cold weather
- Dry, itchy skin and a pale or yellowish complexion
- Dry brittle hair that falls out easily and nails that break or split
- Constipation
- Goiter (swelling in the front of the neck caused by thyroid enlargement)
- Hoarse voice and puffy facial skin
- Unexplained weight gain of 10–20 pounds (4.5–9 kilograms), most of which is fluid
- Sore and aching muscles, most commonly in the shoulders and hips
- In women, extra-long menstrual periods or unusually heavy bleeding
- Weak leg muscles
- Decreased sweating
- Arthritis
- Memory loss or difficulty concentrating
- Slowed heart rate (less than 60 beats per minute) and lowered blood pressure
- Depression

Diagnosis

The diagnosis of hypothyroidism is usually made by tests of the patient's thyroid function following a careful history of the patient's symptoms. The first test is a blood test for thyroid-stimulating hormone, or TSH.

TSH is a hormone produced by the pituitary gland in the brain that stimulates the thyroid gland to produce thyroid hormone. When the thyroid gland is not producing enough hormone, the pituitary gland secretes more TSH; thus a high level of TSH in the blood indicates that the thyroid gland is not as active as it should be.

The TSH test, however, does not always detect borderline cases of hypothyroidism. The doctor may order additional tests to measure the levels of thyroid hormone as well as TSH in the patient's blood. If the doctor thinks that the patient may have Hashimoto disease, he or she may test for the presence of abnormal antibodies in the blood. Because Hashimoto disease is an autoimmune disorder, there will be two or three types of anti-thyroid antibodies in the patient's blood in about 90 percent of cases.

In some cases, the doctor may also order an ultrasound study of the patient's neck in order to evaluate the size of the thyroid gland or take a small sample of thyroid tissue in order to make sure that the gland is not cancerous.

Treatment

Treatment for hypothyroidism consists of a daily dose of a synthetic form of thyroid hormone sold under the trade names of Synthroid, Levothroid, or Levoxyl. The patient is told that the drug must be taken as directed for the rest of his or her life.

In the early weeks of treatment, the patient will need to see the doctor every four to six weeks to have his or her TSH level checked and the dose of medication adjusted. After the doctor is satisfied with the dosage level and the patient's overall health, checkups are done every six to twelve months. The reason for this careful measurement of the medication is that too much of the synthetic hormone increases the risk of osteoporosis in later life or abnormal heart rhythms in the present.

Congenital hypothyroidism or cretinism is also treated with synthetic thyroid hormone. Most hospitals now screen newborns for thyroid problems, because untreated hypothyroidism can lead to lifelong physical and mental developmental disorders.

Prognosis

The prognosis for patients with hypothyroidism is very good, provided they take their medication as directed. They can usually live a normal life with a normal life expectancy. Children with congenital hypothyroidism have a good prognosis if the disorder is caught and treated early. Some develop learning disorders, however, in spite of early treatment.

The chief risks to health are related to a lack of treatment for hypothyroidism. If low levels of thyroid hormone are not diagnosed and treated, patients are at increased risk of goiter, an enlarged heart, and severe depression. In addition, women with untreated hypothyroidism have a higher risk of giving birth to babies with cleft palate and other birth defects.

One rare but potentially life-threatening complication of long-term untreated hypothyroidism is myxedema coma. In this condition, which is usually triggered by stress or illness, the person becomes extremely sensitive to cold, may be unusually drowsy, or lose consciousness. Heart rate, blood pressure, and breathing may all be abnormally low. Myxedema coma requires emergency treatment in a hospital with intravenous thyroid hormone and intensive care nursing.

Prevention

There are no proven ways to prevent hypothyroidism because the disorder has so many possible causes.

The Future

Research in hypothyroidism in the early 2000s has a number of different goals. One is to look for specific genes that may be linked to hypothyroidism. Another area of research is to discover reasons for the high female/male ratio. Still another goal is to discover a cure for the condition that will do away with the need for lifetime treatment with synthetic thyroid hormone.

SEE ALSO Hashimoto disease

For more information

BOOKS

Rosenthal, M. Sara. *The Hypothyroid Sourcebook*. New York: McGraw-Hill, 2002.

Skugor, Mario. *Thyroid Disorders: A Cleveland Clinic Guide*. Cleveland, OH: Cleveland Clinic Press, 2006.

PERIODICALS

Pérez-Peña, Richard. "Cases: Heeding Thyroid's Warnings." *New York Times*, October 7, 2003. Available online at http://query.nytimes.com/gst/fullpage.html?res=980DE0D6133CF934A35753C1A9659C8B63 (accessed June 14,

WORDS TO KNOW

Congenital: Present at birth.

Cretinism: A form of hypothyroidism found in some newborns.

Endocrine system: A system of small organs located throughout the body that regulate metabolism, growth and puberty, tissue function, and mood. The thyroid gland is part of the endocrine system.

Goiter: A swelling in the neck caused by an enlarged thyroid gland.

Hyperthyroidism: A disease condition in which the thyroid gland produces too much thyroid hormone.

Hypothyroidism: A disease condition in which the thyroid gland does not produce enough thyroid hormone.

Metabolism: The chemical changes in living cells in which new materials are taken in and energy is provided for vital processes.

Myxedema: A synonym for hypothyroidism. Myxedema coma is a condition in which a person with untreated hypothyroidism loses consciousness. It is potentially fatal.

2008). The writer of the article was diagnosed with hypothyroidism after several puzzling episodes of memory loss and falling asleep at work.

WEB SITES

American Thyroid Association (ATA). *Hypothyroidism FAQs*. Available online at http://www.thyroid.org/patients/faqs/hypothyroidism.html (updated May 2008; accessed June 14, 2008).

Hormone Foundation. *Hormones and You: Hypothyroidism*. Available online in PDF format at http://www.hormone.org/Resources/Thyroid/upload/bilingual_Hypothyroidism.pdf (updated 2004; accessed June 14, 2008).

Mayo Clinic. *Hypothyroidism (Underactive Thyroid)*. Available online at http://www.mayoclinic.com/health/hypothyroidism/DS00353 (updated June 12, 2008; accessed June 14, 2008).

Virtual Medical Centre. *What Is Hypothyroidism?* Available online at http://www.virtualendocrinecentre.com/diseases.asp?did=143 (accessed June 14, 2008). This is an animation that explains the functions of the thyroid gland as well as the symptoms of hypothyroidism. It takes about a minute and a half to play.

I

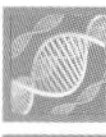
Genetic

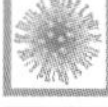
Infection

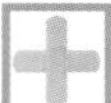
Injury

Multiple

Other

Unknown

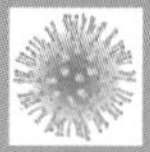

Infectious Diseases

Infectious diseases are a group of illnesses caused by various microbes (organisms too small to be seen without a microscope), which may be bacteria, viruses, fungi, protozoa, parasites, or abnormal proteins called prions. Infectious diseases are contagious. They may spread by physical contact with other infected persons or contaminated objects; by contact with body fluids; by eating or drinking contaminated food or water; by airborne droplets; or by vectors—insects or other animals that transmit disease organisms to humans.

Infectious diseases can spread over a wide geographical area, causing epidemics or pandemics. Some historical pandemics that caused widespread loss of life include the Black Death in the fourteenth century; the smallpox epidemics in Europe and the Americas in the eighteenth century; and the influenza pandemic of 1918–1919.

The microbes that cause infectious diseases are defined as either primary or opportunistic depending on whether they cause disease in people with normal immune systems or whether they can cause disease only in people with weakened immune systems, also called opportunistic infections.

Infectious diseases are still a major cause of death worldwide. According to the World Health Organization (WHO), about 15 million people die each year of infectious diseases—about 26 percent of all deaths. The major killers as of 2008 were pneumonia and influenza, diarrheal diseases, AIDS, and malaria.

SEE ALSO AIDS; Anthrax; Avian influenza; Bronchitis; Chickenpox; Chlamydia; Cold sore; Common cold; Conjunctivitis; Creutzfeldt-Jakob disease; Ear infection; Ebola and Marburg hemorrhagic fevers; Encephalitis; Food poisoning; Genital herpes; Gonorrhea; Hantavirus infection; Hepatitis A; Hepatitis B; Hepatitis C; HPV infection; Infectious mononucleosis; Influenza; Lyme disease; Malaria; Measles; Meningitis; Necrotizing fasciitis; Periodontal disease; Plague; Pneumonia; Polio; Rabies; Rheumatic fever; Rubella; Scarlet fever; Severe acute respiratory syndrome; Smallpox; Sore throat; Staph infection; Strep throat; Syphilis; Tetanus; Tooth decay; Toxic shock syndrome; Toxoplasmosis; Tuberculosis; Ulcers; Urinary tract infection; Warts; West Nile virus infection; Whooping cough

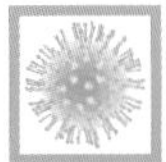

Infectious Mononucleosis

Definition

Infectious mononucleosis is a highly contagious disease caused by the Epstein-Barr virus (EBV) and spread primarily by contact with the saliva of an infected person. Although the disease is sometimes known as the kissing disease because of the role of saliva in spreading the infection, mononucleosis can also be spread through blood and genital secretions (although these forms of transmission are very rare).

Also Known As
Mono, glandular fever, kissing disease

Cause
Epstein-Barr virus (EBV)

Symptoms
Fever, sore throat, swollen lymph nodes

Duration
Usually two to six weeks; sometimes several months

Description

EBV is a very common virus worldwide; most people become infected with it at some point in their lives. Many people become infected with the virus and never develop noticeable symptoms. Those who do develop symptoms typically experience about two weeks of fever, sore throat, and swollen lymph nodes in the neck, throat, or armpits. Although mononucleosis is not a major threat to health, it is a common cause of absence from school or work in teenagers and young adults because it can lead to weeks or months of fatigue and lowered energy.

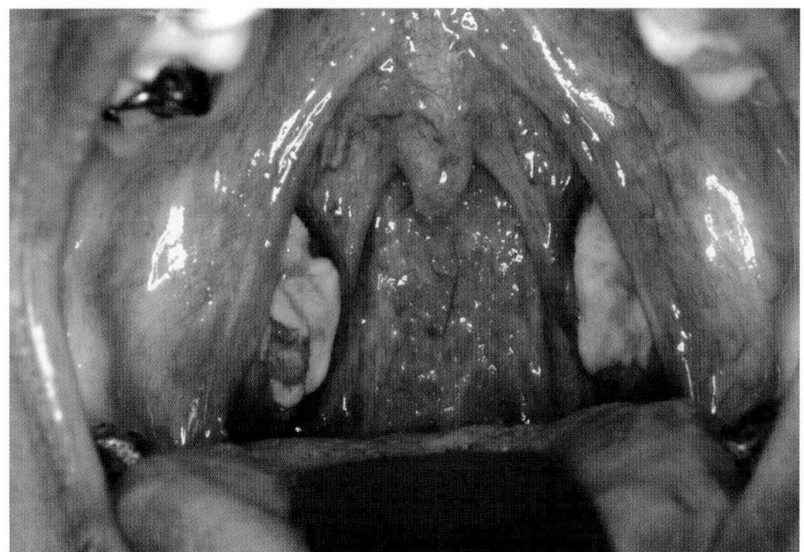

White areas at the back of the throat of a patient with infectious mononucleosis.

Demographics

In the United States, mononucleosis is most common in teenagers and young adults; it is more common in younger children in developing countries. People in any age group can get the disease if they are exposed, however. As many as 95 percent of American adults between thirty-five and forty years of age have been infected, although not all of these have had the symptoms of the illness. When infection with EBV occurs during adolescence or young adulthood, it causes infectious mononucleosis between 35 and 50 percent of the time.

Males and females are equally likely to get mononucleosis, as are people of all races and ethnic groups.

Causes and Symptoms

Infectious mononucleosis is caused by the Epstein-Barr virus, or EBV. The virus is normally transmitted by contact with the saliva of an infected person; it is not ordinarily transmitted through the air. The virus takes about four to six weeks to incubate, and thus infected persons can spread the disease to others over a period of several weeks. After entering the patient's mouth and upper throat, the virus infects B cells, which are a certain type of white blood cell produced in the bone marrow. The infected B cells are then carried into the lymphatic system, where they affect the liver and spleen and cause the lymph nodes to swell and enlarge. The infected B cells are also responsible for the fever, swelling of the tonsils, and sore throat that characterize mononucleosis.

After the symptoms of mononucleosis go away, the EBV virus remains in a few cells in the patient's throat tissues or blood for the rest of the person's life. The virus occasionally reactivates and may appear in samples of the person's saliva, it does not cause new symptoms of illness, it may be transmitted (given) to a susceptible person. Mononucleosis does not cause any problems during pregnancy, such as miscarriages or birth defects.

The primary symptoms of mononucleosis are fever, sore throat, and swollen lymph nodes in the throat, armpit, or neck. Other common symptoms include:

- Swelling or enlargement of the spleen or liver
- General discomfort and mild muscle aches
- Sleepiness and fatigue
- Loss of appetite
- Skin rash
- Swollen tonsils or a yellowish coating on the tonsils
- Night sweats

Less common symptoms of mononucleosis that some patients experience include:

- Headache
- Stiff neck
- Sensitivity to light
- Shortness of breath and chest pain
- Nosebleed
- Hives
- Jaundice

Diagnosis

The diagnosis of mononucleosis is usually based on the results of blood tests combined with the doctor's examination of the patient's throat and neck. The doctor will also tap on or feel the patient's abdomen to see whether the liver and spleen have become enlarged.

A patient infected by EBV will have an increased number of certain white blood cells in the blood sample called atypical lymphocytes, and antibodies to the Epstein-Barr virus. These antibodies can be detected by a test called the monospot test, which gives results within a day but may not be accurate during the first week of the patient's illness. Another type of blood test for EBV antibodies takes longer to perform but gives more accurate results within the first week of symptoms.

Treatment

There is no cure for mononucleosis because it is caused by a virus; it cannot be treated by antibiotics. Treatment consists of self-care at home until the symptoms go away. Patients should rest in bed if possible and drink plenty of fluids. Non-aspirin pain relievers like Advil or Tylenol can be taken to bring down the fever and relieve muscle aches and pains. Throat lozenges or gargling with warm salt water may help ease the discomfort of a sore throat.

Because mononucleosis can affect the spleen, patients should avoid vigorous exercise or contact sports for at least one month after the onset of symptoms or until the spleen returns to its normal size. This precaution will lower the risk of rupture of the spleen.

Prognosis

Mononucleosis rarely causes serious complications. In most patients, the fever goes down in about ten days, but fatigue may last for several weeks or months. Some people do not feel normal again for about three months. A patient who feels sick longer than four months, however, should go back to the doctor to see whether they have another disease or disorder in addition to mononucleosis. In some cases, the patient is diagnosed with chronic fatigue syndrome or CFS. The Epstein-Barr virus does not cause CFS; however, it appears to make some patients with mononucleosis more susceptible to developing chronic fatigue syndrome.

One way to speed complete recovery from infectious mononucleosis is to get plenty of rest early in the disease; the more rest patients get at the beginning, the more quickly they recover.

Severe complications of mononucleosis are unusual but may include rupture of the spleen, which occurs in 0.5 percent of patients—almost all of them males who returned to sports too quickly. Airway obstruction may develop in one patient per thousand, most often a small child. This complication can be treated with steroid medications. Between 1 and 3 percent of patients may develop a form of anemia that can also be treated with steroids.

WORDS TO KNOW

Anemia: A condition in which there are not enough red cells in the blood or enough hemoglobin in the red blood cells.

B cell: A type of white blood cell produced in the bone marrow that makes antibodies against viruses.

Jaundice: A yellowish discoloration of the skin and whites of the eyes caused by increased levels of bile pigments from the liver in the patient's blood.

Prevention

There is no vaccine that can prevent mononucleosis. In addition, the fact that many people can be infected with the virus and transmit it to others without having symptoms of the disease means that mononucleosis is almost impossible to prevent. The best precautionary measure is for patients who have been diagnosed with mono to avoid kissing, or other close personal contact with, others and to wash their drinking glasses, food dishes, and eating utensils separately from those of other family members or friends for several days after the fever goes down. It is not necessary for people with mono to be completely isolated from other people, however.

Because the Epstein-Barr virus remains in the body after the symptoms of mononucleosis go away, people who have had the disease should not donate blood for at least six months after their symptoms started.

The Future

As of 2008 researchers were working on a vaccine against EBV. In December 2007 the *Journal of Infectious Diseases* reported that a vaccine developed in Belgium shows promise in preventing mononucleosis. The vaccine must undergo further clinical trials, however, before it can be definitely shown to be effective and licensed for use in the United States.

SEE ALSO Chronic fatigue syndrome

For more information

BOOKS

Decker, Janet. *Mononucleosis*. Philadelphia: Chelsea House Publishers, 2004.

Hoffmann, Gretchen. *Mononucleosis*. New York: Marshall Cavendish Benchmark, 2006.

Marcovitz, Hal. *Infectious Mononucleosis*. Detroit, MI: Lucent Books, 2008.

PERIODICALS

American Academy of Family Physicians. "Patient Information: Things to Know about Infectious Mononucleosis." *American Family Physician*, October 1, 2004. Available online at http://www.aafp.org/afp/20041001/1289ph.html (accessed June 6, 2008).

Baragona, Steve. "Vaccine Shows Promise in Preventing Mono." News release, *Journal of Infectious Diseases*, December 10, 2007. Available online at http://idsociety.org/Content.aspx?id=8728 (accessed June 6, 2008).

WEB SITES

Mayo Clinic. *Mononucleosis*. Available online at http://www.mayoclinic.com/health/mononucleosis/DS00352 (accessed June 5, 2008).

National Center for Infectious Diseases. *Epstein-Barr Virus and Infectious Mononucleosis*. http://www.cdc.gov/ncidod/diseases/ebv.htm (accessed June 6, 2008).

TeensHealth. *Mononucleosis*. Available online at http://www.kidshealth.org/teen/infections/common/mononucleosis.html (accessed June 6, 2008).

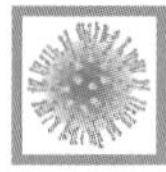

Influenza

Definition

Influenza (flu) is a highly infectious disease of mammals and birds caused by a family of viruses. There are three basic types of influenza virus, known as A, B, and C. Most cases of flu in humans are caused by influenza A.

Description

Influenza is an illness of the nose and throat that has a long history as a troublemaker. It is one of the most highly infectious diseases that affect humans, being the cause of numerous pandemics (large-scale outbreaks), some of which have spread around the civilized world. The first influenza pandemic that is known to have been global in scale took place in 1580; it started in China and spread across Central Asia to Africa and then to Europe, where it nearly wiped out the populations of several major cities in southern Italy and Spain.

While mild cases of influenza are easy to confuse with the common cold, most people will start to feel much sicker with the flu within a few hours of the onset of symptoms. It is not unusual for people with flu to be able to tell the doctor exactly when they first started to feel sick. The

Also Known As
Flu, Spanish fever

Cause
Virus

Symptoms
Chills, fever, headache, muscle aches and pains, sore throat, coughing

Duration
One to two weeks

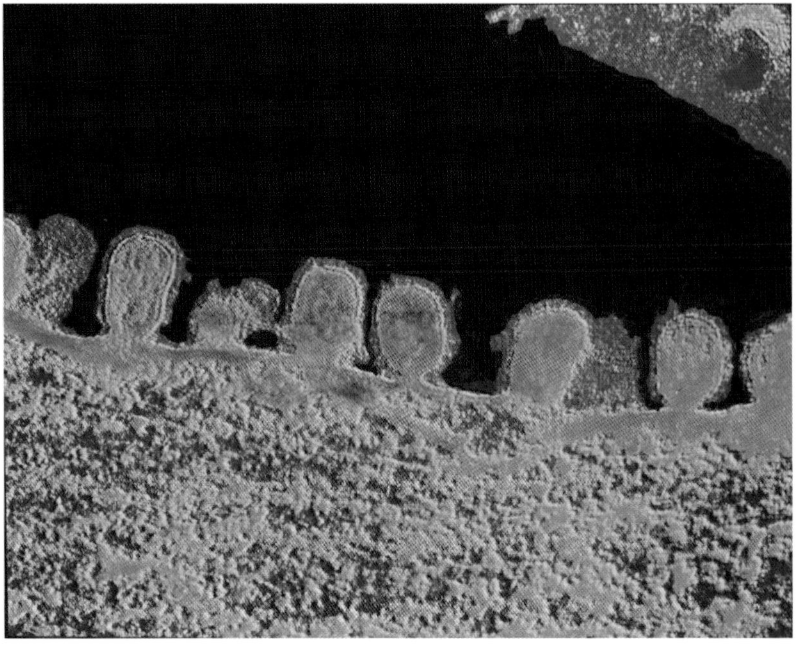

Viruses reproduce by infecting a body cell and forcing the cell to grow more viruses. Here, the new viruses are emerging from the infected cell. © SPL/PHOTO RESEARCHERS, INC.

first sign is usually fever and chills, followed by a sore throat, pain in the muscles, and feeling extremely tired and weak. Some people have a runny nose. Coughing is usually a later symptom.

Most people who get influenza feel better in one or two weeks; however, the disease can cause serious complications because it makes it easier for people to get other infections, such as bacterial pneumonia and ear infections. It also makes chronic health problems like asthma, chronic bronchitis, emphysema, and congestive heart failure worse. The World Health Organization (WHO) estimates that about 300,000 people around the world die each year from complications of influenza. It is important to note that some diseases that are commonly called the flu (like the stomach flu) are not caused by the influenza virus.

Demographics

Millions of people around the world are infected with influenza each year, although the number and the severity of the reported cases vary from year to year, depending on the severity of the particular strain of virus involved. For example, there were more serious cases of flu reported in the United States in the winters of 1999–2000 and 2003–2004 than in the winters of 2001, 2002, and 2005.

The Pandemic of 1918–1919

The influenza pandemic of 1918–1919 is one of the deadliest pandemics in world history. It is estimated that between 2 and 5 percent of the world's population died before the disease ran its course. In the first 25 weeks of the pandemic, 25 million people died—as many as died during the first 25 years of the AIDS pandemic.

An outbreak of influenza at Fort Riley in Kansas in March 1918 is generally considered the beginning of the pandemic. Since 200,000 American soldiers were sent to Europe in late March and April of 1918, some of them carried the deadly virus with them. The virus returned to the United States with a vengeance in the summer and fall of 1918, as well as spreading beyond Europe and North America to Asia and Africa. It was unusual not only for its high death rate—about 2–3 percent of those infected, compared to a usual mortality rate of 0.1 percent (or less)—but also for its demographics. In most flu epidemics, the very young and the very old are most at risk for complications. The pandemic of 1918–1919, however, disproportionately affected young adults; more than half of all deaths were reported in people between the ages of 20 and 40.

The other unusual feature of this particular pandemic was the severity of the symptoms and the rapidity of death. This flu caused people to bleed from the nose, stomach, and intestines. Doctors performing autopsies on flu victims were shocked to find the lungs filled with bloody, foamy fluid. People sometimes collapsed on the street and died within hours. A nurse at Hartford Hospital in Connecticut recounted an incident that was typical of the pandemic. Four Yale students had gotten off the train in Hartford because they did not feel well and walked from the train station to the hospital. By the next morning all four young men were dead.

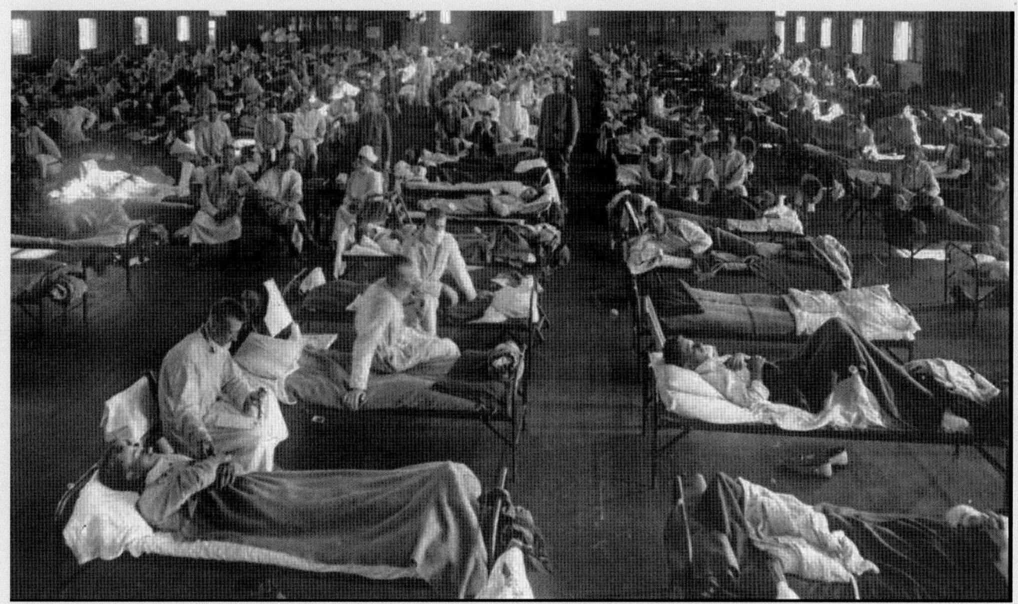

An emergency hospital near Fort Riley, Kansas, during the 1918 influenza pandemic. AP IMAGES.

Flu epidemics usually occur in the winter in temperate climates; however, they can occur at any time of year in countries with tropical climates. Pandemics typically occur every ten to twenty years.

Influenza is most likely to lead to serious complications in infants, the elderly, smokers, people with asthma, people with weakened immune systems, and women in the last three months of pregnancy. The disease affects people of both sexes and all races equally, as far as is known.

Causes and Symptoms

Most cases of flu in humans are caused by either influenza A or B viruses. The influenza A viruses are most likely to cause pandemics in the human population because they infect wild birds and domestic poultry like chickens and turkeys and thus can easily be transmitted to farmers, hunters, and others who raise or study birds. These viruses can also infect horses, dogs, pigs, camels, cats, ferrets, harbor seals, and whales. In addition, influenza A viruses cause more severe disease; viruses of this type are known to have caused the great pandemic of 1918–1919, the Asian flu epidemic of 1957, the Hong Kong flu epidemic of 1968, and the avian (bird) flu of 2007. Influenza viruses change quickly over time, and flu vaccines must be reformulated every year because of this rapid rate of mutation.

Flu is spread by inhaling droplets from an infected person's coughing or sneezing that contain the virus. It can also be transmitted by kissing or by touching food utensils, handkerchiefs, telephone receivers, doorknobs, desk surfaces, and other objects that may have been handled by an infected person. People can transmit the virus for about twenty-four hours before they start to feel sick, which is another reason why the disease spreads so rapidly during flu season. Adults are infectious for about seven days after they feel sick, and children are infectious for about ten days.

When the virus enters the body, it attaches itself to the moist tissues lining the nose, throat, and lungs, where it invades the cells of these tissues and multiplies rapidly.

Typical flu symptoms include:

- Sudden onset of fever and chills (The fever may range from 100°F [37.8°C] to as high as 104°F [40°C].)
- Flushed face and red watery eyes
- Muscle pains and cramps, which can be quite severe in some people

- Headache
- Dry cough and sore throat
- Runny nose
- Weakness and severe fatigue, often requiring complete bed rest

Diagnosis

Most people are likely to consult a doctor when their cough becomes troublesome. In most cases the doctor will make the diagnosis of flu on the basis of the patient's symptoms, because the available medical tests are either too slow for the diagnosis to benefit the patient or not cost-effective. The definitive diagnosis of flu is based on growing samples of the patient's nose or throat secretions in a laboratory; this process takes three to seven days. Rapid diagnostic tests of blood samples require trained laboratory technicians and equipment.

In 2004 the Food and Drug Administration (FDA) approved a new rapid test for flu called the QuickVue test. The test can be used at the patient's bedside. The doctor swabs the inside of the nose with an applicator that is then soaked in a chemical solution for a minute to extract the virus. A special strip is then inserted into the solution and allowed to remain for about ten minutes. If the flu virus is present, a red or pink line will appear on the strip. The QuickVue test is about 80 percent accurate.

Treatment

Most people can care for themselves at home by staying away from others, resting in bed, drinking plenty of fluids, and avoiding the use of alcohol and tobacco. Orange juice or sports drinks are better than plain water for preventing dehydration because they contain electrolytes, which are minerals that the body loses during a high fever along with water from body tissues. Fever and muscle aches and pains should be treated with acetaminophen (Tylenol), ibuprofen (Advil or Motrin), or naproxen (Aleve); aspirin should not be used to bring down fever because of the small risk of Reye syndrome in children. Nasal decongestants can be used to clear a runny or stuffy nose if needed.

Some drugs known as antiviral medications can be given to shorten a flu attack or decrease its severity. Two of these, however, are no longer commonly recommended because the type of influenza A virus most active in the United States since 2005 has developed resistance to these medications. They are Symmetrel and Flumadine. People who need an antiviral medication should ask their doctor for either Relenza or Tamiflu, because the flu virus has not yet developed resistance to these drugs. Antiviral drugs must generally be taken within 48 hours after the start of symptoms in order to be effective, however; they also produce such side effects as nausea and vomiting.

Prognosis

Most people recover from influenza, although some may feel weak and tire easily for several weeks after the acute symptoms go away. People who develop bacterial pneumonia as a complication of influenza, however, are at some risk of death; the average mortality rate for a flu epidemic is about 0.1 percent. The Centers for Disease Control and Prevention (CDC) estimates that between 20,000 and 30,000 people die each year in the United States as a result of influenza.

Prevention

People can lower their risk of getting flu by such common-sense precautions as washing hands with soap and water frequently during flu season; avoiding touching the eyes or face before washing the hands; disposing promptly of soiled tissues; and not sharing personal items with other family members during a flu outbreak. The use of alcohol-based sanitizers on work surfaces and kitchen counters may be helpful in some households.

The most effective means of preventing flu is vaccination. There were two forms of vaccine as of 2008, an injectable vaccine given in the upper arm, and a liquid called FluMist that can be squirted or sprayed into the nose. The flu shot takes about two weeks to produce immunity. It must be given every year in order to protect the person against the newest mutation of the flu virus. The CDC publishes guidelines each year of people who should be vaccinated against flu; these include the elderly, people with HIV infection, those with diabetes and other chronic health conditions, health care workers, young children, and women who are more than fourteen weeks pregnant during flu season. People in North America who should consider vaccination should plan to be vaccinated in September or early October, before the start of the flu season.

WORDS TO KNOW

Pandemic: A disease epidemic that spreads over a wide geographical area and affects a large proportion of the population.

Reye syndrome: A rare but potentially fatal illness that is linked to the use of aspirin in children.

The Future

The high infectiousness of flu viruses, their ability to move back and forth between humans and other animals, and their rapid rate of change mean that it is unlikely that humans will eradicate them any time soon. One promising development, however, is research on a universal vaccine against influenza A viruses. Such a vaccine would eliminate the need to reformulate flu vaccines each year, which is a slow and inefficient process. One such universal vaccine had completed Phase I clinical trials as of early 2008.

SEE ALSO Common cold; Pneumonia; Reye syndrome

For more information

BOOKS

Davidson, Tish. *Influenza.* San Diego, CA: Lucent Books, 2006.

Monroe, Judy. *Influenza and Other Viruses.* Mankato, MN: LifeMatters, 2002.

PERIODICALS

Gladwell, Malcolm. "Contagions: The Scourge You Know." *New Yorker*, October 29, 2001. Available online at http://www.newyorker.com/archive/2001/10/29/011029ta_talk_contagions (accessed April 6, 2008).

WEB SITES

Centers for Disease Control and Prevention (CDC). *Influenza: The Disease.* http://www.cdc.gov/flu/about/disease/index.htm

National Institute of Allergy and Infectious Diseases (NIAID). *Understanding Flu.* http://www3.niaid.nih.gov/healthscience/healthtopics/Flu/understandingFlu/Default.htm (accessed April 5, 2008).

National Library of Medicine/National Institutes of Health online tutorial. *Influenza.* http://www.nlm.nih.gov/medlineplus/tutorials/influenza/htm/index.htm (accessed April 5, 2008). This is a multimedia presentation with voiceover.

Public Broadcasting Service (PBS). *American Experience: Influenza 1918.* http://www.pbs.org/wgbh/amex/influenza/index.html (accessed April 5, 2008). Web site includes a transcript of the television program, a timeline and interactive maps, and reflections by a present-day scientist on the possibility of another pandemic.

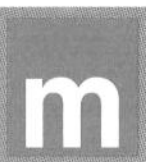

Iron-Deficiency Anemia

Definition

Anemia is a condition in which the blood does not have enough hemoglobin in its red cells. It is a sign of a disease process of some kind rather than a disease by itself. Anemia is the most common blood disorder in the general population. There are many different types of anemias. Some result from blood loss, some from overly rapid destruction of red blood cells (RBCs), and some from the body's failure to produce enough RBCs.

Iron-deficiency anemia is the most common form of anemia. It occurs when people do not get enough iron in their diets, when their bodies do not absorb enough iron from the diet, or when blood loss occurs. Iron is needed for the production of hemoglobin, a substance found in red blood cells that carries oxygen from the lungs to other parts of the body. When there is not enough hemoglobin in the blood, the body's tissues and organs become oxygen-starved, leading to tiredness, loss of a healthy color in the skin, headaches, and other symptoms.

Description

Iron-deficiency anemia varies in severity from person to person. Some people may not have any symptoms—particularly if the loss of iron happens gradually over a long period of time—and may be diagnosed in the course of a routine blood test. Others may tire easily, feel weak, lose weight, or have frequent headaches. Young children and pregnant women can develop serious health problems as a result of iron-deficiency anemia. Children with anemia may develop heart murmurs or experience delays in growth and development. Pregnant women with iron-deficiency anemia have a higher risk of giving birth prematurely or having babies with low birth weight.

Another health problem that can arise as a result of iron-deficiency anemia is a rapid or irregular heartbeat. When the blood is not carrying enough oxygen to meet the needs of the body, the heart will speed up in order to pump more blood to the tissues. Over time, the increased workload on the heart can lead to enlargement of the heart, chest pain, and even heart failure.

Also Known As
Iron-poor blood, sideropenic anemia

Cause
Not enough hemoglobin in the blood

Symptoms
Fatigue, pale complexion, fast heartbeat, headaches, cold hands and feet

Duration
Months to years unless corrected

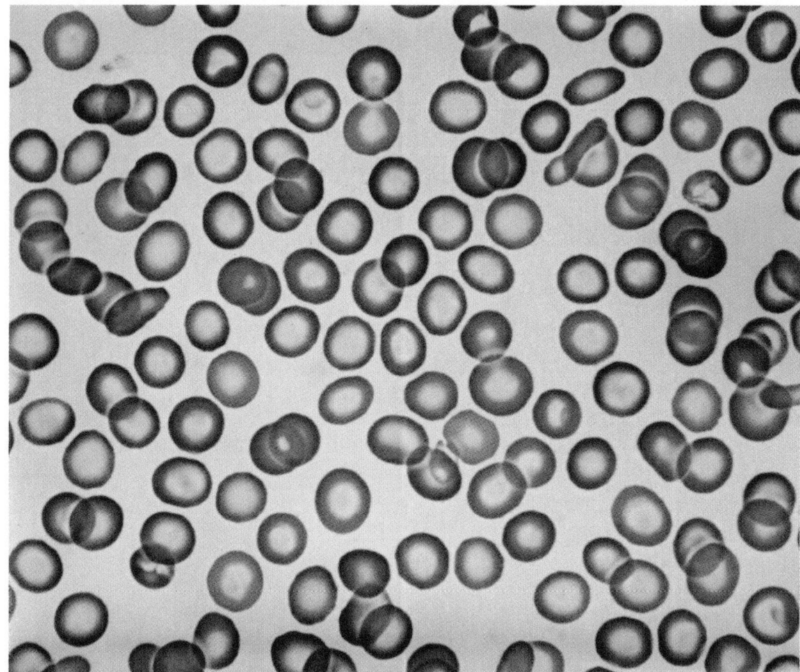

Red blood cells from a patient with iron deficiency anemia. The cells should all be bright red. JOAQUIN CARRILLO FARGA / PHOTO RESEARCHERS, INC.

Demographics

The exact number of people in the United States with iron-deficiency anemia is not known. One estimate is 3.4 million adults and children; however, many researchers think that this figure is much too low. Iron-deficiency anemia in developed countries is most common in women of childbearing age because women lose more iron than men through menstruation and pregnancy. Whereas a healthy male loses about 1 milligram of iron each day, mostly through the digestive tract, women lose between 4 and 100 milligrams of iron with each menstrual period and 500 milligrams of iron with each pregnancy. Most women need to absorb twice as much iron from their diet as men.

In developing countries, iron-deficiency anemia is six to eight times more common than in North America and Europe. One reason for the difference is that people in these countries eat less meat. It is easier for the body to absorb the iron it needs from meat than from vegetables. A second reason is that intestinal parasites—particularly hookworms—are relatively common in developing countries. Intestinal parasites can lead to iron-deficiency anemia because they cause the infected person to lose blood through the digestive tract.

When the Doctor Recommends Iron Pills

Iron supplements can cause heartburn, constipation, or stomach cramps. To lower the risk of these side effects, people who are taking iron tablets or capsules as treatment for iron-deficiency anemia may want to try the following tips:

- Take the pills or capsules with food.
- Do not take the iron supplement at bedtime if it causes stomach upset.
- Add foods rich in fiber to the diet or take a stool softener if constipation is a problem.
- Start with a low dose of the iron supplement—perhaps just one pill or capsule per day—and work up gradually to the full dose recommended by the doctor.
- If one type of iron formula causes problems, talk to the doctor about a different formula. Some people find that iron in capsule form is easier on their digestion than pills.

Risk factors for iron-deficiency anemia include:

- Sex. Twenty percent of women of child-bearing age have iron-deficiency anemia compared to 2 percent of men.
- Age. Infants or children who are not getting enough iron in their diet are at risk, particularly those who are given cow's milk rather than being breastfed and older children going through rapid growth spurts. Elderly people are also at increased risk of anemia because aging reduces the ability to taste food, leading to loss of appetite and possible malnutrition.
- Premature or low-birth-weight babies.
- Eating a strict vegetarian diet.
- Undiagnosed peptic ulcers, colon cancer, or other diseases that can cause loss of blood through the digestive tract.
- Kidney disorders that must be treated with dialysis. The process of dialysis shortens the life span of red blood cells.

Causes and Symptoms

Iron-deficiency anemia can be caused by a lack of iron in the diet, by the body's inability to absorb iron, or by the loss of blood through the digestive tract, menstruation, or pregnancy. People's diets may not contain enough iron because they are malnourished in general or because they do not eat meat, fish, or dairy products. Diseases that affect the small intestine, such as celiac disease or Crohn's disease, are the most common cause of failure to absorb iron, because the small intestine is the part of the digestive system where iron is taken into the bloodstream from partially digested food. Blood loss through the digestive tract may have several causes, ranging from colorectal cancer or peptic ulcers to intestinal parasites or long-term use of aspirin.

People with mild anemia may not have any symptoms. The most common symptoms that appear in persons with moderate iron-deficiency anemia are tiring easily, pale skin, weakness, shortness of breath, headache, lightheadedness, and cold hands or feet. Less common symptoms include:

- Loss of appetite and unintended weight loss
- Sore tongue
- Brittle fingernails
- Unusual cravings for ice, starch, dirt, or other substances that are not food (a condition called pica)
- Bloody or tarry-looking stools

Diagnosis

Iron-deficiency anemia is often diagnosed as the result of a routine blood test during blood donation or a yearly medical checkup. The blood test may reveal either that there is a low level of hemoglobin in the person's blood cells or that the blood has a low hematocrit (a measurement of the ratio of red blood cells to liquid serum in the person's blood). Normal hemoglobin levels for the general population are between 12 and 16 grams per deciliter (g/dL) of blood. A normal hematocrit level is between 36 and 46 percent for women and 46 to 56 percent for men. A patient who has a hemoglobin level below 12 g/dL or a hematocrit below 36 in women or 46 in men will be diagnosed as having iron-deficiency anemia.

Other measurements that may be taken from a blood sample are the amount of iron itself in the blood serum; the amount of ferritin, a protein that helps the body store iron; and the level of transferrin, a protein that carries iron in the blood. A low level of ferritin and a high level of transferrin point to a diagnosis of iron-deficiency anemia.

A colonoscopy or an ultrasound study may be ordered if the doctor suspects that the patient's anemia is caused by blood loss through the digestive system.

Treatment

The usual treatment for iron-deficiency anemia caused by an iron-poor diet is a combination of adding iron-rich foods to the patient's diet plus dietary supplements containing iron. Red meat, especially beef and liver, is the best source of iron in the diet. Other iron-rich foods include chicken, turkey, pork, fish, and shellfish; eggs; pasta or cereals that are fortified with iron; beans and nuts; dried fruits; and green leafy vegetables like spinach. The doctor may also recommend adding citrus fruits and other fruits and vegetables rich in vitamin C (mangos, apricots, strawberries, cantaloupe, watermelon, broccoli, tomatoes, peppers, cabbage, and potatoes) to the daily menu. Vitamin C helps the body absorb the iron that is present in meat and other foods.

Dietary supplements may include multivitamins containing iron and vitamin C, or iron compounds in pill or capsule form to be taken with meals. Because iron supplements can cause constipation or heartburn, patients may need to make some adjustments at mealtimes (see sidebar).

Patients whose anemia is caused by intestinal parasites will be given medications to kill the parasites. Those with colorectal cancer or other disorders of the small intestine are usually treated with surgery. Peptic ulcers are treated with a combination of antibiotics and Pepto-Bismol or drugs that block the production of stomach acid.

Patients with severe anemia may require hospital treatment, including blood transfusions and iron injections.

Prognosis

Iron-deficiency anemia is easily treated and has an excellent prognosis when the patient's only problem is lack of iron in the diet. Most people's hematocrit will return to normal after two months of iron therapy. Iron supplements should be continued for another six to twelve months, however, to build up the body's reserves of iron in the bone marrow. In general, older adults take longer to regain normal hemoglobin and hematocrit levels than younger people. The patients with the poorest prognosis are those whose anemia is caused by colorectal cancer.

Prevention

Iron-deficiency anemia can usually be prevented simply by eating a well-balanced diet that includes iron-rich foods and foods containing vitamin C. Other preventive measures include:

- Taking iron supplements if following a vegetarian diet.
- Avoiding extreme weight-reduction diets or food fads.
- Breastfeeding a baby for the first year of life rather than giving cow's milk.
- Women who are pregnant or menstruate heavily should check with their doctor about the possible need for iron supplements as well as eating an iron-rich diet.

WORDS TO KNOW

Anemia: A condition in which a person's blood does not have enough volume, enough red blood cells, or enough hemoglobin in the cells to keep body tissues supplied with oxygen.

Hematocrit: The proportion of blood volume occupied by red blood cells.

Hemoglobin: An iron-containing protein in red blood cells that carries oxygen from the lungs to the rest of the body.

Pica: An abnormal craving for substances that are not normally considered food, like soil, chalk, paper, or ice cubes.

- Older adults should also have periodic blood tests, particularly if they take high doses of aspirin or other over-the-counter pain relievers for arthritis, or if they are losing their appetite for food.

The Future

Iron-deficiency anemia is likely to continue to be a common health problem in all age groups in the United States because it has so many different potential causes, ranging from poor diet to stomach and intestinal disorders. Researchers are presently trying to develop simpler tests for diagnosing the causes of iron-deficiency anemia. They are studying the safety of a newer iron-containing formula that would be easier to digest than current pills and capsules.

SEE ALSO Celiac disease; Colorectal cancer; Crohn disease; Heart failure; Lead poisoning; Prematurity; Restless legs syndrome; Sickle cell anemia; Thalassemia; Ulcers

For more information

BOOKS

Iron Disorders Institute. *Guide to Anemia*. Nashville, TN: Cumberland House Publishing, 2003.

PERIODICALS

Brody, Jane E. "'Tired Blood' Warning: Ignore It at Your Peril." *New York Times*, September 23, 2003, updated by Eric Sabo, October 22, 2007. Available online at http://health.nytimes.com/ref/health/healthguide/esn-anemia-ess.html (accessed October 6, 2008).

WEB SITES

American Academy of Family Physicians (AAFP). *Anemia: When Low Iron Is the Cause*. Available online at http://familydoctor.org/online/famdocen/home/common/blood/009.html (updated August 2006; accessed October 6, 2008).

Mayo Clinic. *Iron Deficiency Anemia*. Available online at http://www.mayoclinic.com/health/iron-deficiency-anemia/DS00323 (updated March 7, 2007; accessed October 6, 2008).

National Heart, Lung, and Blood Institute (NHLBI). *What Is Iron-Deficiency Anemia?* Available online at http://www.nhlbi.nih.gov/health/dci/Diseases/ida/ida_whatis.html (updated May 2006; accessed October 6, 2008).

Office of Dietary Supplements, National Institutes of Health (NIH). *Dietary Supplement Fact Sheet: Iron*. Available online at http://ods.od.nih.gov/factsheets/iron.asp (updated August 24, 2007; accessed October 6, 2008). This fact sheet is a guide to choosing a well-balanced diet; it also contains information about dietary supplements containing iron.

TeensHealth. *Anemia*. Available online at http://kidshealth.org/teen/diseases_conditions/blood/anemia.html (updated June 2007; accessed October 6, 2008).

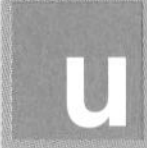

Irritable Bowel Syndrome

Definition

Irritable bowel syndrome or IBS is a chronic (long-term) disorder of the digestive tract characterized by changes in bowel habits—constipation, diarrhea, or a combination of both—along with abdominal cramps and bloating or gassiness. It is not contagious, inherited, or a forerunner of cancer.

Also Known As
IBS, mucous colitis, nervous indigestion, spastic colon

Cause
Unknown; may be triggered by infection or emotional stress

Symptoms
Abdominal cramps, constipation, diarrhea, gassiness

Duration
Years

Description

IBS is a functional disorder of the digestive tract, which means that it affects the workings of the digestive system rather than its structure. IBS is a common disorder around the world. People with IBS experience cramping or bloating in the abdomen after a meal followed by an urgent need to defecate. The patient typically notices that the stools are more frequent, looser, and may contain mucus. There are four basic patterns: the patient has mostly diarrhea; the patient is mostly constipated; the constipation alternates with diarrhea; or the patient has a mixture of the two conditions. About 75 percent of patients change from one subtype to another within a year, however.

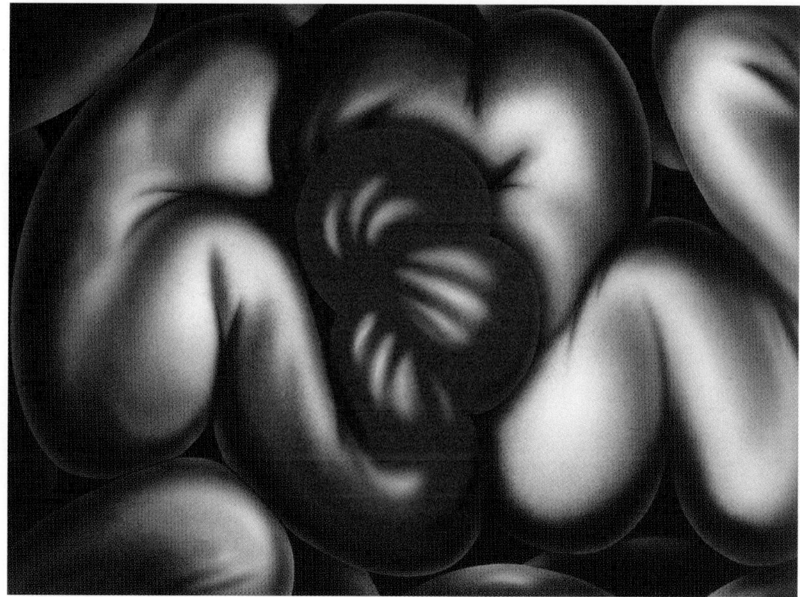

Image of irritable bowel syndrome, in which the intestine in the center is suffering from cramping. DAVID GIFFORD / PHOTO RESEARCHERS, INC.

IBS is a chronic rather than an acute disorder with rapid onset. It does not usually get worse over time and is not accompanied by weight loss, loss of appetite, fever, or blood in the stools. Patients with these symptoms usually have other digestive disorders.

Patients with IBS are likely to have certain other disorders at the same time. These include fibromyalgia, lactose intolerance, food allergies, migraines or other recurrent headaches, depression, and backache.

Demographics

IBS is common in the general American population, affecting as many as a fifth of the adult population. Only 10 to 20 percent of people with symptoms of IBS consult a doctor, however. Most of those seeking treatment are adults but many report that their symptoms began in childhood. Half of all patients diagnosed with IBS state that their symptoms started before age thirty-five. Patients who are over forty when their symptoms begin are less likely to have IBS and more likely to have another digestive problem.

The gender ratio of IBS varies from country to country. In the United States and Europe, women are two to three times more likely than men to have the disorder, but in India, 70 percent of IBS patients are men. The reasons for this difference are not yet known. Some doctors in the United States think that women are more likely than men to seek help for their symptoms rather than being more likely to develop it.

IBS is thought to be equally common in all racial and ethnic groups in Europe and the United States, although some researchers state that the disorder is less common among Asian Americans.

Causes and Symptoms

The cause of IBS is not known. There are, however, several theories about the possible causes of the disorder. These include:

- Infections. Some researchers think that IBS may be caused by a bacterial infection. Evidence for this includes signs of inflammation in the small bowel of some patients with IBS as well as the fact that some patients diagnosed with IBS did not have symptoms until they had a gastrointestinal infection.
- Emotional trauma. Some studies indicate that a significant number of women diagnosed with IBS are survivors of physical or sexual abuse.
- Abnormal patterns of contraction of the muscles in the walls of the intestines. During the process of digestion, the muscular walls of the intestines push food along the digestive tract by rhythmic contractions. In some patients with IBS, the contractions are too close together or too far apart, leading to the cramping sensations and diarrhea or constipation of IBS.
- Unusual sensitivity of the nerve endings in the intestines. Some researchers think that the intestinal tissues in patients with IBS are more sensitive to stretching than those in most people, or that there are more intense connections between the central nervous system and the intestines in patients with IBS.

In addition to cramping, bloating, and changes in bowel habits, patients with IBS may have the following symptoms:

- Feeling a need to defecate even when there is nothing in the bowel or rectum.
- Feeling that the bowel has not been completely emptied after a movement.
- Finding that cramps and gassiness are relieved by a bowel movement.
- Visible swelling or bloating of the abdomen.
- Finding mucus in the stools.

Diagnosis

IBS is a diagnosis of exclusion, which means that the doctor must rule out other possible causes of the symptoms. There is no single laboratory test or imaging study that can confirm a diagnosis of IBS. There are several sets of diagnostic criteria drawn up by various professional groups that the doctor can use. Most of these criteria state that the patients must have had abdominal pain or bloating for at least twelve weeks in the past year; that the pain is relieved by a bowel movement; and that the patient has noticed changes in the shape, frequency, or appearance of the stools.

If the patient is over fifty, the doctor may order tests to rule out the possibility of colon cancer. Other tests may be ordered if the patient has fever, weight loss, blood in the stools, or persistent pain, as these symptoms are not characteristic of IBS.

Treatment

There is no cure for IBS. Patients may be treated with a combination of medications, dietary adjustments (described more fully in the section on prevention), and psychotherapy. In some cases the doctor may ask the patient to keep a food diary to see whether certain foods make the symptoms worse. Patient education is a very important part of treatment for this disorder, as there are steps that patients can take to manage their symptoms and reduce the frequency of flare-ups.

The specific medications prescribed depend on the patient's most bothersome symptoms. They may include:

- Fiber supplements like Metamucil or Citrucel. These are taken with fluids to relieve constipation.
- Antispasmodic drugs. These are given to slow down the contractions of the intestines. They include drugs like Bentyn and Levsin.
- Antidepressants. Drugs like Paxil and Prozac are reported to help patients with severe constipation. They are also given to IBS patients with coexisting depression.
- Antidiarrheal medications. Imodium and Lomotil are the drugs most often recommended for treating severe diarrhea.
- There are also some newer drugs that are available only for patients who do not respond to other treatments. Lotronex and Tegaserod are drugs approved only for temporary use in women with severe IBS symptoms. Both drugs have potentially serious side effects and

have not been approved by the Food and Drug Administration (FDA) for treating men.

There are no surgical treatments for IBS. Some alternative therapies that some patients find helpful include acupuncture and herbal remedies, particularly peppermint tea or capsules. Peppermint is a natural antispasmodic that relaxes the intestinal muscles.

Prognosis

IBS is a bothersome condition but it is not life-threatening and will not cause or lead to cancer. Patients with IBS have the same life expectancy as others of their age or sex in the general population.

Prevention

People with IBS cannot completely prevent occasional episodes of diarrhea or constipation with any medications presently available, but they can minimize the severity of their symptoms in a number of ways:

- Psychotherapy or counseling. Some people find their symptoms are helped by learning to avoid overreacting to normal life stressors.
- Getting regular exercise. Exercise helps to maintain bowel function as well as lower stress levels.
- Avoiding foods that produce cramping or gas. These include coffee, spicy foods, beans, onions, broccoli, and cabbage.
- Practicing eating slowly and avoiding overeating.
- Quitting smoking and reducing or eliminating alcoholic beverages.
- Practicing yoga, meditation, relaxation techniques, or deep breathing.
- Cutting back on cola drinks and other carbonated beverages.
- Adding wheat bran or other foods high in fiber to the diet.
- Hypnosis. Some patients with IBS report significant symptom relief when they are taught self-hypnosis aimed at relaxing the muscles of the abdomen.

The Future

IBS is likely to continue to be a common problem among American adults. Current research includes clinical trials of several new drugs for IBS; investigations of alternative therapies, including traditional Chinese

WORDS TO KNOW

Antispasmodic: A type of drug given to relieve the cramping of the intestines or other muscles.

Lactose intolerance: An inability to digest lactose, the form of sugar found in milk and milk products.

medicine, St. John's wort (a herbal remedy), and massage therapy; and imaging studies to see whether the brains of patients with IBS are different from those of people without the disorder.

SEE ALSO Celiac disease; Crohn disease; Fibromyalgia; Lactose intolerance; Ulcerative colitis

For more information

BOOKS

Bonci, Leslie. *American Dietetic Association Guide to Better Digestion*. New York: John Wiley and Sons, 2003.

Darnley, Simon, and Barbara Millar. *Understanding Irritable Bowel Syndrome*. Hoboken, NY: John Wiley and Sons, 2003.

Magee, Elaine. *Tell Me What to Eat If I Have Irritable Bowel Syndrome*. New York: Rosen Publishing Group, 2009.

WEB SITES

American College of Gastroenterology. *Understanding Irritable Bowel Syndrome*. Available online in PDF format at http://www.acg.gi.org/patients/ibsrelief/IBS.pdf (updated May 8, 2003; accessed August 19, 2008).

KidsHealth. *Irritable Bowel Syndrome*. Available online at http://kidshealth.org/kid/health_problems/stomach/ibs.html (updated October 2007; accessed August 19, 2008).

Mayo Clinic. *Irritable Bowel Syndrome*. Available online at http://www.mayoclinic.com/health/irritable-bowel-syndrome/DS00106 (updated May 9, 2008; accessed August 19, 2008).

National Institute of Diabetes and Digestive and Kidney Diseases (NIDDK). *Irritable Bowel Syndrome*. Available online at http://digestive.niddk.nih.gov/ddiseases/pubs/ibs/index.htm (updated September 2007; accessed August 19, 2008).

K

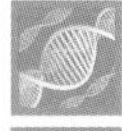
Genetic

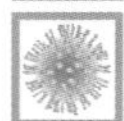
Infection

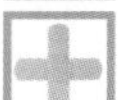
Injury

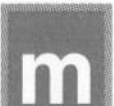
Multiple

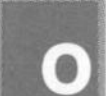
Other

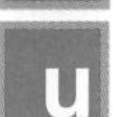
Unknown

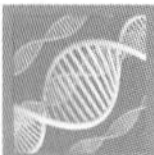

Klinefelter Syndrome

Definition

Klinefelter syndrome is a condition caused by one or more extra X chromosomes in males. It is the second most common health condition caused by an extra sex chromosome. Klinefelter syndrome is named for Dr. Harry Fitch Klinefelter (1912–1990), an endocrinologist at Massachusetts General Hospital in Boston, who first described it in 1942. The genetic cause of the syndrome was not discovered until 1959.

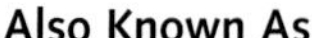

Also Known As
XXY syndrome; 47, XXY syndrome

Cause
An extra X chromosome in a male's genetic makeup

Symptoms
Small genitals, sparse body and facial hair, enlarged breasts, unusual height, infertility

Duration
Lifelong

Description

Many men with an XXY chromosome arrangement tend to be taller than their father or brothers, to have a rounded body type with a tendency to be overweight, to develop enlarged breasts resembling those of a woman, to have a smaller than average penis and testicles, and to lack facial or body hair. On the other hand, many other men who are XXY do not develop these features; some live out their lives without ever knowing that they have an extra X chromosome. For this reason, many doctors no longer use the term "Klinefelter syndrome" but prefer to describe males with the extra chromosome simply as "XXY males."

Demographics

Klinefelter syndrome affects only males. It is thought to occur in one in every 500–1,000 boy babies. About 3,000 affected males are born each

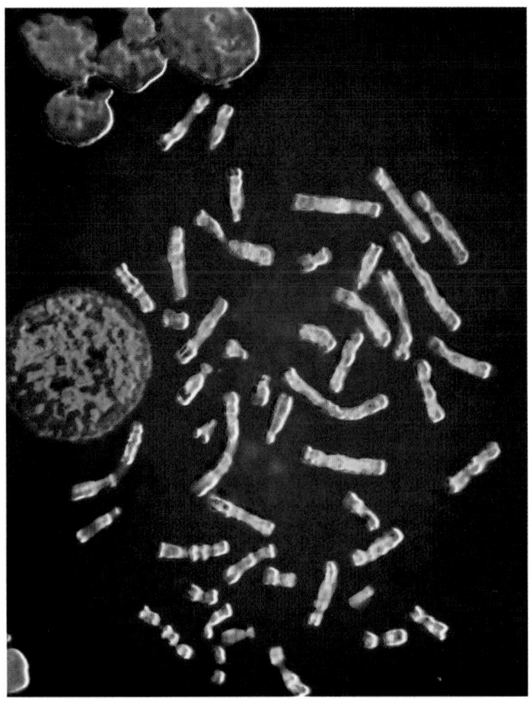

Chromosomes of a person with Klinefelter syndrome. There is an extra X chromosome, resulting in 47 chromosomes, rather than the normal 46. CNRI / PHOTO RESEARCHERS, INC.

year in the United States. The rate of Klinefelter syndrome is five to twenty times higher in boys with mental retardation than in the general population of newborns. It appears to be equally common in all races and ethnic groups.

Causes and Symptoms

Klinefelter syndrome is caused by a type of genetic error called nondisjunction. Ordinarily, the process of cell division that leads to the formation of germ cells (sperm and eggs) results in a cell with only half the number of chromosomes—twenty-three, instead of forty-six. In nondisjunction, the division of sex chromosomes does not occur, resulting in either an egg with two X chromosomes or a sperm with both an X and a Y chromosome. If a normal sperm carrying a Y sex chromosome fertilizes an egg with two Xs, or a sperm carrying both an X and a Y chromosome fertilizes a normal egg, an XXY male will be conceived. According to researchers, about half the time the extra chromosome comes from the baby's father and the other half of the time from the mother. A mother who is thirty or older has a slightly increased risk of having an XXY son.

Klinefelter syndrome is characterized by a range of psychosocial as well as physical problems. Not all XXY males will have all these difficulties, and many have them only in mild form.

- Smaller than normal testes and penis, with lower than normal levels of male sexual hormones.
- Thin or absent body and facial hair.
- High-pitched voice.
- Rounded body shape, enlarged breasts, rapid weight gain in adolescence.
- Developmental and learning disabilities. These include delayed speech, difficulty paying attention, mild difficulties with short-term memory, and problems with learning to read.
- Depression and emotional distress caused by low-self-esteem.

- Taller than average height after puberty with disproportionately long arms and legs.
- Infertility (inability to father children).

XXY males are at increased risk of certain autoimmune disorders, including rheumatoid arthritis and lupus. They are also at increased risk of breast cancer and osteoporosis.

Diagnosis

Diagnosis of Klinefelter syndrome depends in part on the severity of the patient's symptoms. As has been noted, many XXY males are only mildly affected by their extra X chromosome and may never be diagnosed. Although babies can be diagnosed with the syndrome before birth, the two most common symptoms that bring XXY males to the doctor's office for testing are enlarged breasts and infertility, both of which become matters of concern after puberty. Some XXY boys are diagnosed during the elementary school years because they have speech problems and other learning difficulties.

The diagnosis is made by taking a karyotype, or chromosome test. To perform a karyotype, the doctor takes a small sample of the patient's blood. The white blood cells are isolated and cultured in a special solution and examined under a microscope to see what the chromosomes look like.

The doctor may also test a sample of blood for hormone levels. XXY males have low levels of testosterone, a male sex hormone, in their blood serum.

One Man's Story

An XXY male who was born in 1961 and grew up in the 1970s tells about the difference that having a karyotype (chromosome test) made in his life. He was diagnosed with Klinefelter syndrome in junior college. Before his diagnosis, he had problems in school related to low energy levels as well as gaining large amounts of weight: "The major problem faced by me, and by every other Klinefelter's Syndrome victim, is that maturity and learning go from normal to very, very slow after puberty kicks into action. It takes energy to learn, and I didn't have any.... I could not keep up physically, nor could I keep up intellectually. In some things, like computers, I worked well, for I could sit in one place and learn. If I had to move around, go visit the library, do research, exercise, or make any effort at all, I was muted by a weakness that was always labeled as fat and lazy."

After testosterone therapy, the writer had much more energy, joined his parents in their business for several years, was able to return to college eventually and complete his degree in 2003. He married and was able to lose weight after obesity surgery. He summarizes the benefits of his diagnosis and treatment by reaching out to other XXY males: "I keep meeting people with Klinefelter's who are not taking testosterone and remaining weak and immature in many ways. Don't avoid testosterone. It matured more than my physical form. It matured my mind."

Treatment

Treatment of Klinefelter syndrome may involve an educational evaluation as well as medical treatment:

- Hormone injections. Injections of androgens (male sex hormones) are given to XXY males, preferably beginning at puberty, in order to help them gain muscle strength, develop facial hair and a deeper voice, enlarge the testes, raise overall energy levels, and protect against osteoporosis. In many cases hormone treatment improves the boy's mood and self-esteem as well.

- Surgery. XXY males with noticeably enlarged breasts may have surgery to remove the extra breast tissue. Surgical treatment reduces the man's risk of breast cancer as well as removing a cause of social embarrassment.
- Speech therapy and language therapy. Most doctors recommend that XXY boys have a complete educational evaluation, preferably in elementary school, so that their learning difficulties (if any) can be treated before they develop behavioral problems or become depressed.
- Physical therapy. Some XXY boys benefit from exercises that help them improve their muscle strength and coordination.

Most doctors consider mid-to-late adolescence the best time to tell an XXY boy about his condition. At that age most are able to understand the cause of the syndrome and its implications, and to decide whether they want to share the information with anyone else.

Prognosis

Most XXY males can live productive lives with normal life expectancy; many complete college and graduate school. In 1996 a technique was developed for extracting sperm from the male testicle and injecting it into a female egg; since that date, at least sixty children around the world have been conceived and born using sperm from men with Klinefelter syndrome. Men who are able to father children this way do not have any greater risk of producing an XXY son than men in the general population.

Prevention

There is no known way to prevent Klinefelter syndrome because it is caused by a random genetic error.

The Future

It is unlikely that Klinefelter syndrome will become more common in the general population in the future because nondisjunction is a random

WORDS TO KNOW

Androgen: The generic term for the group of male sex hormones produced by the body.

Germ cell: A cell involved in reproduction. In humans the germ cells are the sperm (male) and egg (female). Unlike other cells in the body, germ cells contain only half the standard number of chromosomes.

Karyotype: A photomicrograph of the chromosomes in a single human cell. Making a karyotype is one way to test for genetic disorders.

Nondisjunction: A genetic error in which one or more pairs of chromosomes fail to separate during the formation of germ cells, with the result that both chromosomes are carried to one daughter cell and none to the other. If an egg or sperm with a paired set of chromosomes is involved in the conception of a child, the child will have three chromosomes in its genetic makeup, two from one parent and one from the other.

Testosterone: The principal male sex hormone.

genetic error. What is likely, however, is that earlier diagnosis and better understanding of the syndrome will help XXY males do well in school and the adult workplace and lower their risk of depression and other setbacks. The knowledge that most XXY males benefit from hormonal treatment, surgery, and various supportive educational measures and can have normal lives is certainly encouraging.

SEE ALSO Breast cancer; Lupus; Osteoporosis; Rheumatoid arthritis

For more information

BOOKS

Bock, Robert. *Understanding Klinefelter Syndrome: A Guide for XXY Males and Their Families*, rev. ed. Bethesda, MD: National Institute of Child Health and Human Development, 2006.

Morales, Ralph. *Out of Darkness: An Autobiography: Living with Klinefelter Syndrome*. Louisville, KY: Chicago Spectrum Press, 2002.

PERIODICALS

Brody, Jane. "Personal Health: The Havoc of an Undetected Extra Chromosome." *New York Times*, August 31, 2004. Available online at http://query.nytimes.com/gst/fullpage.html?res=9504EEDD1731F932A0575BC0A9629C8B63 (accessed April 6, 2008).

WEB SITES

American Association for Klinefelter Syndrome Information and Support (AAKSIS). *A Guide to Klinefelter Syndrome*. Available online in PDF format at http://www.aaksis.org/Documents2/Klinefelter_Brochure_.pdf (accessed April 6, 2008).

Brager, David. "I'm Not Fat, I'm Deformed: Klinefelter's Syndrome & Me." *David Brager's Homepage.* http://www.geocities.com/dibragerowtcom/klinefel.html (accessed April 6, 2008). This is one man's personal account of his life before and after his diagnosis.

Genetics Home Reference. *Klinefelter Syndrome.* http://ghr.nlm.nih.gov/condition=klinefeltersyndrome#resources (accessed April 6, 2008).

Knowledge Support and Action (KS&A). *Klinefelter Syndrome.* http://www.genetic.org/knowledge/support/action/199/ (accessed April 6, 2008). KS&A is a nonprofit organization that was formed in 1989 to help people born with extra X or Y chromosomes. This portion of the KS&A website contains basic information about Klinefelter syndrome as well as links to articles, research reports, and other materials related to the condition.

National Human Genome Research Institute (NHGRI). *Learning about Klinefelter Syndrome.* http://www.genome.gov/19519068 (accessed April 6, 2008).

L

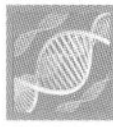
Genetic

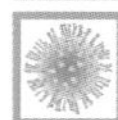
Infection

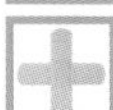
Injury

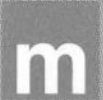
Multiple

Other

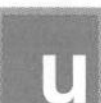
Unknown

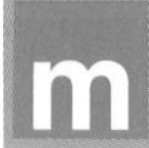

Lactose Intolerance

Definition

Lactose intolerance occurs when a person cannot digest lactose, a sugar found in milk and other dairy products. Lactose intolerance develops when lactase, an enzyme that is needed to break down milk sugar into simpler sugars, is less available or absent.

Also Known As
Lactase deficiency

Cause
Underproduction of lactase, a digestive enzyme

Symptoms
Intestinal gas, bloating, nausea, and diarrhea

Duration
May last a few weeks or be lifelong

Description

Lactose intolerance is a very common chronic digestive disorder in which a person's intestinal tract lacks the ability to make lactase, an enzyme that breaks down lactose, or milk sugar, into two simpler sugars that the body can use. A person can have a lactase deficiency without having the symptoms of lactose intolerance.

Lactose intolerance is not the same as being allergic to cow's milk. An allergy to cow's milk concerns a person's immune system, whereas lactose intolerance has to do with the process of digestion.

Lactose intolerance may be caused by any of three different factors. One is normal aging. As people get older, their small intestine produces lower amounts of lactase. After the lactase production drops below a certain point, the person may experience the symptoms of lactose intolerance.

A second cause of lactose intolerance is diseases of the intestines or surgical procedures in which part of the small intestine is removed. These disorders or operations may affect the part of the small intestine that secretes lactase. The third cause of lactose intolerance is genetic. A few people inherit lactose intolerance from both parents and are affected from birth.

The symptoms of lactose intolerance usually begin within half an hour to two hours after drinking milk or eating a meal high in dairy products. The person typically experiences diarrhea, which is the most common symptom of lactose intolerance, along with a gassy, bloated feeling, abdominal cramps, and possibly nausea. The severity of the symptoms is not necessarily related to the amount of milk or dairy products that were consumed but rather to the person's age, ethnicity, and the speed of his or her digestive processes.

Foods to Watch

Foods that are naturally high in lactose (in addition to milk) include butter and sometimes margarine; buttermilk; cottage cheese, cream cheese, and ricotta cheese; half and half, light cream, and whipping cream; ice milk, sherbet, ice cream, evaporated milk, and dry powdered milk; milk chocolate; whey; and yogurt.

Foods that contain hidden lactose include hot dogs, cold cuts, bologna, sausages, pancakes, creamy salad dressings, creamed soups, breaded meats, commercial pie crust and pie fillings, caramels, fudge and other chocolate candies, prepared cakes and sweet rolls, powdered coffee creamers, imitation dairy products, party dips, cream-based cordials, certain breads, sauces and gravies, frosting, certain prepared or processed foods, some prescription medications, and some over-the-counter medications.

Demographics

In most cases, lactose intolerance is part of the normal human developmental process. Most mammals stop producing lactase after they are weaned because they are eating solid food instead of drinking milk from the mother. Humans begin to slow down the production of lactase some time around age three to five years; thus most human adults are at some risk of developing lactose intolerance.

It is noteworthy, however, that the levels of lactose intolerance vary quite widely among different ethnic groups. In some groups, almost 100 percent of the adult population may be lactose intolerant. In the United States and Canada, lactose intolerance is estimated to affect between 20 and 60 percent of the adult population. In terms of specific ethnic groups, people of Dutch, Swedish, German, or other northern European descent have low rates of lactose intolerance (about 5 percent); persons of southern European ancestry have rates between 18 and 25 percent; African Americans have a rate around 45 percent; persons from Japan or southeastern Asia have rates above 95 percent; and Native Americans are almost 100 percent lactose intolerant.

One theory that has been proposed to explain these differences is the long-standing differences among human societies in milk consumption after childhood. In Asia and Africa, children were rarely given milk after being weaned; in these societies, lactase production generally falls by 90 percent by the time the child is four years old. In societies in which milk consumption continues into adult life, however, a mutation on chromosome 2 that bypasses the normal shutdown of lactase production became widespread in the population. Thus members of these groups can continue to consume milk and dairy products throughout their adult lives. Some researchers have traced the mutation back as far as 4500 BCE in both Sweden and the Middle East.

Causes and Symptoms

Lactose intolerance results from a drop in or disruption of the production of lactase in the small intestine. Lactase is produced by specialized cells in the membrane that lines the villi, which are small finger-like projections on the walls of the small intestine. The production of the enzyme may drop at a certain age or because a disease or radiation treatment for cancer has damaged the villi of the small intestine.

The symptoms of lactose intolerance are diarrhea, bloating, nausea, and a gassy feeling within thirty minutes to two hours following a meal high in dairy products. They do *not* include fever, bleeding from the digestive tract, or weight loss in adults. People who have these symptoms should be checked by their doctors for other disorders of the intestines.

Diagnosis

Diagnosis of lactose intolerance is based on a patient's history, particularly a detailed history of the patient's consumption of dairy products. Many people underestimate the amount of milk or products containing lactose that they consume; they may not think of yogurt or ice cream, for example, as milk products. After getting a complete picture of the patient's diet, the doctor will usually suggest cutting out dairy products for a week or so in order to see whether the symptoms improve. If they do, further testing may be unnecessary.

There are three tests that can be used, one of which is generally given only to infants and small children. It is a test that measures the acidity of the child's stool sample. Undigested lactose ferments inside the intestine and forms an acid that can be measured in the stool sample.

The most common diagnostic test used in adults is the hydrogen breath test. The patient is asked to drink a liquid containing a high level of lactose. The doctor then measures the amount of hydrogen in the breath at certain intervals. Undigested lactose reaches the colon and ferments, causing hydrogen and other gases to be released, absorbed by the intestines, and eventually exhaled. Large amounts of exhaled hydrogen indicate that the patient's body is not digesting lactose completely and that the patient is probably lactose intolerant.

The third type of diagnostic test involves taking a small sample of tissue from the lining of the small intestine and measuring the amount of lactase present in the tissue sample. This type of test requires a specialized laboratory to evaluate the results, however, and is rarely used outside clinical research.

Treatment

There are several treatment options for lactose intolerance:

- Completely eliminating milk and dairy products from the diet. This change in diet usually requires careful reading of labels on other foods because many processed foods contain milk or milk solids (see sidebar). In addition, some drug manufacturers use lactose as a binding substance to carry the active ingredient in the medication. The patient may need to check with the doctor or pharmacist about any prescription medications they may be using to see if the drugs were formulated with lactose.
- Eliminating dairy products from the diet for a time and then gradually reintroducing small amounts of them. Some people can tolerate small amounts of yogurt or milk after avoiding them completely for a few weeks.
- Using specially manufactured lactose-free milk products or soy products and other plant-based substitutes for milk.
- Taking dietary supplements that contain lactase. Products like Lactaid, DairyEase, and Lactogest can be purchased without a prescription.

People who are concerned about the risk of osteoporosis (brittle bones) can take calcium supplements to keep their bones strong rather than getting their calcium from milk. Patients should ask their doctors how much calcium they should be getting from other sources. Most adults should not take more than 1,200–1,500 milligrams of calcium per day.

WORDS TO KNOW

Chronic: Recurrent or long-term

Congenital: Present from birth.

Lactase: An enzyme that breaks down lactose into simpler sugars during the process of digestion.

Lactose: A complex sugar found in milk and other dairy products. It is sometimes called milk sugar.

Villi (singular, villus): Small finger-like projections along the walls of the small intestine that increase the surface area of the intestinal wall.

Prognosis

Most people recover completely by removing milk products from the diet or by substituting reduced-lactose or lactose-free dairy products for those that contain lactose.

Prevention

There is no way to prevent congenital or adult-onset lactose intolerance.

The Future

Lactose intolerance is not a life-threatening condition. Most people can manage quite well by using milk substitutes, watching the amount of milk and other dairy products that they consume, or by taking over-the-counter lactase supplements. There are also a number of cookbooks with lactose-free recipes or recipes that use milk substitutes.

SEE ALSO Celiac disease; Crohn disease; Irritable bowel syndrome; Osteoporosis

For more information

BOOKS

Dobler, Merri Lou. *Lactose Intolerance Nutrition Guide.* Chicago: American Dietetic Association, 2003.

Goldberg, Phyllis Z. *How to Tolerate Lactose Intolerance: Recipes and a Guide for Eating Well without Dairy Products.* Springfield, IL: Charles C. Thomas, 1998.

PERIODICALS

Brody, Jane. "Personal Health: Debate over Milk: Time to Look at Facts." *New York Times*, September 26, 2000. Available online at http://query.nytimes.com/gst/fullpage.html?res=9C03E3D91E3BF935A1575AC0A9669C8B63&sec=&spon=&pagewanted=all (accessed May 3, 2008).

WEB SITES

International Foundation for Functional Gastrointestinal Disorders (IFFGD). *Lactose Intolerance: Definition, Symptoms and Treatment.* Available online in PDF format (free download) at http://www.iffgd.org/store/viewproduct/122 (updated September 2007; accessed May 4, 2008).

Mayo Clinic. *Lactose Intolerance.* Available online at http://www.mayoclinic.com/health/lactose-intolerance/DS00530 (updated February 16, 2008; accessed May 4, 2008).

National Institute of Diabetes and Digestive and Kidney Diseases (NIDDK). *Lactose Intolerance.* Available online in PDF format at http://digestive.niddk.nih.gov/ddiseases/pubs/lactoseintolerance/lactoseintolerance.pdf (updated March 2006; accessed May 4, 2008).

TeensHealth. *Lactose Intolerance.* Available online at http://www.kidshealth.org/teen/nutrition/diets/lactose_intolerance.html (updated September 2006; accessed May 4, 2008).

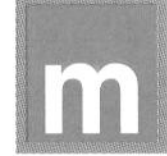

Laryngitis

Definition

Laryngitis is defined as inflammation or irritation of the larynx, which is the voice box that lies at the base of the throat just above the windpipe. It is a condition or symptom rather than a distinctive disease. Acute laryngitis is defined as lasting three weeks or less; laryngitis that lasts longer than three weeks is called chronic laryngitis.

Also Known As
Losing one's voice, dysphonia

Cause
Overuse of the voice, infection, or throat irritation

Symptoms
Hoarseness, difficulty speaking, sore throat, dry cough

Duration
Seven to ten days (acute); over three weeks (chronic)

Description

Laryngitis occurs when the vocal folds (or vocal cords) swell as a result of infection or another cause of inflammation. The vocal folds are two bands of tissue that stretch across the larynx. Under normal circumstances, when a person wants to speak, the vocal folds tighten. Air from the lungs is forced through the smaller space between the bands of muscle, causing them to vibrate. Lengthening, shortening, tightening, and loosening of the cords allows a person to control the pitch of the voice. When the vocal folds swell up due to irritation or inflammation, they cannot vibrate easily, which causes the voice to sound hoarse, raspy, or faint.

Demographics

Laryngitis is so common in the general population that no exact statistics are kept. Most people treat acute laryngitis at home without visiting a doctor, particularly if the voice problem seems to be a side effect of a cold or the flu. According to one study, acute laryngitis is most common in adults between the ages of eighteen and forty. It appears to affect both sexes and all races equally. Chronic laryngitis is more common in adults over fifty and in people whose occupations expose them to irritating chemicals.

People who smoke, people with asthma, firefighters, and singers or public speakers are at greater risk of laryngitis than the general population.

Home Care for Laryngitis

Acute laryngitis caused by a cold or the flu can usually be treated at home:

- Keep the air in the house moist by using a humidifier.
- Moisten the tissues of the throat by breathing in the steam from a hot shower or holding the heat over a bowl of hot steaming water.
- Drink plenty of fluids.
- Use throat lozenges, a salt-water gargle, or chewing gum to help keep the throat moist.
- Give the voice as much complete rest as possible.
- Avoid whispering; whispering is harder on the vocal folds than normal speech.

Causes and Symptoms

The most common single cause of acute laryngitis is an upper respiratory infection caused by a virus, most often a cold or influenza virus. Other viruses, such as those that cause chickenpox, mumps, or measles, can also cause laryngitis.

Other causes of laryngitis include:

- Infections caused by bacteria or fungi
- Irritation of the throat caused by smoking
- Drying of the tissues lining the throat caused by asthma inhalers, overuse of decongestants, or antihistamines
- Exposure to dust, chemicals, smoke, fumes, or other irritating substances in a person's workplace
- High levels of alcohol consumption
- Air pollution
- Gastroesophageal reflux disease (GERD; a disorder in which acid from the stomach flows backward up the esophagus and into the throat, irritating the throat tissues.)
- Repeated episodes of sinus infection
- Throat cancer

In addition to a hoarse or faint voice, people with laryngitis may complain of soreness in the throat, a tickling sensation, a dry cough, difficulty breathing, or discomfort when swallowing food.

Diagnosis

Acute laryngitis is usually diagnosed by taking the patient's history—particularly recent exposure to colds or flu—and an examination of the throat and neck. The doctor will usually feel the outside of the neck for signs of swollen lymph glands and will look down the patient's throat using a mirror or with a device called a laryngoscope. If the patient has acute laryngitis, the vocal folds will look red, swollen, and covered with fluid secretions. Laboratory studies are not usually needed.

If the patient has chronic laryngitis, the doctor will examine him or her for signs of GERD or refer the patient to an otolaryngologist. Otolaryngologists are doctors who specialize in diagnosing disorders of the ears, nose, and throat. The patient may need some special examinations to evaluate the possibility of throat cancer.

Treatment

People can often treat acute laryngitis at home with some simple remedies (see sidebar). It is not usually necessary to take antibiotics for acute laryngitis, as several studies have shown that these drugs do not speed up the patient's recovery. If the laryngitis does not clear up after two weeks, however, the patient should have the throat checked again.

Chronic laryngitis caused by GERD is usually treated by drugs that lower the production of stomach acid, by changes in the patient's diet, and by raising the head of the bed during sleep. The laryngitis usually clears up once the abnormal backward flow of stomach acid into the throat stops.

Laryngitis caused by overuse of the voice is usually treated by complete vocal rest for several days. Even if the patient is a professional singer, cheerleader, or public speaker, trying to use the voice during an episode of laryngitis can make the condition worse.

Prognosis

Acute laryngitis caused by an infection usually clears up completely in about a week. The prognosis of chronic laryngitis depends on the cause of the condition. People with chronic laryngitis caused by GERD or by overuse of the voice will usually recover without complications if they follow the doctor's advice about diet and vocal rest. The prognosis of

WORDS TO KNOW

Chronic: Recurrent or long-lasting.

Larynx: The medical name for the voice box located at the base of the throat.

Otolaryngologist: A doctor who specializes in diagnosing and treating diseases of the ears, nose, and throat.

Pitch: The highness or lowness of the voice or a musical note.

Vocal folds: Twin folds of mucous membrane stretched across the larynx. They are also known as vocal cords.

throat cancer depends on the stage of the cancer at the time it is diagnosed. Fortunately, throat cancer is a very rare cause of laryngitis.

Prevention

Some measures can be taken to reduce the risk of getting laryngitis:

- Quitting smoking (or not starting in the first place) and avoiding secondhand smoke.
- Taking precautions against colds and flu; for many people, these measures include an annual flu shot.
- Avoiding the overuse of antihistamines or decongestants when treating a cold at home.
- Avoiding breathing irritating household cleansers and other chemicals.
- Avoiding overuse of the voice, including loud yelling or screaming.

The Future

Laryngitis is a common health problem that is likely to continue to be common, if only because it is so often associated with colds and other common respiratory ailments. Laryngitis related to occupational hazards is also likely to continue to be a common health problem.

SEE ALSO Asthma; Common cold; Gastroesophageal reflux disease; Influenza; Smoking; Sore throat

For more information

BOOKS

Beers, Mark J., ed. *Merck Manual of Medical Information*, 2nd home ed. Whitehouse Station, NJ: Merck Medical Laboratories, 2003.

WEB SITES

KidsHealth. *Laryngitis*. Available online at http://www.kidshealth.org/kid/ill_injure/sick/laryngitis.html (accessed April 19, 2008).

Mayo Clinic. *Laryngitis*. Available online at http://www.mayoclinic.com/health/laryngitis/DS00366/DSECTION=1 (accessed April 20, 2008).

University of Michigan Health System. "Laryngitis." *Adult Health Advisor*, 2005. Available online at http://www.med.umich.edu/1libr/aha/aha_chronlar_crs.htm (accessed April 20, 2008).

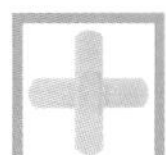

Lead Poisoning

Definition

Lead poisoning is a form of chronic (long-term) damage to the nervous system and other body organs. It is caused by inhaling dust containing lead or eating or drinking material contaminated with lead.

Description

Lead poisoning has been a source of human illness and premature death since people first began to use lead in pottery, plumbing, cosmetics, jewelry, metal cookware, and even medicines. The oldest known lead mine, opened about 6500 BCE, is located in present-day Turkey. Lead poisoning was first identified around 200 BCE by Nicander of Colophon, a Greek doctor. The metal was popular in the ancient world, however, because it is easily worked, it has a low melting point, and it does not rust. The most common sources of lead poisoning from ancient Rome through the Middle Ages were drinking vessels made of pewter, a metal made mostly of tin with small amounts of copper and lead added; and wine, which was often sweetened by a compound of lead called lead acetate or sugar of lead.

Lead poisoning in humans is often slow to develop because of the small quantities of the metal that can cause health problems. Lead harms the body by preventing the body from using iron, zinc, and calcium in the production of hemoglobin (a pigment found in red blood cells) and in other important body processes. In addition, lead is not easily removed from the body. After it enters the body through the lungs or the digestive tract, it travels first to the blood and other internal organs and then is stored in the bones and teeth. Lead in the blood and soft tissues is

Also Known As
Lead toxicity, plumbism

Cause
Inhaling or ingesting lead from paint, soil, or other objects

Symptoms
Muscle weakness, anemia, damage to brain and nervous system, infertility, joint pain

Duration
May be lifelong

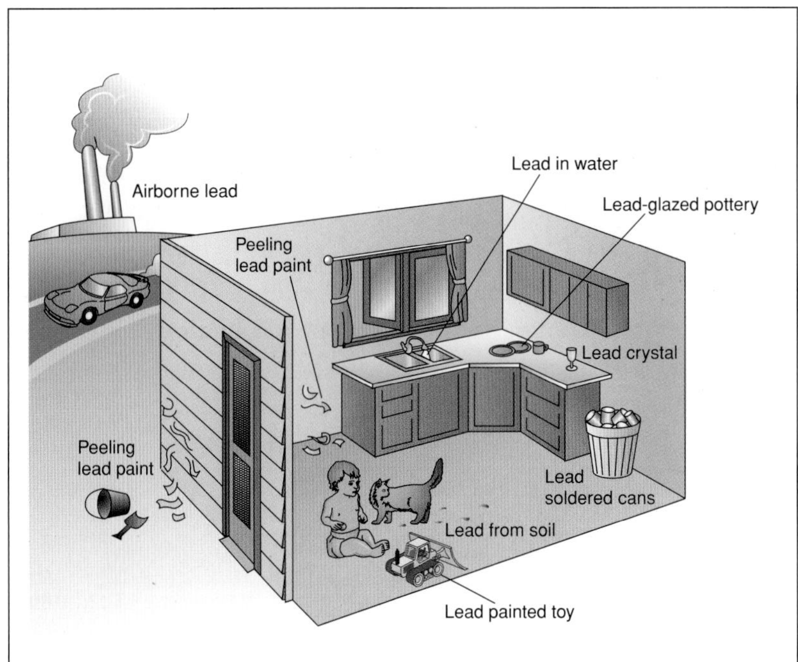

Illustration showing various sources of lead that can cause lead poisoning. THE GALE GROUP.

gradually filtered by the kidneys over a period of sixty to seventy days but may remain in the bones and teeth for several years.

Demographics

In the United States, lead poisoning is most likely to affect children below the age of five years and adults in certain high-risk occupations. About 1.5 million workers are exposed to lead in the workplace. The number of children with risky blood levels of lead, or BLLs, has decreased 68 percent since 1991. As of 2002, the most recent survey year, 1.6 percent of American children between one and five years of age had BLLs above 10 micrograms of lead per deciliter (about 3.5 ounces) of blood.

Children of any race living in cities or near highways with high levels of auto exhaust fumes are at greater risk of high BLLs than children living in rural areas. African American children are at greater risk than either Hispanic or Caucasian children. Boys and girls are at equal risk.

Causes and Symptoms

The basic cause of lead poisoning is inhaling, swallowing, or otherwise being exposed to lead in paint, soil, or lead-based products in the environment. Although lead is no longer used in the manufacture of paints, gasoline, and other products, people can still be exposed to dangerous amounts of lead. In the United States, the most common sources of exposure to lead include:

- Houses built before the 1960s and painted before 1978. House paint was made with lead until 1978, but many older houses have layers of paint that were applied before lead-free paints were available. Stripping or sanding away older paint can be dangerous, too, because the removal process releases fine dust particles containing lead into the air. Children can breathe in this dust or take in lead by swallowing paint chips or dust from lead-based paint.
- Toys and furniture that were painted before 1976.
- Plumbing, pipes, and faucets.
- Storage batteries.
- Children's toys made outside the United States, including paint sets and art supplies.
- Soil contaminated by long years of car exhaust, such as soil along the sides of highways or near gas stations.
- Lead bullets, fishing sinkers, and curtain weights.
- Homemade illegal whiskey ("moonshine").
- Pewter pitchers, goblets, and dinnerware.
- Lead-based costume jewelry.
- Hobbies that involve soldering, glazing pottery, making jewelry, or making items out of stained glass.

Other sources of lead poisoning in some ethnic groups in the United States are folk remedies for various ailments. These include the practice of eating soil, certain traditional medicines imported from Southeast Asia, and a folk remedy called litargirio, sold in Hispanic grocery stores.

The symptoms of lead poisoning usually develop gradually over time rather than coming on suddenly. In many cases the symptoms are not specific to lead poisoning and may be mistaken for the symptoms of other disorders. In children, whose nervous systems are more vulnerable to lead, symptoms of lead poisoning include irritability, loss of appetite and weight, tiredness, abdominal cramps, vomiting, constipation, a pale complexion due to anemia, impulsive behavior, seizures, lowered IQ, and learning difficulties.

Symptoms of lead poisoning in adults may include:

- Pain, numbness, or tingling sensations in the arms and legs
- Difficulty conceiving in women or abnormal sperm in men
- Headache and memory problems
- Abdominal cramps and constipation
- Mood disorders and personality changes
- Muscle pains and weakness
- Hypertension (high blood pressure)
- Cataracts

Diagnosis

Most cases of lead poisoning are detected by screening people at risk rather than because the doctor suspects that the symptoms are caused by lead. The diagnosis of lead poisoning is based on a blood test called the blood lead level or BLL. The test can be given to measure the effects of treatment for lead poisoning as well as to screen people for exposure to harmful amounts of lead.

The blood test results are evaluated according to standards set by the American Academy of Pediatrics and the Centers for Disease Control and Prevention (CDC). The BLL is measured in micrograms of lead per deciliter of blood (mcg/dL). A deciliter is about a fifth of a pint. The definition of what is considered a dangerous level of blood lead has changed over the years. In 1997 the blood lead level of concern for children was decreased from 25 micrograms per deciliter to 10 micrograms per deciliter.

Not everyone needs to be screened for possible lead poisoning. The CDC recommends screening for adults employed in certain occupations, particularly metal working, glass working, lead plating, ore refining, auto repair, road repair, and construction. Children in the following categories should be screened for possible lead poisoning:

- Children whose families are receiving federal assistance
- Children who live in or regularly visit a house or apartment built before 1950, or before 1978 if the house has been or is undergoing remodeling
- Children who have a sibling or playmate diagnosed with lead poisoning
- Children from refugee or immigrant families

The CDC divides the results of the BLL test into six groups or classes:

- Class I: Less than 10 mcg/dL
- Class IIA: 10–14 mcg/dL
- Class IIB: 15–19 mcg/dL
- Class III: 20–44 mcg/dL
- Class IV: 45–69 mcg/dL
- Class V: 70 mcg/dL or higher (This blood lead level is considered a medical emergency.)

Treatment

Mild cases of lead poisoning (Classes I through III) can often be treated simply by removing the source of the lead. Children should have their BLL retested a month later to make sure their blood lead level is dropping.

People with higher BLLs are usually treated with chelation therapy. This is a type of treatment in which the person is given a drug that binds with the lead in the body so that it can be excreted in the urine. People in Class III and some in Class IV are given a drug called succimer, which is taken by mouth. People with BLLs above 50 mcg/dL are usually treated with a drug called EDTA, which must be given intravenously.

Children who have developed anemia as a result of lead poisoning may be given iron supplements.

Prognosis

The prognosis for recovery from lead poisoning depends on the patient's age and the level of lead in his or her body. Adults with low levels of lead often recover without problems. Those with higher levels have a greater risk of long-lasting health problems and must be monitored carefully by their doctor. Their nerves and muscles may no longer function well. Moreover, other body systems may be harmed to various degrees, including the kidneys and blood vessels. People who survive toxic lead levels may suffer some permanent brain damage. However, death from lead poisoning is rare in the early 2000s because of the widespread use of chelation therapy.

Some people also develop complications after chelation therapy, as treatment with chelating drugs does not always reverse nerve damage. Depression, increased aggressiveness, impotence, and infertility have been reported in adults.

WORDS TO KNOW

Chelation therapy: Treatment of lead poisoning by administering medications that help the body excrete the lead in the urine.

Pewter: A metal made mostly of tin and small quantities of copper. Modern pewter is no longer made with lead.

Plumbism: The medical name for lead poisoning.

Prevention

The National Institute for Environmental Health Sciences (NIEHS) recommends the following measures to reduce people's exposure to lead:

- People who think they may have lead paint in their homes should get advice on safe paint removal from the Housing and Urban Development (HUD) at 800-RID-LEAD or the National Information Center at 800-LEAD-FYI.
- Parents who work in occupations where they are exposed to lead should change clothes before coming home.
- Everyone should wash their hands before meals.
- People should have the household tap water tested for lead levels. If it is high, filter it or use bottled water for drinking and cooking.
- Throw out old painted toys if it is unclear whether the paint contains lead.
- The home should be kept as dust-free as possible.
- Avoid using candies, canned goods, or folk medications produced outside the United States.

The Future

Lead poisoning is likely to continue to be a public health problem for some time. One reason is that lead is not biodegradable. This means that lead persists in the outside environment for a long time. There are still many older buildings that were painted with lead-based paints before 1978, and many people are still unaware of the dangers of removing old paint without safeguards. In addition, it is difficult to control the entry and sale of folk medicines containing lead in the United States.

SEE ALSO Cataracts; Depression; Hypertension

For more information

BOOKS

Bothell, Joan, Mary-Margaret Gaudio, and Maureen T. Mulroy. *How Mother Bear Taught the Children about Lead.* Storrs, CT: University of Connecticut Cooperative Extension System, 2003. Developed by the Penobscot Indian Nation and the Environmental Protection Agency, this is a 29-page illustrated storybook for young readers about the dangers of lead. It can be downloaded in PDF format at http://kids.niehs.nih.gov/bear/fullbook.pdf (accessed May 5, 2008).

Legal Services of New Jersey. *Lead Poisoning: What It Is and What You Can Do about It.* New Brunswick, NJ: Legal Services of New Jersey, 2006.

PERIODICALS

Brody, Jane E. "Personal Health: Dally No Longer; Get the Lead Out." *New York Times*, January 17, 2006. Available online at http://query.nytimes.com/gst/fullpage.html?res=9B03E4D6143FF934A25752C0A9609C8B63&sec=&spon=&pagewanted=all (accessed May 5, 2008).

WEB SITES

Agency for Toxic Substances and Disease Registry (ATSDR). *Lead Webcast for the Community.* Available online at http://www.atsdr.cdc.gov/csem/lead/community/index.html (accessed May 5, 2008). This is a ten-minute webcast with PowerPoint presentation about lead poisoning and its treatment.

Centers for Disease Control and Prevention (CDC). *Childhood Lead Exposure.* Available online at http://www.cdc.gov/Features/ChildhoodLead/ (updated November 2, 2007; accessed May 5, 2008).

Mayo Clinic. *Lead Poisoning.* Available online at http://www.mayoclinic.com/health/lead-poisoning/FL00068 (updated March 15, 2007; accessed May 5, 2008).

National Institute of Environmental Health Sciences (NIEHS). *Lead and Your Health.* Available online in PDF format at http://www.niehs.nih.gov/health/topics/agents/lead/docs/lead.pdf (updated April 2006; accessed May 5, 2008).

Learning Disorders

Learning disorders is a term used to describe childhood school-related problems related to academic and functional skills, including being able to read, write, spell, speak, listen, think a problem through logically, and organize information. Learning disorders are sometimes called learning disabilities. They can be caused by a number of factors, ranging from heredity and damage to the child's brain before birth to premature birth or accidents after birth.

A learning disorder is not the same thing as mental retardation or having low intelligence. Many children diagnosed with learning disorders have average or above-average intelligence. Some doctors categorize learning disorders according to whether the child's problem is caused by:

- Problems taking in information through the senses (vision problems or hearing loss).
- Problems organizing information in the mind. This skill includes relating new information to facts previously learned and being able to put facts together to form a larger picture of the subject.
- Memory problems.
- Problems with speech or motor activities (drawing or handwriting).

Specific learning disorders include dyslexia, the most common learning disorder; writing disorder; mathematics disorder; motor (movement) skill disorder; and disorders of speaking and listening. Treatment of learning disorders is focused on identifying them and working with the child to overcome them as early as possible.

SEE ALSO Dyslexia; Fetal alcohol syndrome; Hearing loss; Prematurity

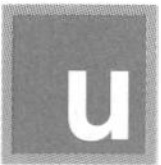

Leukemia

Definition and Description

Leukemia is the name of a group of cancers that affect white blood cells. It takes its name from the abnormally high numbers of white blood cells found in patients' blood before treatment. It is not a single disease; there are four major types of leukemia, two that are considered acute (they worsen rapidly) and two that are chronic (they progress slowly). These four types are:

- Chronic lymphocytic leukemia (CLL). A lymphocytic leukemia is one in which the cancer affects white blood cells (WBCs) called lymphocytes. The abnormal but relatively mature cells multiply, keeping normal cells from doing their job of fighting infections.

Also Known As
Cancer of the blood

Cause
Unknown

Symptoms
Fatigue, easy bruising and bleeding, swollen lymph glands, frequent infections

Duration
Years

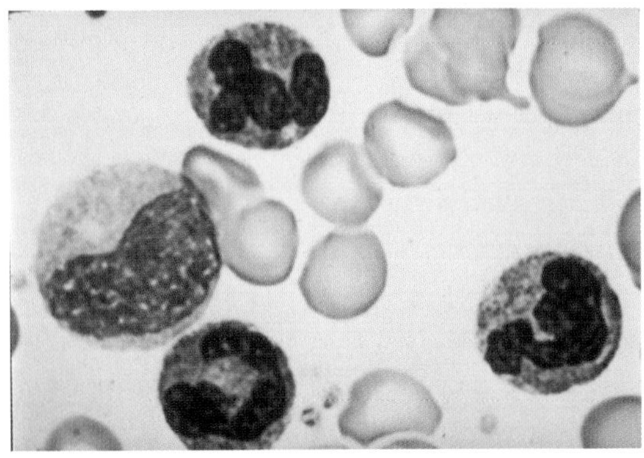

Magnified image of leukemia cells in blood. © PHOTOTAKE INC. / ALAMY.

CLL is related to another type of cancer called lymphoma, which is a cancer that affects the lymphatic system. CLL is a common adult leukemia; it progresses slowly and many patients feel well for years without treatment.

- Chronic myeloid leukemia (CML). A myeloid leukemia is one that affects bone marrow cells that normally produce platelets (small cells that affect the blood's ability to clot), and a few types of white blood cells called neutrophils. CML is associated with an abnormality in chromosome 9 called the Philadelphia chromosome. This abnormality occurs when a portion of the genetic material in chromosome 9 is exchanged with a portion of the genetic material in chromosome 22. Ninety-five percent of patients with CML have this genetic alteration. Like CLL, CML is a slowly developing form of leukemia; patients diagnosed with it may have few or no symptoms for months or years before the disease grows worse.
- Acute lymphocytic leukemia (ALL). ALL is the most common type of leukemia in young children and can be rapidly fatal if not treated. In ALL, the patient's bone marrow produces a large number of immature malignant lymphocytes that crowd out healthy blood cells, both red and white. Children with ALL are vulnerable to infection and easy bleeding. The abnormal WBCs can also collect in certain areas of the body, including the central nervous system and spinal cord. This buildup can cause such symptoms as severe headaches, difficulty breathing, a swollen liver and spleen, and dizziness.
- Acute myeloid leukemia (AML). AML is caused by the rapid multiplication of abnormal and immature neutrophils or similar cells that build up within the bone marrow and interfere with the production of normal cells. It worsens quickly if not treated, but it may respond well to therapy, at least in the beginning. Unfortunately, many patients with AML suffer relapses.

Demographics

There are about 31,000 cases of leukemia diagnosed in the United States each year, 2,000 in children and 29,000 in adults. Of the four major types of leukemia, about 14,000 cases of CLL are diagnosed each year, almost all of them in adults over fifty-five; 4,400 cases of CML, mostly in adults; 3,800 cases of ALL, almost all in children; and 11,000 cases of AML, which affects both adults and children.

Two-thirds of patients with CLL are men; ALL is slightly more common in men and boys than in women and girls; and about 60 percent of patients with AML are men.

ALL is more common in Italy, the United States, Switzerland, and Costa Rica than in other countries; AML is more common in Caucasians in the United States than in other ethnic groups. CLL is more common in Jewish people of Eastern European descent than in other ethnic groups.

Causes and Symptoms

The causes of leukemia are not completely understood. What is known is that there are several risk factors for these forms of cancer.

- Exposure to high levels of radiation, most often from radiation used to treat other forms of cancer or from nuclear accidents.
- Exposure to certain chemicals, such as benzene or formaldehyde. This type of exposure is most likely to affect adults.
- Chemotherapy for other forms of cancer. Adults treated with certain types of cancer-killing medications may develop leukemia later on.
- Down syndrome. People with this particular genetic disorder have higher rates of leukemia than people in the general population.
- Chromosomal abnormalities such as the Philadelphia chromosome.

It is important to keep in mind, however, that most people with these risk factors do not develop leukemia, and that many people who do suffer from leukemia have none of these risk factors.

The early symptoms of leukemia may develop gradually rather than suddenly and are often mistaken for the symptoms of other diseases. About 20 percent of patients with chronic leukemia do not have any noticeable symptoms at the time they are diagnosed—most often as the result of a routine blood test. Common symptoms of leukemia include:

- Fever and night sweats
- Feeling tired much of the time
- Getting frequent colds and other infections

- Headaches
- Pain in the bones or joints
- Swelling or pain in the abdomen from enlargement of the spleen
- Cuts or sores taking an unusually long time to heal
- Swelling of the lymph nodes in the neck or armpit
- Unintentional weight loss
- Soft tissue bruising easily, with frequent purple areas or pinpoint bruises under the skin
- Gums and open cuts bleeding easily
- Shortness of breath
- Nausea or vomiting
- In some cases, confusion, dizziness, seizures, or blurred vision

Diagnosis

The diagnosis of leukemia is complicated by the fact that most of its early symptoms are nonspecific; that is, they occur in many other diseases. The diagnosis is made by a combination of blood tests to check the patient's white blood cell number and kind, followed by a bone marrow biopsy. To do the biopsy, a hematologist (doctor who specializes in the diagnosis and treatment of blood disorders) draws a sample of bone marrow (usually from the hip bone) through a needle after the patient has been given a local anesthetic. The biopsy is necessary to confirm the diagnosis because some diseases other than leukemia can cause an abnormally high number of white blood cells, and some leukemias can only be found in early stages in the bone marrow.

In some cases the doctor will also order a chest x ray or a spinal tap to check for signs of leukemia. In a spinal tap, a small amount of cerebrospinal fluid is removed from the spinal column through a needle. It is done to see whether the disease has spread to the brain or spinal cord.

Treatment

Treatment for leukemia varies according to the type of disease:

- CLL: Low-grade forms of CLL may not be given any form of treatment because patients do not benefit from therapy in the early stages of the disease. Patients are usually treated when their RBC count or platelet count starts to drop, the lymph nodes become painful, or the number of abnormal WBCs starts to rise sharply. Patients are usually treated with combination chemotherapy; younger patients sometimes benefit from bone marrow transplantation.

- CML: There are several anticancer drugs that can be used to treat CML, but in recent years the standard treatment is a drug called Gleevec, which has relatively few side effects and can be taken by mouth at home. About 90 percent of patients can be maintained on Gleevec for five years without the disease becoming worse. If the drug stops working, bone marrow transplantation is an option; however, the procedure is risky as 30 percent of CML patients die shortly after the operation.
- ALL: Treatment of ALL is focused on preventing the disease from spreading into the central nervous system. It generally has four phases: a beginning phase of chemotherapy to stop the production of abnormal WBCs in the bone marrow; a second phase of medication therapy to eliminate remaining leukemia cells; a third phase of radiation or chemotherapy to prevent the disease from spreading to the brain and spinal cord; and maintenance treatment with chemotherapy to prevent the disease from recurring. ALL can also be treated by bone marrow transplantation.
- AML: AML is treated primarily by chemotherapy in two stages: an induction phase in which the patient is given drugs to reduce the number of cancerous blood cells to an undetectable level; and a second or consolidation phase to eliminate any remaining abnormal cells.

Treatment for leukemia also includes antibiotics to help fight infections when needed, since patients with this type of cancer are vulnerable to infection. The doctor will also provide advice about nutrition and refer the patient to a dietitian if necessary to make sure that the patient is eating a healthy diet and is not losing weight.

Although chemotherapy is the mainstay of treatment for leukemia, in some cases the doctor may recommend surgery to remove the spleen if it has become enlarged. This operation is usually done to control pain and avoid pressure on other organs in the patient's abdomen.

Prognosis

The prognosis of leukemia depends on the specific type. In general, females have a better prognosis than males.

- CLL: The five-year survival rate is 75 percent.
- CML: The five-year survival rate is 90 percent.
- ALL: Survival rates vary depending on the patient's age. The five-year survival rate is 85 percent for children but only 50 percent for adults.
- AML: The five-year survival rate is 40 percent.

Prevention

There is no known way to prevent leukemia because the causes of this group of cancers are still not known.

The Future

Leukemia is one type of cancer in which survival rates have increased dramatically since the 1960s. In 1960 the overall five-year survival rate for all types of leukemia was about 14 percent; it is over 50 percent as of the early 2000s.

Cancer research in general is a rapidly expanding field. Many new medical centers devoted entirely to cancer research and treatment have been established across the United States. Doctors are testing new approaches to cancer treatment as well as new anticancer drugs, doses, and treatment schedules. Other researchers are working on improving the technique of bone marrow transplantation as a way to treat leukemia, as well as improved methods of diagnosing the disease.

SEE ALSO Down syndrome; Lymphoma

For more information

BOOKS

Ball, Edward D., and Alex Kagan. *100 Questions and Answers about Leukemia*, 2nd ed. Sudbury, MA: Jones and Bartlett Publishers, 2008.

Klosterman, Lorrie. *Leukemia.* New York: Marshall Cavendish Benchmark, 2005.

Sullivan, Nanci A. *Walking with a Shadow: Surviving Childhood Leukemia.* Westport, CT: Praeger, 2004.

WEB SITES

eMedicine Health. *Leukemia.* Available online at http://www.emedicinehealth.com/leukemia/article_em.htm (updated October 21, 2005; accessed on June 6, 2008).

Mayo Clinic. *Leukemia.* Available online at http://www.mayoclinic.com/health/leukemia/DS00351 (updated April 5, 2008; accessed on June 7, 2008.)

WORDS TO KNOW

Acute: Referring to a disease or symptom that is severe or quickly worsens.

B cell: A type of white blood cell produced in the bone marrow that makes antibodies against viruses.

Bone marrow: The soft spongy tissue inside the long bones of the body where blood cells are formed.

Chronic: Referring to a disease or symptom that goes on for a long time, tends to recur, and usually gets worse slowly.

Hematologist: A doctor who specializes in diagnosing and treating disorders of the blood.

Lymphocyte: The medical term for white blood cells. A lymphocytic anemia is one that affects the cells in the bone marrow that give rise to white blood cells.

Lymphoma: A type of cancer that affects the lymphatic system.

Myeloid: Relating to bone marrow.

Philadelphia chromosome: A genetic abnormality in chromosome 9 associated with CML. Its name comes from the location of the University of Pennsylvania School of Medicine, where it was discovered in 1960.

Platelet: A type of small blood cell that is important in forming blood clots.

National Cancer Institute (NCI). *What You Need to Know about Leukemia.* Available online in PDF format at http://www.cancer.gov/pdf/WYNTK/WYNTK_leukemia.pdf (updated April 2003; accessed on June 6, 2008).

National Library of Medicine (NLM). *Leukemia.* Available online at http://www.nlm.nih.gov/medlineplus/tutorials/leukemia/htm/index.htm (accessed on June 6, 2008). This is an online tutorial with voiceover; viewers have the option of a self-playing version, a text version, or an interactive version with questions.

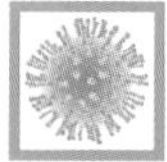

Lice Infestation

Definition

A lice infestation is a condition in which lice are present on a person's scalp, body (or clothes), or pubic area. It is called an infestation rather than an infection because the parasites live on or near the skin and outside of the body rather than in the internal organs. Lice are tiny insects that can spread from one person to another through close contact;

through sharing such personal items as clothing, hats, combs, or hairbrushes; or through lying on a bed, pillow, or carpet that has been in contact with someone with lice.

Description

The three types of lice that infest humans are somewhat different in size and outward appearance. Head lice are 1–2 millimeters long, white or gray in color, and have flattened abdomens. The female louse lays her nits (eggs) close to the base of a hair shaft and attaches them to it with a sticky, glue-like substance. The glue is what makes it so difficult to remove the nits from the hair shaft.

Body or clothing lice are generally larger than head lice, between 2 and 4 millimeters long. The body louse lives in the seams of clothing, emerging at night to feed on the person's body. Pubic lice are smaller and broader, about 1.2 millimeters long. They have larger front claws, which is why pubic lice are sometimes called "crabs." The claws enable pubic lice to cling to the coarse hairs in the human groin and armpit areas.

Demographics

The demographics of lice infestation vary depending of the type of lice involved. On the whole, lice infestations are common in the general population. There are at least 12 million cases in the United States each year, although this figure is only an estimate. Head lice infestations are often not reported because people find them socially embarrassing—even though the Centers for Disease Control and Prevention (CDC) states that: "Personal hygiene or cleanliness in the home or school has nothing to do with getting head lice." The number of all three types of lice infestations in North America has increased in recent years.

Head lice are most common in schoolchildren between the ages of three and eleven, and their families. Girls are more likely to be infested than boys because they are more likely to share clothing and other personal items with friends. It can be difficult to prevent a child from picking up head lice at school because of the amount of close contact among children and their belongings.

Body lice infest both children and adults. There is no difference in frequency between men and women. Homeless people and others who live in crowded conditions without opportunities to bathe or shower regularly are at greatest risk of getting body lice. Because the body louse lives in clothing, infestations occur in colder climates. Pubic lice are most

Also Known As
Pediculosis, crabs

Cause
Wingless parasitic insects that live on the head or body, or in the pubic hair

Symptoms
Itching; small red bumps on scalp or neck; visible lice or nits (eggs)

Duration
Can last from initial infestation until effective treatment; may be recurrent

common in people between the ages of fourteen and forty who are sexually active.

There is some seasonal difference in lice infestations in temperate climates. Head lice infestations are more common during the warmer months while body and pubic lice infestations are more common in the fall and winter.

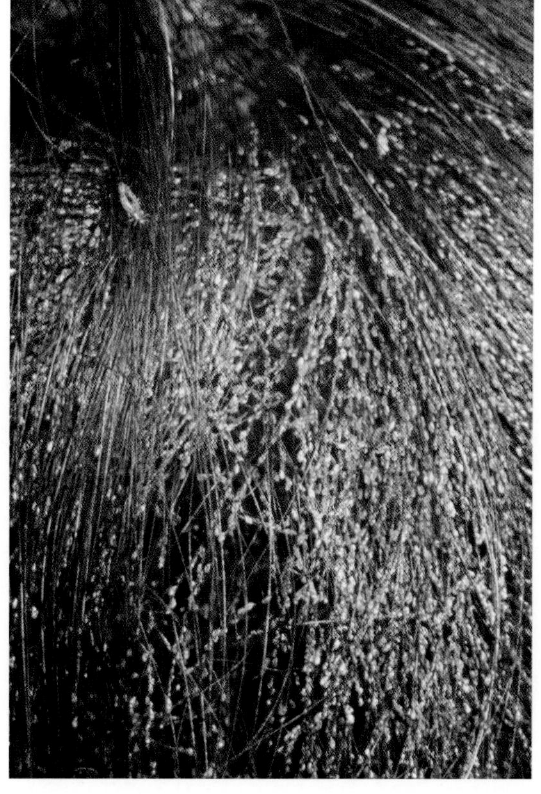

Human hair infested with lice and nits. ST. BARTHOLOMEW'S HOSPITAL/PHOTO RESEARCHERS, INC.

Causes and Symptoms

The cause of lice infestations is the presence of head, body, or pubic lice on a person's body or in his or her clothing. The life cycle of lice helps to explain some of the symptoms of an infestation. When the nit or egg hatches, about eight or ten days after being laid, it produces an immature louse called a nymph. The nymph needs blood to survive. It has sucking mouth parts on its head that can pierce the skin and draw blood to feed on. Human lice must feed about five times a day to survive, otherwise they become dehydrated and die. The nymph becomes a mature adult about ten days after hatching. Its complete life cycle is between thirty and thirty-five days in length.

The symptoms of a lice infestation depend on the area of the body that is affected:

- Head lice: itchy scalp due to an allergic reaction to the bites of the lice; small red bumps on the head or neck; sensation of something moving over the scalp; an irritated rash caused by scratching the itchy parts of the scalp.
- Body lice: itching and a rash caused by an allergic reaction to the bites of the lice. A long-term infestation may cause discoloration of the skin of the waist area and upper thighs. There may also be open sores caused by scratching the itching areas; these raw areas can become infected by other disease organisms.
- Pubic lice: itching in the genital area or other body areas with coarse hair (armpits, mustache area, eyebrows, eyelashes), and visible nits or lice crawling in the affected area.

A Poem to a Louse

Most people would not think of a head louse as a pleasant topic for a poem. But one of the best-known poems by Robert Burns (1759–1796), Scotland's national poet, is about seeing a louse crawling up and down a lady's bonnet during a church service. The poem, written in 1786, is a commentary on class snobbery.

In the poem, Burns appears to criticize the louse for its "impudence" in choosing "sae fine a lady" for its host. He tells the creature to "gae somewhere else and seek your dinner/On some poor body." But it is obvious by the end of the poem that he is poking some fun at the well-dressed lady, proud of her expensive bonnet, who is totally unaware that a parasite she would associate with poor people has attached itself to her own head. Burns wrote in Scots dialect rather than standard modern English.

Diagnosis

The diagnosis of lice infestation is usually made by examining the skin, hair, pubic area, or clothing of the affected person. The doctor can collect nits from the hair by using a fine-toothed comb or remove lice from the body with a piece of cellulose tape. The organisms can then be studied under the microscope to determine the type of lice involved.

Another test that can be performed involves the use of a Wood's lamp, which is a device that uses ultraviolet light to detect lice, fungal infections, and a few other types of skin infections. The patient is taken into a dark room while the doctor shines the lamp on the area that may be infested. If lice or nits are present, they will glow greenish-yellow.

Treatment

Treatment of head lice requires washing the infested person's clothing and bedding in hot water at 130°F (54.5°C) two days prior to treatment. Clothing that is not washable should be dry-cleaned. Combs and brushes should be soaked in rubbing alcohol for an hour or washed in soap and hot water. These steps are necessary to lower the risk of reinfestation. Toys or other personal items can also be cleared of lice by sealing them inside a plastic bag for at least two weeks; the lice will die from lack of air and food.

The treatment itself consists of applying an over-the-counter or prescription shampoo to the scalp that contains a drug that kills lice. The product directions should be followed exactly regarding how long the product should be left on the hair and whether it should be rinsed out afterward. Following the application, a fine-toothed or special nit comb should be used to comb nits out of the hair. This combing should be repeated every two to three days for three weeks to make sure all the lice and nits are gone. Retreatment with the medicated shampoo may be necessary.

Another treatment that has been found effective in treating head lice is a drug called Mectizan (ivermectin), which was originally

WORDS TO KNOW

Crabs: A slang term for pubic lice.

Host: An organism that is infected by a virus, bacterium, or parasite.

Infestation: A condition in which a parasite develops and multiplies on the body of its host rather than inside the body.

Nits: The eggs of lice.

Wood's lamp: A special lamp that uses ultraviolet light to detect certain types of skin infections and infestations. It was invented in 1903 by physicist Robert Wood.

developed to treat intestinal parasites. The person needs to take only one dose of the drug.

Body lice are treated by removing all the infested person's clothing and either destroying or washing them in hot water followed by at least twenty minutes in a dryer on the hot setting. The person must take a shower and change into clean clothing. A lice-killing shampoo may be applied to the hairy parts of the person's body.

Pubic lice are treated by applying a shampoo, mousse, or lotion containing a drug called pyrethrin. These products can be purchased over the counter at a pharmacy and should be used exactly as directed on the container. There is also a drug called Ovide that requires a doctor's prescription that can also be used to treat pubic lice. Pubic lice in the eyebrows must be treated by applying a prescription ointment, as Ovide and the over-the-counter products should not be used close to the eyes.

Prognosis

The prognosis for treatment of lice is extremely good provided care is taken afterward to prevent reinfestation. Head lice and pubic lice are not known to spread other diseases. Body lice, however, are dangerous because they can transmit three potentially fatal illnesses: typhus, relapsing fever, and trench fever.

Prevention

Practicing good personal hygiene, avoiding sharing personal items with others, and prompt treatment of lice infestations are the best ways of preventing the spread of lice.

The Future

Lice are not likely to disappear from the human scene any time soon. Scientists estimate that lice have been infesting humans for at least 3 million years. It is possible that researchers will discover more effective shampoos or soaps to get rid of lice, but for the time being, the best medicine is prevention.

For more information

BOOKS

Hirschmann, Kris. *Lice*. Farmington Hills, MI: Kidhaven Press, 2004.

Somervill, Barbara A. *Lice: Head Hunters*. New York: PowerKids Press, 2008.

PERIODICALS

Martin, Guy. "Secret Shame Dept.: The Lice Lady." *New Yorker*, January 28, 2002. Available online at http://www.newyorker.com/archive/2002/01/28/020128ta_talk_martin (accessed April 11, 2008). This is a brief article about a woman in New York City who specializes in removing head lice from infested children. It offers an interesting commentary on the social embarrassment related to lice.

Nagourney, Eric. "Remedies: Researchers Devise New Weapon for Head Lice." *New York Times*, November 7, 2006. Available online at http://www.nytimes.com/2006/11/07/health/07reme.html?_r=1&adxnnl=1&oref=slogin&adxnnlx=1207983942-MstifzAXSWAkVQov04eGlQ (accessed April 11, 2008).

Wade, Nicholas. "In Lice, Clues to Human Origin and Attire." *New York Times*, March 8, 2007. Available online at http://www.nytimes.com/2007/03/08/science/08louse.html (accessed April 12, 2008).

WEB SITES

Centers for Disease Control and Prevention (CDC). *Parasitic Disease Information: Lice Infestation*. Available online at http://www.cdc.gov/ncidod/dpd/parasites/lice/default.htm (accessed April 8, 2008).

Nemours Foundation. *KidsHealth: Hey! A Louse Bit Me!*. Available online at http://www.kidshealth.org/kid/ill_injure/bugs/louse.html (last updated September 2007; accessed April 12, 2008).

Lung Cancer

Definition

Lung cancer is the uncontrolled growth of malignant cells in one or both lungs. There are two major types of lung cancer, small cell lung cancer (SCLC) and non-small cell lung cancer (NSCLC). NSCLC is the more common of the two types, accounting for about 87 percent of cases. It develops in the cells of the tissues that line the lungs. SCLC, which is sometimes called oat cell cancer, accounts for the other 13 percent. It develops out of the hormone-producing cells in the lungs and grows more quickly than the NSCLC type of lung cancer. Small cell lung cancer is also more likely to spread to other parts of the body.

Both types of lung cancer may be either primary or secondary. A primary lung cancer is one that starts in the lung and metastasizes (spreads) to other parts of the body—most commonly to the adrenal glands, bones, liver, and brain. A secondary lung cancer is one that began in another organ and spread to the lungs. For example, breast cancer is a type of cancer that frequently spreads to the lungs.

Description

Lung cancer was a rare disease before smoking tobacco products became widespread; it was not even recognized as a distinct illness until 1761. It is now known to begin when tobacco smoke or some other irritant damages the cells of the lung tissue. The body can repair this damage for some time; eventually, however, the injured cells begin to multiply abnormally, forming a tumor in the lung tissue. The tumor may grow large enough to put pressure on the airway, causing the coughing and difficult breathing that are characteristic of advanced-stage lung cancer.

Another development that can occur is that the cancerous cells in the lung tissue can enter the blood and lymph vessels that supply the lungs. The circulation of the blood and lymphatic fluid can then carry the cancerous cells to other parts of the body. It is possible for the primary lung cancer to metastasize to other organs before coughing or other symptoms appear in the patient's lungs.

Many lung cancers are richly supplied with blood vessels close to the surface of the tumor. If the surface of the tumor is fragile, it may break off and cause bleeding into the airway. The blood may then be coughed up by the patient. Another complication that can develop is pneumonia. If the lung cancer is large enough to partially block the airway, mucus and tissue fluid may build up in the lung tissue behind the blockage, thus making it easier for bacteria to multiply and cause infectious pneumonia.

Demographics

Lung cancer is the leading cause of cancer deaths worldwide; about 1.3 million people die each year from the disease, 162,000 of them in the

Also Known As
Bronchogenic carcinoma

Cause
Smoking, exposure to asbestos or radon, or unknown causes

Symptoms
Shortness of breath, coughing up blood, chest pain, hoarse voice, wheezing

Duration
Years

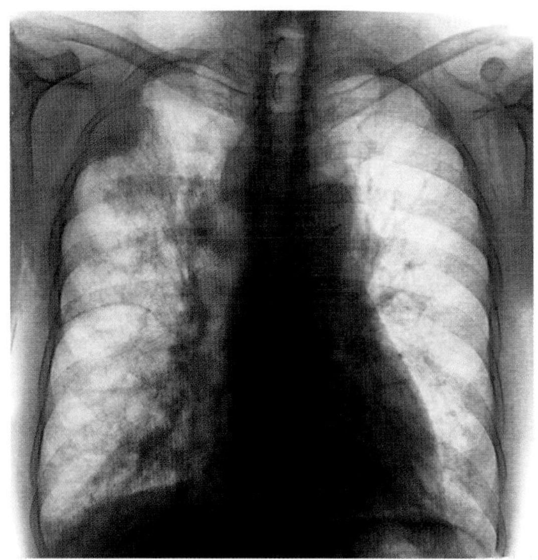

Chest x ray of a patient with lung cancer.

United States. Fewer than half of newly diagnosed lung cancer patients live beyond a year after diagnosis; and only 14 percent survive for five years. Lung cancer represents 15 percent of all cancer diagnoses in North America and 29 percent of all cancer deaths.

Lung cancer is a highly preventable disease. Although some risk factors for lung cancer cannot be changed, avoiding tobacco would reduce deaths by about 80 percent. Men who smoke are twenty-three times more likely to develop lung cancer than men who have never smoked; women who smoke have a risk thirteen times greater than that of nonsmokers. In addition to active smoking, the risk factors for lung cancer include:

- Exposure to secondhand tobacco smoke. Nonsmokers who share housing or office space with heavy smokers have an increased risk of lung cancer.
- Exposure to radon. Radon is an invisible, odorless gas produced by the breakdown of uranium in soil and rock. Between 9 and 14 percent of deaths from lung cancer are caused by exposure to radon.
- Occupational exposure to asbestos, uranium, and coke (a fuel used in iron manufacturing).
- Air pollution.
- Age. Lung cancer is almost entirely a disease of older adults. The average age at diagnosis in the United States is seventy years.
- Sex. Men are more likely than women to develop lung cancer; however, the rates for women have risen sharply in recent years because of the increase in smoking among women starting in the 1960s. Nonsmoking women are more likely to develop lung cancer, however, than nonsmoking men.
- Race. African Americans of either sex are more likely to develop and die from lung cancer than any other ethnic group in the United States. On the other hand, Native Americans have one of the lowest rates. The reasons for these differences are not yet known.

- Family history. People with a parent or sibling diagnosed with lung cancer are at increased risk of developing the disease themselves even if they do not smoke.
- Personal history of bronchitis or repeated episodes of pneumonia. Some researchers think that a history of lung disease is a risk factor for eventual lung cancer.

Causes and Symptoms

The largest single cause of lung cancer is exposure to tobacco smoke, followed by such other irritants as radon, asbestos, and air pollution. The causes of lung cancer in nonsmokers are not yet fully understood. Some researchers think that damage to chromosomes 3, 5, 13, and 17 increases a nonsmoker's risk of small cell lung cancer. Another theory concerns human papillomavirus, which has been shown to cause lung cancer in animals. These scientists think that human papillomavirus (HPV, a sexually transmitted virus) infection may trigger lung cancer in some people by causing uncontrolled cell division in lung tissue.

Lung cancer often does not have symptoms in its early stages. A primary lung cancer may produce the following symptoms:

- Fatigue
- Coughing that does not go away
- Coughing up blood
- Chest pain
- Shortness of breath
- Loss of appetite and unintended weight loss
- Coughing up large quantities of mucus

A lung cancer that has spread to other organs may produce bone pain, abdominal or back pain, headache, weakness, seizures, or speech difficulties.

Diagnosis

Lung cancers are sometimes diagnosed relatively early when a person develops pneumonia and the doctor discovers a cancerous tumor. In most cases, however, the tumor is diagnosed when the person develops the symptoms of advanced-stage lung cancer.

There is no universally accepted screening test for lung cancer. Some doctors think that a newer type of computed tomography (CT) scan called a spiral CT scan is a useful way to screen for lung cancer. In a spiral CT scan, the patient lies on a table while the scanner rotates around them. Other doctors, however, think that this test does not yet distinguish clearly enough between lung cancer and other less serious lung problems to justify using it as a screener.

The tests that are most commonly used to detect lung cancer and determine whether it is SCLC or NSCLC include:

- Imaging studies, usually a CT scan of the lungs or an x-ray image of the chest.
- Sputum sample. The patient is asked to cough up some sputum (mucus or phlegm), which can be studied under a microscope for the presence of cancer cells.
- Tissue biopsy. Samples of suspicious tissue may be obtained in one of several ways. The doctor may use an instrument called a bronchoscope (a lighted tube passed down the throat and into the lungs), or make an incision at the base of the neck and remove a tissue sample from the space behind the breastbone. A third technique involves inserting a needle through the chest wall directly into the suspected tumor to remove a sample of tissue.
- Thoracentesis. This is procedure in which the surgeon inserts a needle through the chest wall in order to withdraw some tissue fluid from the space between the lung and the chest wall. As with a sputum sample, the fluid can be checked for cancer cells.

After determining whether the cancer is small cell or non-small cell in type, the next step is staging. Staging is a description of the location of the cancer, its size, how far it has penetrated into healthy tissue, and whether it has spread to other parts of the body. SCLC and NSCLC tumors are staged differently because these two types of lung cancer are treated differently.

- SCLCs are staged in two stages, limited and extensive. A limited-stage SCLC is found only in one lung and its nearby tissues. An extensive tumor is found outside the lung in which it started or in distant organs.
- NSCLCs are staged in an occult (hidden) stage, in which the cancer is detectable only in cells from a sputum sample without

a visible tumor; and five stages graded from 0 to IV in which there is a visible tumor. The grade of the tumor is based on its size and on whether it has spread to the lymph nodes or nearby tissues. In stage 0, for example, the cancer is found only in the innermost lining of the lung. In stage IV, the cancer has spread from one lung to the other lung, or has spread to the brain, bones, liver, or other organs.

Treatment

Treatment of lung cancer depends on which type it is and its stage.

SCLCs: Limited-stage small cell lung cancers, which account for about 30 percent of those diagnosed, can usually be treated with radiation therapy. Extensive SCLCs cannot be completely treated with radiation therapy alone and usually require a combination of radiation therapy and chemotherapy.

NSCLCs: Patients diagnosed with non-small cell lung cancers may have surgery, chemotherapy, radiation therapy, or a combination of treatments. The treatment choices are different for each stage. Surgery, for example, may involve removing only a wedge-shaped portion of a lung, an entire lobe of a lung, or the complete lung.

Prognosis

The prognosis for lung cancer is poor. It has one of the lowest five-year survival rates of all cancers—about 14 percent as of 2008. For SCLCs, the overall five-year survival rate is 5 percent, with patients diagnosed with extensive disease having a five-year survival rate of less than 1 percent. The average length of survival time for patients with limited-stage disease is 20 months.

For patients with NSCLCs, those with stage I disease treated with surgery have a five-year survival rate of 67 percent; the five-year survival rate of patients with stage IV disease is less than 1 percent.

Prevention

There are some preventive measures that people can take to lower their risk of lung cancer:

- Don't smoke or quit smoking.
- Avoid secondhand smoke.

WORDS TO KNOW

Occult: The medical term for a cancer that is too small to produce a visible tumor.

Radon: A colorless and odorless gas produced by the breakdown of uranium known to cause lung cancer.

Targeted therapy: A newer type of cancer treatment that uses drugs to target the ways cancer cells divide and reproduce or the ways tumors form their blood supply.

- Have the home tested for radon. The American Lung Association or the local public health authorities can provide information on radon testing.

The Future

Lung cancer is likely to be a serious health problem throughout the world as people who started smoking heavily in the 1960s are now getting to the age when lung cancer is usually diagnosed. In the United States, as of 2008 the National Institutes of Health (NIH) is conducting or sponsoring over 2,300 studies related to lung cancer.

SEE ALSO Bronchitis; HPV infection; Pneumonia; Smoking

For more information

BOOKS

American Cancer Society (ACS). *Quick Facts Lung Cancer: What You Need to Know—Now / from the Experts at the American Cancer Society*. Atlanta, GA: American Cancer Society, 2007.

Gilligan, David, and Robert Rintoul. *Your Guide to Lung Cancer*. London, UK: Hodder Arnold, 2007.

Sheen, Barbara. *Lung Cancer*. Detroit, MI: Lucent Books, 2008.

PERIODICALS

Fink, Sheri. "New Therapies Aim at Lung Tumors, Case by Case." *New York Times*, October 25, 2006. Available online at http://health.nytimes.com/ref/health/healthguide/esn-lungcancer-ess.html (accessed on September 28, 2008).

Grady, Denise, and Brent McDonald. "CT Screening for Lung Cancer." *New York Times*, October 31, 2006. Available online at http://video.on.nytimes.com/index.jsp?fr_story=cde8a179a490d9a9fe977c6df92fb8fe3b88a538 (accessed on September 28, 2008).

WEB SITES

American Lung Association (ALA). *Lung Cancer.* Available online at http://www.lungusa.org/site/apps/nlnet/content3.aspx?c=dvLUK9O0E&b=2060245&content_id={6F0688E6-33A8-4323-8367-ECACED27CDDC}¬oc=1 (updated October 2007; accessed on September 28, 2008).

American Society of Clinical Oncology Cancer Net. *Lung Cancer.* Available online at http://www.cancer.net/patient/Cancer+Types/Lung+Cancer (updated December 2007; accessed on September 28, 2008).

Mayo Clinic. *Lung Cancer.* Available online at http://www.mayoclinic.com/health/lung-cancer/DS00038 (updated November 10, 2007; accessed on September 28, 2008).

National Cancer Institute (NCI). *What You Need to Know about Lung Cancer.* Available online at http://www.cancer.gov/cancertopics/wyntk/lung/allpages (updated July 26, 2007; accessed on September 28, 2008).

National Library of Medicine (NLM). *Lung Cancer.* Available online at http://www.nlm.nih.gov/medlineplus/tutorials/lungcancer/htm/index.htm (accessed on September 28, 2008).

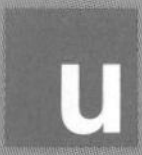

Lupus

Definition

Lupus, an autoimmune disease, is caused by vascular inflammation (vasculitis) that results in significant damage to a number of different body systems and organs, including the joints, skin, kidneys, heart, lungs, and brain. For this reason it is sometimes called a multisystem disease. Its symptoms vary from patient to patient, ranging from mild conditions that can be managed by medications to life-threatening emergencies.

There are four major types of lupus:

- Systemic lupus erythematosus or SLE. This is the form of the disease most commonly meant by lupus. SLE can occur in childhood but is most common in people between the ages of fifteen and forty-five.
- Discoid lupus. Discoid lupus is a skin disorder in which the patient develops thick raised patches of scaly reddened skin on the face or scalp. A small percentage of patients with discoid lupus later develop SLE.
- Drug-induced lupus. This is a form of lupus triggered by medications. It goes away when the patient stops taking the drugs. Drug-induced lupus is more common in men than in women.

Also Known As
Systemic lupus erythematosus, SLE

Cause
Unknown

Symptoms
"Butterfly" rash on face, unexplained fever, swollen joints, muscle pain, kidney disease

Duration
Years

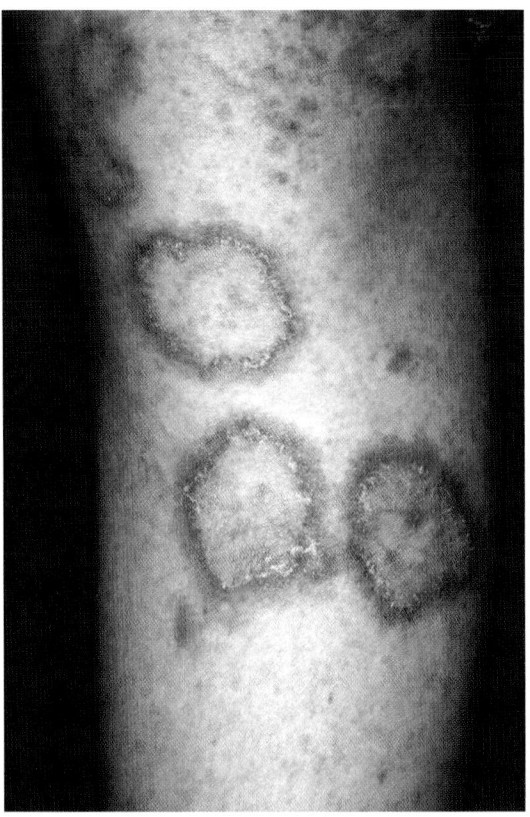

Skin rash on a patient with lupus. © SCOTT CAMAZINE / ALAMY

- Neonatal lupus. This is a rare form of lupus that sometimes occurs in babies born to mothers with SLE, Sjögren syndrome, or no disease at all.

Description

The causes of lupus, a complex disease, are not understood. It is difficult to diagnose because its symptoms are easy to confuse with those of many other disorders and because there is no symptom profile that applies to all patients with lupus. What is known is that lupus is a chronic inflammatory disease in which the body's immune system turns against its own tissues, producing what are called autoantibodies. Autoantibodies are protein molecules that target the person's own cells, tissues, or organs, causing inflammation and tissue damage. In lupus, the autoantibodies damage the blood vessels in such vital organs as the kidneys.

The inflammation of body tissues in lupus leads to a variety of symptoms that may come and go over time as well as vary from patient to patient. These include aches and pains in joints and muscles, skin rashes, sensitivity to sunlight, unexplained fever, swollen glands, extreme fatigue, hair loss, mouth ulcers, chest pains, easily bruised tissues, and emotional disorders. Periods when the symptoms are absent or low-key are called remissions, and periods when the symptoms return or increase in severity are called flares.

Demographics

Lupus is primarily a disease of women of childbearing age. It is rarely diagnosed in children except for the neonatal form. In the United States, lupus affects about one person in every 2,000. According to the Lupus Foundation of America, between 1.5 and 2 million people in the United States may have a form of lupus. The actual number may be higher because the diagnosis is often missed by doctors. Around the world, the rate of lupus varies from country to country, from twelve cases per

100,000 people in Great Britain to thirty-nine per 100,000 in Sweden. In New Zealand, there are fifty cases per 100,000 population among Polynesians, compared with only 14.6 cases per 100,000 among white New Zealanders.

In the United States, lupus is three times more common among African Americans than among Caucasians. It is also more common among Hispanics, Asian Americans, and Native Americans. Like many other autoimmune diseases, lupus strikes women nine times more frequently than men. Among males with lupus, older men are more likely to get the disease than younger men. The fact that women of childbearing age are the group most likely to develop lupus is the reason why some researchers think that female sex hormones may be involved in the disease.

Men and Lupus

Like osteoporosis, breast cancer, and rheumatoid arthritis, lupus is a disease that is largely considered a problem for women. But the 10 percent of lupus patients who are male have some difficulties that female patients do not, precisely because of the gender ratio. According to the Lupus Foundation of America, men with lupus are often worried about being seen as less masculine because of the diagnosis, even though they can still be sexually active and have children. In addition to its feminine image, lupus can cause emotional distress for men by limiting their ability to earn a living or to do chores around the house requiring physical labor. Loss of independence, coupled with such physical changes as hair loss and weight gain, can be a heavy blow to a man's self-esteem.

Researchers are also looking into whether lupus in older men is more severe than in women in the same age groups. Some studies have suggested that men with SLE have a higher risk than women of severe damage to the blood vessels, nerves, and kidneys. Currently male patients with lupus are given the same therapies as women.

Causes and Symptoms

Researchers believe that lupus is the end result of a combination of genetic, hormonal, and environmental factors. At least ten different genes have been identified that increase a person's risk of developing lupus, and the disease is known to run in families. There is no single lupus gene, however. Other factors that are being studied as possible triggers of lupus include sunlight, stress, certain drugs, and viruses.

The symptoms of lupus may appear in almost any body system:

- Skin: Butterfly-shaped facial rash (also called a malar rash); rash elsewhere on body; ulcers in the mouth, nose, or vagina; loss of hair on head; sensitivity to sun exposure. About 90 percent of patients with lupus have symptoms affecting the skin and hair.
- Bones and muscles: Arthritis, muscle cramps, pains in the hands and wrists.
- Blood: Anemia, low white blood cell count, problems with normal blood clotting, Raynaud's phenomenon (loss of blood flow to fingers and toes due to stress or cold exposure).

- Heart and lungs: Inflammation of the lining of the heart (pericariditis) and lungs (pleuritis). About 50 percent of patients with lupus develop some form of lung disease.
- Nervous system: Seizures, psychotic episodes, memory loss, depression, anxiety. These affect about 15 percent of patients with lupus.
- Kidneys and liver: Kidney disease and eventual kidney failure. About 50 percent of patients with lupus have kidney problems.
- Other: Unexplained fever, weight loss or gain, fatigue.

Diagnosis

There is no single test that can provide a definitive diagnosis of lupus. The disease is not easy to diagnose because it usually develops slowly over a period of years, its symptoms often come and go, and none of them are unique to lupus. The American College of Rheumatology compiled a list of eleven criteria in 1982 to help distinguish lupus from other diseases. Seven of these are symptoms:

- Butterfly (malar) rash on face
- The raised red patches of discoid lupus
- Skin rash triggered or worsened by sun exposure
- Ulcers in the nose or mouth
- Arthritis
- Inflammation of the tissues lining the inside of the lungs or heart
- Seizures or convulsions in the absence of other causes for these events

The other four criteria are test results:

- Abnormally high levels of protein and red or white blood cell fragments in the urine
- Abnormally low red or white blood cell counts
- Presence of antinuclear antibodies (ANA) and anti-double strand DNA in the blood
- Other positive blood tests that indicate an autoimmune disorder

A person should meet four or more of these criteria for the doctor to suspect lupus. The symptoms do not all have to occur at the same time.

Treatment

There is no cure for lupus. The symptoms of the disease are managed by medications tailored to the location and the severity of the individual patient's symptoms. The patient's doctor may prescribe drugs from any of the following groups:

- Nonsteroidal anti-inflammatory drugs (NSAIDs). These drugs include aspirin and such non-aspirin pain relievers as Aleve and Motrin. They can be used to treat joint pain, bring down fever, and other inflammatory symptoms of mild lupus.
- Antimalarial drugs. There is no known connection between lupus and malaria; however, some drugs used to treat malaria appear to prevent lupus flares as well as treat symptoms.
- Corticosteroids. This group of drugs includes prednisone, one of the drugs prescribed most frequently to treat lupus. Corticosteroids act to bring down inflammation rapidly. Unfortunately, they also have serious side effects, including weight gain resulting from increased appetite, weakened bones, high blood pressure, damage to the arteries, and an increased risk of infections and diabetes. Doctors try to minimize these side effects by prescribing the lowest dose necessary to control symptoms for the shortest possible time.
- Immunosuppressants. These are drugs that work by reducing the overactivity of the immune system that is involved in lupus. Immunosuppressants are generally given only to patients with severe flares that are damaging organ function, or in order to reduce a patient's dose of corticosteroids.

Prognosis

The prognosis for lupus is variable depending on the severity of the symptoms. In general, patients whose kidneys or central nervous systems are affected by the disease have a worse prognosis. Men with lupus have a slightly worse prognosis than women.

The overall life expectancy for patients with lupus has improved since the 1950s, when less than 50 percent of patients were still alive five years after diagnosis. For patients diagnosed with SLE in the United States, Canada, and Europe, 95 percent are alive at five years after diagnosis, 90 percent at ten years, and 78 percent at twenty years. The overall death rate for patients diagnosed with lupus is three times that of the general American population.

WORDS TO KNOW

Flare: A period of worsened symptoms in lupus.

Malar rash: The medical term for the butterfly-shaped facial rash found in lupus.

Neonatal: The medical term for newborn.

Raynaud's phenomenon: Discoloration of the fingers and toes caused by blood vessels going into spasm and decreasing the flow of blood to the affected digits.

Remission: A period of decreased or absent lupus symptoms.

Prevention

There is no way to prevent lupus because the causes of the disease have not been clearly identified.

The Future

Researchers are focusing on new treatments for lupus as well as genetic studies of ethnic groups and families at increased risk of the disease. The Lupus Foundation of America has links to registries for individuals and families with lupus and lupus-related conditions at http://www.lupus.org/webmodules/webarticlesnet/templates/new_aboutfaq.aspx?articleid=384&zoneid=19. The National Institute of Arthritis and Musculoskeletal and Skin Diseases (NIAMS) is presently conducting studies of lupus in African Americans and Native Americans to look for possible genetic factors associated with the high rates of lupus in these groups.

SEE ALSO Chronic fatigue syndrome; Fibromyalgia; Sjögren syndrome

For more information

BOOKS

Abramovitz, Melissa. *Lupus*. Detroit, MI: Lucent Books, 2008.

Isenberg, David, and Susan Manzi. *Lupus*. New York: Oxford University Press, 2008.

Wallace, Daniel J. *The Lupus Book: A Guide for Patients and Their Families*, 4th ed. New York: Oxford University Press, 2009.

PERIODICALS

"Cancer Drug Velcade Might Work in Lupus: Study." *Reuters*, June 8, 2008. Available online at http://www.reuters.com/article/healthNews/idUSL0491213620080608?feedType=RSS&feedName=healthNews (accessed June 24, 2008).

Pierce, Andrea. "Uncovering the Mysteries of Immunity, and of Lupus." *New York Times*, May 12, 2008. Available online at http://health.nytimes.com/ref/health/healthguide/esn-lupus-ess.html (accessed June 23, 2008).

WEB SITES

Lupus Foundation of America. *Introduction to Lupus*. Available online at http://www.lupus.org/webmodules/webarticlesnet/templates/new_aboutintroduction.aspx?amp;articleid=71&zoneid=9s (accessed June 24, 2008).

Mayo Clinic. *Lupus*. Available online at http://www.mayoclinic.com/health/lupus/DS00115 (updated June 5, 2008; accessed June 23, 2008).

National Institute of Arthritis and Musculoskeletal and Skin Diseases (NIAMS). *Handout on Health: Systemic Lupus Erythematosus*. Available online at http://www.niams.nih.gov/Health_Info/Lupus/default.asp (updated August 2003; accessed June 23, 2008).

National Library of Medicine (NLM). *Lupus*. Available online at http://www.nlm.nih.gov/medlineplus/tutorials/lupus/htm/index.htm (accessed June 24, 2008). This is an online tutorial with voiceover. Viewers have the option of a self-playing version, a text version, or an interactive version with questions.

TeensHealth. *Lupus*. Available online at http://kidshealth.org/teen/diseases_conditions/bones/lupus.html (updated June 2008; accessed June 24, 2008).

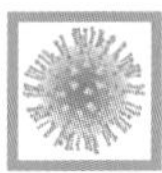

Lyme Disease

Definition

Lyme disease is an infectious disease caused by a spirochete (spiral-shaped bacterium) transmitted to humans by the bite of an infected deer tick. The alternate name of Lyme disease—borreliosis—comes from the scientific name of the bacterium, *Borrelia burgdorferi*. Lyme disease can be classified as an infectious arthritis because the body's immune response to the bacterium produces inflammation and arthritis-like joint or muscle pain in some people.

Lyme disease is considered a zoonosis, or disease transmitted by animals to humans, as well as an emerging infectious disease. Household pets (cats and dogs) that are allowed outdoors can be infected with Lyme disease as well as humans. Typical symptoms of Lyme disease in animals include joint soreness, limping or lameness, fever, and loss of appetite.

Also Known As
Borreliosis

Cause
Spirochete (spiral-shaped bacterium)

Symptoms
Fever, headache, fatigue, rash, joint pains, meningitis

Duration
Weeks to years

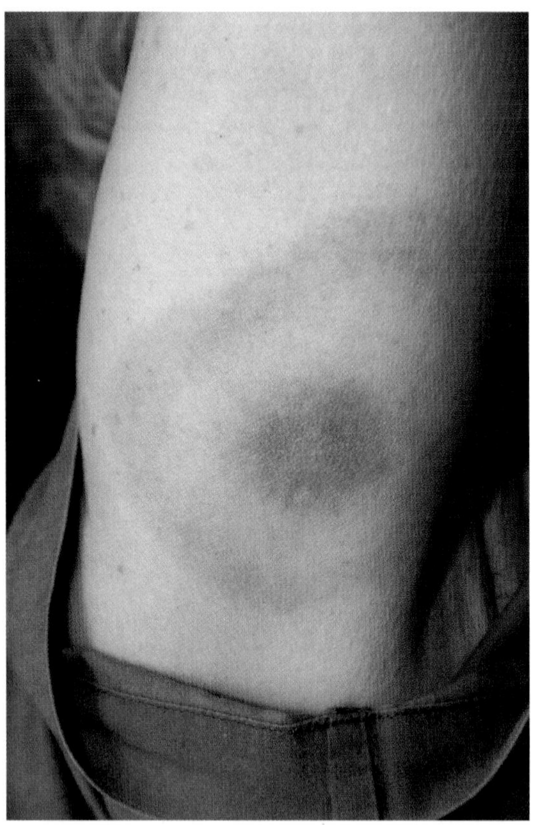

A patient's arm with the bull's eye rash typical of Lyme disease. AP IMAGES.

Description

An infectious disease, Lyme disease is caused by a spiral-shaped bacterium that lives inside deer ticks. The tick transmits the disease from one animal to another or from animals to humans when it feeds on their blood. The symptoms of the disease vary from person to person. Not everyone who gets Lyme disease has all the symptoms or has them with equal severity.

The first stage of Lyme disease is often (though not always) marked by a red rash known as erythema chronicum migrans, or EM, at the site of the tick bite. The rash may have a circular or bull's-eye appearance. It occurs in about 80 percent of patients within three to thirty days after the bite. The rash expands over the next few days to cover as much as 12 inches (30 centimeters) of skin. Patients may also have flulike symptoms, including fatigue, chills, low-grade fever, headache, muscle and joint aches, and swollen lymph nodes. In some cases, these flu-like symptoms may be the only indication of Lyme infection.

If the infection is not treated, patients may develop a second stage of symptoms that can include heart palpitations, fatigue, headaches, temporary paralysis of facial muscles, meningitis, or dizziness.

Some patients experience a third stage of the disease, marked by arthritis-like pain in the joints and muscles, numbness in the arms and legs, loss of memory, and other neurological symptoms.

Demographics

The Centers for Disease Control and Prevention (CDC) reported 23,305 cases of Lyme disease in the United States in 2005. Most occurred in the coastal Northeast, the Mid-Atlantic States, Wisconsin and Minnesota, and northern California. Most cases of Lyme disease occur in the spring and summer months when ticks are most active and people are spending more time outside. In both the United States and Europe, the age groups most likely to be affected are children between the ages of five and nine years, and adults between fifty and fifty-nine. Among children, boys are

The Long History of Lyme Disease

Lyme disease is named for Old Lyme, the town in Connecticut where an outbreak of the disease among children in the early 1970s was described by a physician at nearby Yale University. The infectious form of arthritis, however, had been described as far back as the early 1900s in Europe. In 1909, Swedish doctor Arvid Afzelius described a patient with a rash now known as erythema chronicum migrans—or simply erythema migrans (EM)—an early symptom of the disease. By 1934 other European doctors had noted that patients with the strange circular rash eventually developed arthritis-like joint pain and in some cases, psychiatric or neurological symptoms. They had also traced the rash to tick bites.

After World War II, European doctors found that newly developed antibiotics were quite effective in treating the tick-borne disease. The first known case of EM in the United States was reported in 1970 by a doctor in Wisconsin who was treating a patient bitten by a tick while hunting. The first cluster of cases of Lyme disease in the United States occurred in 1976 at a U.S. naval base in Connecticut. The following year saw cases involving the school children of Old Lyme. At that time, the disease was called Lyme arthritis. In 1982 Willy Burgdorfer, a researcher with the Rocky Mountain Laboratories of the National Institutes of Health, identified the cause of Lyme disease while gathering black-legged ticks in Montana. The organism was named *Borrelia burgdorferi* in his honor. Researchers have shown two other Borrelia species cause the European form of Lyme disease.

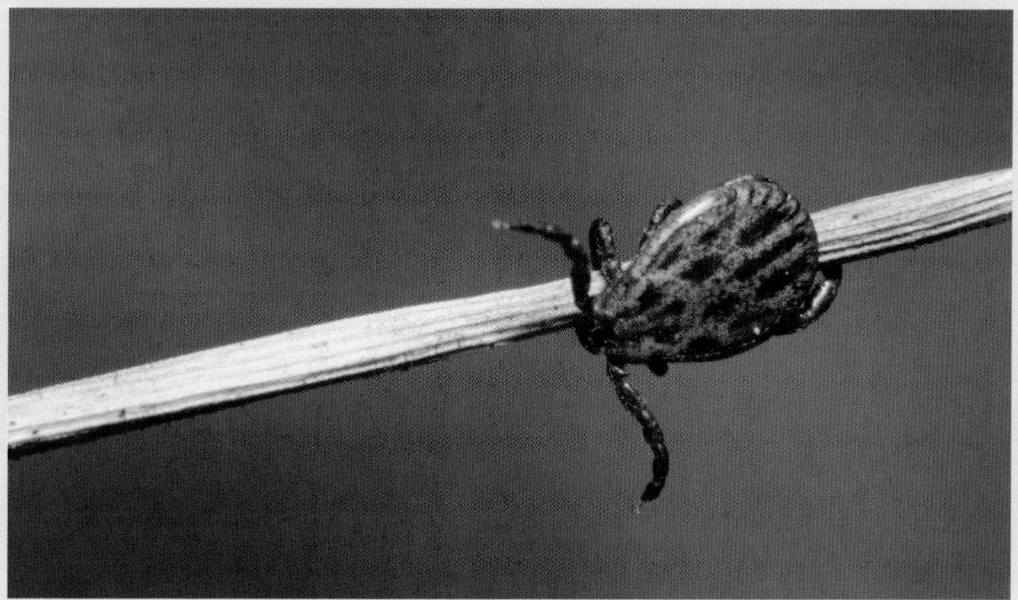

Tick capable of carrying the bacteria that causes Lyme disease. SHUTTERSTOCK.

more likely to be infected than girls, but in the older age group, women are slightly more likely than men to get Lyme disease. In 1998, Caucasians accounted for 76 percent of reported cases of Lyme disease in the United States, but it is not known whether this statistic indicates greater susceptibility to the disease or simply regional differences in reporting.

Causes and Symptoms

The cause of Lyme disease is a spirochete carried from one animal or human host to another by several varieties of ticks found in the United States. These ticks have a two-year life cycle. They are born in the summer as larvae and feed only once, on the blood of field mice. The next spring, the larva becomes a nymph and feeds again on a mouse's blood. In the fall, the nymph becomes an adult tick and feeds on the blood of a white-tailed deer. If the tick has picked up the spirochete from the mice or the deer, it can transmit the disease to a human at this point.

It takes one to three days for the tick to transmit *B. burgdorferi* to a human because it takes time for the bacterium to multiply inside the tick after it has bitten a person. Once feeding begins, the bacteria inside the tick multiply rapidly and move into the salivary glands of the tick after one to two days or so. The tick then injects the bacteria into the human as it continues its feeding. This time delay is one reason why prompt removal of a tick is usually effective in preventing Lyme disease and most other tick-borne infections.

Diagnosis

The diagnosis of Lyme disease is complicated by several factors. The first is that only 20 percent of patients are aware that they have been bitten by a tick. If they do not develop the characteristic EM rash, the diagnosis may be delayed. Second, the ticks that carry Lyme disease also often carry other diseases like ehrlichiosis or babesiosis, so that a person may have another tick-borne infection alongside or instead of Lyme disease. Third, most of the symptoms of Lyme disease can be caused by a variety of other disorders, including rheumatoid arthritis, complications of gonorrhea, lupus, or gout.

The CDC recommends as of 2007 that doctors look for three factors when evaluating a patient who might have Lyme disease:

- A history of possible exposure to ticks in parts of the United States known to have a higher than average rate of Lyme disease

- Physical symptoms that include EM
- A blood test that shows the patient has antibodies to *B. burgdorferi*

Even so, blood tests are not 100 percent accurate, particularly if they are given before the patient's body has had time to develop antibodies to the spirochete. In most parts of the United States, an initial blood test for antibodies is followed up by a second test known as a Western blot test to confirm the diagnosis.

Diagnosis

Early-stage Lyme disease can be effectively treated with a fourteen- to twenty-one-day course of antibiotics taken by mouth. These drugs usually clear the infection and reduce the risk of later complications. Second- or third-stage Lyme disease is treated with either a thirty-day course of an oral antibiotic or fourteen to twenty-eight days of an intravenous antibiotic.

Prognosis

The prognosis of Lyme disease is difficult to estimate because of the fact that EM is sometimes misdiagnosed. Further, many patients do not return for follow-up visits, which complicates the doctor's ability to measure the effectiveness of treatment or record the length of time that the patient had symptoms. In general, children who are treated early with antibiotics have an excellent prognosis for complete recovery. Adults are more likely to develop chronic muscle and joint pain or fatigue, but generally recover given time and appropriate treatment. Although there have been a few fatal cases of Lyme disease in humans as of 2008, the overall mortality rate is extremely low.

Prevention

A vaccine effective against Lyme disease was released in 1998 but was taken off the market because of the possible side effects reported by some patients and because it was not widely used. Although research into a better vaccine is ongoing, there was no vaccine available against the disease as of mid-2008. Preventive measures against Lyme disease are important because of the lack of an effective vaccine. The CDC recommends the following precautions:

- Stay away from wooded, brushy, and grassy areas, especially in May, June, and July. These are the months when ticks are most likely to feed on humans and pets.

- Wear light-colored clothing (which allows the ticks to be seen more easily); shoes that cover the entire foot; long pants tucked into socks or shoes; and long-sleeved shirts tucked into pants. Also wear a hat for additional protection.
- Use insect repellent containing a chemical called DEET on clothes and exposed skin other than the face. Another repellent that can be used on clothing is permethrin, which kills ticks on contact.
- When hiking in the woods, walk in the center of the trail or path; avoid brush and tall grasses.
- Remove clothing after being outside; wash it in hot water and dry it in a dryer on a high setting.
- Check the body for ticks after being outside, particularly the hair, the groin area, and the armpits.
- Check pets allowed outdoors for ticks in their fur, and give them tick-repellent collars. There is a vaccine to protect dogs against Lyme disease; there is, however, no vaccine for cats as of 2008. Cats appear to be much less likely to get the disease than dogs, which can develop fatal kidney problems from Lyme disease.
- Remove a tick properly if one is found on the body. Grasp the tick near its head or mouth, as it is critical to remove the head intact. Do not crush the tick but pull it backward from the skin slowly and carefully. Take the tick to a doctor or local public health department so that it can be tested to see if it is a Lyme disease-related tick.

The Future

Lyme disease is likely to become more common in North America in the years ahead because of the rising number of deer, mice, and other small rodents that can be infected by *B. burgdorferi*, and the increased amount of contact between humans and these animals in wooded areas. This increased contact is partly due to the growing popularity of woodland hiking and fishing and partly to the building of new houses in tick-infested areas. The CDC reports that Lyme disease was one of the fastest-growing infectious diseases in the United States as of 2008 and that it has spread from the regions where it was first noticed to forty-nine of the fifty states. Researchers are working on developing a new vaccine against Lyme disease. In addition, other scientists are trying to learn more

WORDS TO KNOW

Babesiosis: A malaria-like disease that can be transmitted by ticks.

Ehrlichiosis: A tick-borne disease found primarily in dogs that can also be transmitted to humans.

Emerging infectious disease (EID): A disease that has become more widespread around the world in the last twenty years and is expected to become more common in the future.

Endemic: A term applied to a disease that maintains itself in a particular area without reinforcement from outside sources of infection.

Erythema chronicum migrans (EM): The medical name for the distinctive rash that is often seen in early-stage Lyme disease.

Larva: The immature form of a deer tick.

Meningitis: Inflammation of the membranes covering the brain and spinal cord.

Nymph: The second stage in the life cycle of the deer tick.

Spirochete: A spiral-shaped bacterium. Lyme disease is caused by a spirochete.

Tick: A small bloodsucking parasitic insect that carries Lyme disease and several other diseases.

Zoonosis: A disease that animals can transmit to humans.

about the bacterium that causes the disease in order to develop better ways to diagnose and treat it.

SEE ALSO Lupus; Rheumatoid arthritis

For more information

BOOKS

Edlow, Jonathan A. *Bulls-Eye: Unraveling the Medical Mystery of Lyme Disease*, 2nd ed. New Haven, CT: Yale University Press, 2004.

Lang, Denise, and Kenneth B. Liegner. *Coping with Lyme Disease: A Practical Guide to Dealing with Diagnosis and Treatment*, 3rd ed. New York: Henry Holt, 2004.

PERIODICALS

Food and Drug Administration (FDA) Consumer Update. "Beware of Ticks … and Lyme Disease," June 27, 2007. Available online at http://www.fda.gov/consumer/updates/lymedisease062707.html (accessed May 24, 2008).

WEB SITES

American College of Physicians (ACP). "Lyme Disease: A Patient's Guide." Available online at http://www.acponline.org/clinical_information/resources/lyme_disease/patient/ (updated 2008; accessed May 23, 2008).

American Lyme Disease Foundation. "Lyme Disease." Available online at http://www.aldf.com/lyme.shtml (updated 2006; accessed May 23, 2008).

Centers for Disease Control and Prevention (CDC). "Learn about Lyme Disease." Available online at http://www.cdc.gov/ncidod/dvbid/lyme/index.htm (accessed May 23, 2008).

Centers for Disease Control and Prevention (CDC). "National Lyme Disease Risk Map." Available online at http://www.cdc.gov/ncidod/dvbid/lyme/riskmap.htm (updated 2004; accessed May 23, 2008).

Patient Education Institute, National Library of Medicine. "Lyme Disease." Available online at http://www.nlm.nih.gov/medlineplus/tutorials/lymedisease/htm/lesson.htm (accessed May 23, 2008). This is an interactive tutorial with voiceover about Lyme disease.

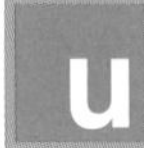

Lymphoma

Definition

Lymphoma refers to a varied group of cancers of the blood that develop from white blood cells in the lymphatic system. The lymphatic system is a group of organs and tissues that are part of the immune system and also help to form new blood cells. It includes lymph nodes, small organs composed of lymphoid tissue located at various points throughout the body that are joined by lymphatic vessels; the spleen, a small organ on the left side of the abdomen that produces lymphocytes and stores red blood cells; the bone marrow, which produces new red and white blood cells; and the thymus gland just below the neck, which produces one type of lymphocyte, the T cell.

Two major types of lymphoma were defined in the early 1980s—Hodgkin disease, sometimes called Hodgkin lymphoma or HL; and non-Hodgkin lymphoma or NHL. HL was named for Thomas Hodgkin (1798–1866), a British doctor who first described it in 1832, and was the first form of lymphoma to be officially defined, in 1963. Researchers focused on Hodgkin disease relatively early because it can be treated effectively by radiation therapy. Other forms of lymphoma were then grouped under the general heading of non-Hodgkin lymphoma or NHL in 1982. This entry will focus on non-Hodgkin lymphoma or NHL.

Also Known As
Lymphocytic lymphoma, non-Hodgkin lymphoma, NHL

Cause
Unknown

Symptoms
Swollen lymph nodes, night sweats, fever, weight loss, lack of energy

Duration
Lifelong unless treated

Description

Like Hodgkin disease, non-Hodgkin lymphoma begins in the lymphocytes, or white blood cells in the immune system. About 85 percent of

NHLs originate in B cells, which are lymphocytes produced in the bone marrow. Most of the remaining 15 percent develop from T cells produced in the thymus gland. What happens is that the abnormal B or T cells start to multiply uncontrollably, often within the lymph nodes, causing swelling and pain. The lymphoma can spread from the lymph nodes to the lymphatic vessels, tonsils, adenoids, spleen, thymus, and bone marrow. A non-Hodgkin lymphoma can also spread outside the lymphatic system to such other organs as the liver.

Non-Hodgkin lymphomas vary considerably in their speed of development and danger to survival. The 1982 classification categorized NHLs as low-grade, intermediate-grade, or high-grade depending on their aggressiveness and the organs affected by the cancer. Low-grade lymphomas are sometimes called indolent lymphomas because they grow slowly and cause relatively few symptoms. Intermediate-grade and high-grade lymphomas grow and spread more rapidly and cause severe symptoms.

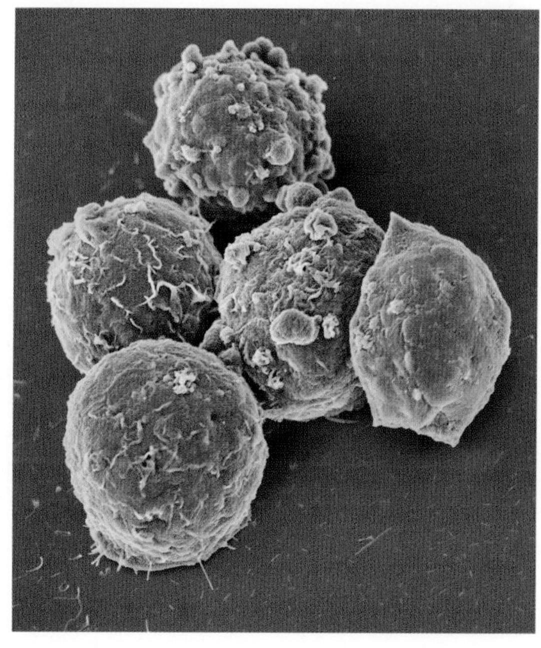

Image of lymphoma cells grown in a laboratory. STEVE GSCHMEISSNER / PHOTO RESEARCHERS, INC.

Demographics

Non-Hodgkin lymphoma accounts for about 4 percent of all cancer diagnoses in the United States. It is seventh in frequency among all cancers and is five times more common than Hodgkin disease. About 64,000 Americans are diagnosed with NHLs each year, and 18,700 die from this form of cancer. The five-year survival rate for non-Hodgkin lymphomas is 63 percent.

Non-Hodgkin lymphomas usually affect older adults; they are most likely to occur in people over sixty. Low-grade lymphomas account for 37 percent of NHLs in patients aged thirty-five to sixty-four but account for only 16 percent of cases in patients younger than thirty-five. Low-grade lymphomas are extremely rare in children.

Men are slightly more likely than women to develop non-Hodgkin lymphomas; the gender ratio is 1.4:1. Caucasians are more likely to develop NHLs than either African Americans or Asian Americans.

Risk factors (other than age) for non-Hodgkin lymphoma include:

- Exposure to certain chemicals, particularly benzene and certain weed-killing chemicals
- Exposure to radiation, including nuclear reactor accidents as well as radiation treatment for cancer
- Taking drugs that suppress the immune system, including chemotherapy for cancer as well as drugs given to prevent rejection of a transplanted organ
- Certain infections, including AIDS and infection with a bacterium associated with stomach ulcers
- Autoimmune diseases, including lupus and rheumatoid arthritis
- Extreme obesity

Causes and Symptoms

Non-Hodgkin lymphomas are caused by the uncontrolled multiplication of abnormal B or T cells. What triggers the formation of the abnormal cells is not completely understood but is thought to be related to the activation of abnormal genes called oncogenes. Oncogenes are genes that have the potential to trigger normal cells into becoming cancerous.

The most common symptoms of NHLs are:

- Swollen but painless lymph nodes in the neck, groin, or armpit areas
- Fever
- Unexplained or unintended weight loss
- Soaking night sweats
- Coughing or difficulty breathing
- Chest pain
- Fatigue that does not go away
- Itchy skin
- Pain, swelling, or a feeling of fullness in the abdomen

A few patients may have no symptoms at all in the early stages of the disease other than swollen lymph nodes.

Diagnosis

The diagnosis of NHLs can be complicated because none of the symptoms of lymphomas are unique to this type of cancer. The first step in diagnosing non-Hodgkin lymphoma is to rule out other diseases that can cause swollen lymph nodes. In addition to examining the patient's lymph nodes as part of a physical examination, the doctor will order blood and urine tests to see whether an infection might be the cause of the patient's symptoms. The doctor will also ask how long the symptoms have been present; while the flu can cause fever and fatigue, for example, those symptoms should go away after a week or two.

The next step in diagnosis is imaging studies, including a chest x ray and a computed tomography (CT) scan or magnetic resonance imaging (MRI) study of the chest, abdomen, or pelvic area. These tests can identify the location and size of tumors within the lymph nodes in those parts of the body. A newer type of imaging test that may be ordered to detect lymphoma is a positron emission tomography (PET) scan. In a PET scan, a radioactive substance called a tracer is injected into the patient's circulation. The radioactive material tends to concentrate in tissues that show an increased level of metabolic activity, which often means a tumor.

In addition to imaging studies, the doctor will collect a tissue sample called a biopsy to be examined under the microscope in a specialized laboratory. If the swollen lymph node is close to the surface of the skin, the doctor can remove the tissue sample through a hollow needle. If the lymph node lies deeper within the body, a surgeon may be called in to remove the tissue by making an incision.

To determine whether the lymphoma has spread, the doctor may also order a bone marrow biopsy. In this test, the patient is given a local anesthetic and a sample of bone marrow is removed from the hip bone through a hollow needle.

Treatment

The first step in treating any kind of cancer is called staging. Staging is a description of the location of the cancer, its size, how far it has penetrated into healthy tissue, and whether it has spread to other parts of the body. Non-Hodgkin's lymphoma is classified into four stages:

- Stage I: The disease is limited to one lymph node group or one tissue or organ (such as the spleen or liver).
- Stage II. The disease involves two or more lymph node groups on the same side of the diaphragm, or in one part of an organ and the lymph nodes near that organ.

- Stage III. The disease has spread to lymph node groups on both sides of the diaphragm and may involve a part of an organ or tissue near those groups.
- Stage IV. The disease has spread to several parts of one or more organs in addition to the lymph nodes.

The treatment of non-Hodgkin lymphoma depends on the subtype to which the tumor belongs and its stage of development.

- If the patient has an indolent NHL without symptoms, the doctor may recommend watchful waiting rather than beginning treatment right away, as all forms of cancer therapy have some side effects.
- Early-stage NHLs are treated with either radiation therapy or a combination of radiation and chemotherapy. Chemotherapy for lymphoma usually involves a combination of drugs rather than a single agent. It may be given either intravenously or by mouth.
- Early-stage lymphomas may also be treated with biological therapy, which involves vaccines and other drugs intended to boost the functioning of the patient's immune system. Biological therapy is also given to offset some of the side effects of radiation and chemotherapy.
- Aggressive lymphomas are treated with a combination of chemotherapy and biological therapy.
- Patients whose cancers return after therapy are given high doses of radiation, chemotherapy, or both, followed by stem cell transplantation. This procedure involves giving the patient stem cells after chemotherapy in order to help the patient's bone marrow recover and begin to produce healthy blood cells again.

Prognosis

The prognosis of non-Hodgkin lymphoma depends on the specific tumor type and location; the patient's age; severity of symptoms; the patient's ability to tolerate intensive chemotherapy; and whether the disease has spread beyond the lymph nodes. In general, patients older than sixty, patients with weakened immune systems, and patients with T-cell lymphomas have worse prognoses than younger patients, patients who are otherwise healthy, and patients with B-cell lymphomas.

About 70 percent of patients with intermediate- or high-grade lymphomas at the time of diagnosis either fail to respond to treatment or

WORDS TO KNOW

Biological therapy: An approach to cancer treatment that is intended to strengthen the patient's own immune system rather than attack the cancer cells directly.

Diaphragm: A sheet of muscle extending across the bottom of the rib cage that separates the chest from the abdomen.

Indolent: The medical term for a tumor or disease that grows or develops slowly.

Lymph nodes: Small rounded masses of lymphoid tissue found at various points along the lymphatic vessels.

Lymphocyte: A type of white blood cell that fights infection. Lymphocytes are divided into two types, T cells (produced in the thymus gland) and B cells (produced in the bone marrow).

Oncogene: A gene that has the potential to cause a normal cell to become cancerous.

Staging: Measuring the severity or spread of a cancer.

Stem cell: A type of body cell that has the ability to differentiate into various types of specialized cells.

Thymus: A small organ located behind the breastbone that is part of the lymphatic system and produces T cells.

have a recurrence of their cancer. About 5 percent of patients with recurrent cancer will survive for two years after the recurrence.

Prevention

There is no way to prevent non-Hodgkin lymphoma because its causes are still unknown, and some potential risk factors may not yet have been identified.

The Future

Researchers are looking for an explanation for the rise in the number of cases of NHLs in the United States since the 1970s. The figure nearly doubled between the 1970s and early 2000s. Although some of the increase can be explained by improved diagnostic techniques, there appear to be other factors involved that have not yet been identified.

Other scientists are studying various innovative treatments for non-Hodgkin lymphoma, including new anticancer drugs, new types of biological therapy, and improved methods of stem cell transplantation.

SEE ALSO Hodgkin disease; Leukemia

For more information

BOOKS

Adler, Elizabeth M. *Living with Lymphoma: A Patient's Guide*. Baltimore, MD: Johns Hopkins University Press, 2005.

Holman, Peter, Jodi Garrett, and William D. Jansen. *100 Questions and Answers about Lymphoma*. Sudbury, MA: Jones and Bartlett, Publishers, 2004.

PERIODICALS

Jaret, Peter. "Non-Hodgkin's Lymphoma on the Rise, Along with Hopes for a Cure." *New York Times,* May 2, 2008. Available online at http://health.nytimes.com/ref/health/healthguide/esn-lymphoma-ess.html (accessed on August 27, 2008).

WEB SITES

American Cancer Society (ACS). *Overview: Lymphoma, Non-Hodgkin Type*. Available online at http://www.cancer.org/docroot/CRI/CRI_2_1x.asp?dt=32 (updated October 25, 2007; accessed on August 27, 2008).

Lymphoma Research Foundation. *About Lymphoma*. Available online at http://www.lymphoma.org/site/pp.asp?c=chKOI6PEImE&b=2249267 (accessed on August 27, 2008).

National Cancer Institute (NCI). *What You Need to Know about Hodgkin Lymphoma*. Available online at http://www.cancer.gov/cancertopics/wyntk/hodgkin/allpages (updated February 5, 2008; accessed on August 27, 2008).

National Cancer Institute (NCI). *What You Need to Know about Non-Hodgkin Lymphoma*. Available online at http://www.cancer.gov/cancertopics/wyntk/non-hodgkin-lymphoma/allpages (updated February 12, 2008; accessed on August 27, 2008).

Where to Learn More

Books

Abramovitz, Melissa. *Lupus*. Detroit, MI: Lucent Books, 2008.

American Cancer Society (ACS). *Quick Facts Lung Cancer: What You Need to Know—Now / from the Experts at the American Cancer Society*. Atlanta, GA: American Cancer Society, 2007.

Bernard, Amy B. *West Nile Virus*. Brockton, MA: Western Schools, 2005.

Bloom, Ona, and Jennifer Morgan. *Encephalitis*. Philadelphia: Chelsea House Publishers, 2006.

Currie-McGhee, Leanne K. *AIDS*. Detroit, MI: Lucent Books, 2009.

Davidson, Tish. *Influenza*. San Diego, CA: Lucent Books, 2006.

Decker, Janet, and Alan Hecht. *Anthrax*, 2nd ed. New York: Chelsea House, 2008.

Germ Wars: Battling Killer Bacteria and Microbes. New York: Rosen Publishing Group, 2008.

Goldsmith, Connie. *Meningitis*. Minneapolis, MN: Twenty-First Century Books, 2008.

Jones, Phill. *Sickle Cell Disease*. New York: Chelsea House, 2008.

Kiesbye, Stefan, ed. *Teen Smoking*. Detroit, MI: Greenhaven Press, 2008.

Marcovitz, Hal. *Infectious Mononucleosis*. Detroit, MI: Lucent Books, 2008.

Marcus, Bernard A. *Malaria*. Philadelphia: Chelsea House Publishers, 2004.

Marr, Lisa. *Sexually Transmitted Diseases: A Physician Tells You What You Need to Know*, 2nd ed. Baltimore, MD: Johns Hopkins University Press, 2007.

Michaud, Christopher. *Gonorrhea*. New York: Rosen Publishing Group, 2007.

Nardo, Don. *Human Papillomavirus (HPV)*. Detroit, MI: Lucent Books, 2007.

Peirce, Jeremy. *Attention-Deficit/Hyperactivity Disorder*. New York: Chelsea House, 2008.

Raabe, Michelle. *Hemophilia*. New York: Chelsea House, 2008.

Saffer, Barbara. *Measles and Rubella*. Detroit: Lucent Books, 2006.

Sheen, Barbara. *Allergies*. Detroit: Lucent Books, 2008.

Sheen, Barbara. *Food Poisoning*. Detroit, MI: Lucent Books, 2005.

Sheen, Barbara. *Toxic Shock Syndrome*. San Diego, CA: Lucent Books, 2006.

Sherman, Irwin W. *Twelve Diseases That Changed Our World*. Washington, DC: ASM Press, 2007.

So, Po-Lin. *Skin Cancer*. New York: Chelsea House, 2008.

Stewart, Gail B. *Fetal Alcohol Syndrome*. Detroit, MI: Lucent Books, 2005.

Winheld, Josh. *Worth the Ride: My Journey with Duchenne Muscular Dystrophy*. Beach Haven, NJ: Little Treasure Books, 2008.

Wyborny, Sheila. *Alcoholism*. Detroit, MI: Lucent Books, 2008.

Web Sites

Alliance for a Healthier Generation. *Healthy Schools Program*. http://www.healthiergeneration.org/schools.aspx (accessed December 15, 2008).

Alzheimer's Association. *Just for Kids & Teens*. http://www.alz.org/living_with_alzheimers_just_for_kids_and_teens.asp (accessed December 15, 2008).

American Cancer Society. *Learn About Cancer*. http://www.cancer.org/docroot/LRN/lrn_0.asp (accessed December 15, 2008).

American Hearth Association. *For Kids*. http://www.americanheart.org/presenter.jhtml?identifier=3028650 (accessed December 15, 2008).

American Lung Association. *Sudden Infant Death Syndrome Fact Sheet (SIDS)*. http://www.lungusa.org/site/apps/nlnet/content3.aspx?c=dvLUK9O0E&b=2060727&content_id={DD8EAC73-1371-4129-9D82-0220D296D5E9}¬oc=1 (accessed December 15, 2008).

Asthma Society of Canada. *About Asthma*. http://www.asthma.ca/adults/about/ (accessed December 15, 2008).

Centers for Disease Control and Prevention. *BAM! Body and Mind*. http://www.bam.gov/ (accessed December 15, 2008).

Centers for Disease Control and Prevention. *Rabies*. http://www.cdc.gov/ncidod/dvrd/kidsrabies/ (accessed December 15, 2008).

KidsHealth, The Nemours Foundation. *About Sexually Transmitted Diseases (STDs)*. http://kidshealth.org/teen/sexual_health/stds/std.html (accessed December 15, 2008).

KidsHealth, The Nemours Foundation. *Diseases and Conditions*. http://kidshealth.org/teen/diseases_conditions/ (accessed December 15, 2008).

KidsHealth, The Nemours Foundation. *Everyday Illnesses and Injuries*. http://kidshealth.org/kid/ill_injure/index.html (accessed December 15, 2008).

KidsHealth, The Nemours Foundation. *Health Problems of Grown-Ups*. http://kidshealth.org/kid/grownup/index.html (accessed December 15, 2008).

KidsHealth, The Nemours Foundation. *Kids's Health Problems*. http://kidshealth.org/kid/health_problems/index.html (accessed December 15, 2008).

MedlinePlus. *Infectious Diseases*. http://www.nlm.nih.gov/medlineplus/infectiousdiseases.html (accessed December 15, 2008).

MedlinePlus. *Obesity in Children*. http://www.nlm.nih.gov/medlineplus/obesityinchildren.html (accessed December 15, 2008).

MedlinePlus. *Severe Acute Respiratory Syndrome (SARS)*. http://www.nlm.nih.gov/medlineplus/severeacuterespiratorysyndrome.html (accessed December 15, 2008).

National Center for Chronic Disease Prevention and Health Promotion *Diabetes Public Health Resource: The Eagle's Nest*. http://www.cdc.gov/diabetes/eagle/ (accessed December 15, 2008).

National Institute of Arthritis and Musculoskeletal and Skin Diseases. *Arthritis*. http://www.niams.nih.gov/Health_Info/Arthritis/arthritis_rheumatic_qa.asp (accessed December 15, 2008).

Office on Women's Health, U.S. Department of Health and Human Services. *girlshealth.gov*. http://www.girlshealth.gov/index.cfm (accessed December 15, 2008).

Providence Health and Services. *Childhood Diseases*. http://www.providence.org/healthlibrary/contentViewer.aspx?hwid=hn-3564009&serviceArea= generic (accessed December 15, 2008).

U.S. Food and Drug Administration. *Health Information for Teens*. http://www.fda.gov/oc/opacom/kids/html/7teens.htm (accessed December 15, 2008).

U.S. Food and Drug Administration. *Preventing Tick-borne Disease*. http://www.fda.gov/fdac/features/696_flea.html#prevent (accessed December 15, 2008).

List of Organizations

Academy for Eating Disorders
111 Deer Lake Rd., Ste. 100
Deerfield, IL 60015
Phone: (847) 498-4274
Fax: (847) 480-9282
E-mail: info@aedweb.org
Internet: http://www.aedweb.org/

American Academy of Child and Adolescent Psychiatry
3615 Wisconsin Ave. NW
Washington, DC 20016-3007
Phone: (202) 966-7300
Fax: (202) 966-2891
Internet: http://www.aacap.org/

American Academy of Pediatrics
141 Northwest Point Blvd.
Elk Grove Village, IL 60007-1098
Phone: (847) 434-4000
Fax: (847) 434-8000
E-mail: kidsdocs@aap.org
Internet: http://www.aap.org/

Alzheimer's Association
225 N. Michigan Ave.,
17th Floor
Chicago, IL 60601-7633
Phone: (312) 335-8700
Fax: (866) 699-1246
E-mail: info@alz.org
Internet: http://www.alz.org/

American Academy of Sleep Medicine
One Westbrook Corporate Center,
Ste. 920
Westchester, IL 60154
Phone: (708) 492-0930
Fax: (708) 492-0943
Internet: http://www.aasmnet.org/

American Cancer Society
1599 Clifton Rd. NE
Atlanta, GA 30329
Phone: (800) ACS-2345
Internet: http://www.cancer.org/

American Diabetes Association
1701 N. Beauregard St.
Alexandria, VA 22311
Phone: (800) 342-2383
E-mail: AskADA@diabetes.org
Internet: http://www.diabetes.org/

American Foundation for AIDS Research
120 Wall St., 13th Fl.
New York, NY 10005-3908
Phone: (212) 806-1600
Fax: (212) 806-1601
Internet: http://www.amfar.org/

American Heart Association
7272 Greenville Ave.
Dallas, TX 75231
Phone: (800) 242-8721
Internet: http://www.americanheart.org/

American Lung Association
61 Broadway, 6th Fl.
New York, NY 10006
Phone: (212) 315-8700
Phone: (800) 586-4872
Internet: http://www.lungusa.org/

American Medical Association
515 N. State St.
Chicago, IL 60610
Phone: (800) 621-8335
Internet: http://www.ama-assn.org/

American Obesity Association
8630 Fenton St., Ste. 814
Silver Spring, MD 20910
Phone: (301) 563-6526
Fax: (301) 563-6595
Internet: http://www.obesity.org/

American Parkinson Disease Association
135 Parkinson Ave.
Staten Island, NY 10305
Phone: (718) 981-8001
Phone: (800) 223-2732
Fax: (718) 981-4399
E-mail: apda@apdaparkinson.org
Internet: http://www.apdaparkinson.org/

Arthritis Foundation
PO Box 7669
Atlanta, GA 30357-0669
Phone: (800) 283-7800
Internet: http://www.arthritis.org/

Autism Society of America
7910 Woodmont Ave., Ste. 300
Bethesda, MD 20814-3067
Phone: (301) 657-0881
Phone: (800) 328-8476
Internet: http://www.autism-society.org/

Centers for Disease Control and Prevention (CDC)
1600 Clifton Rd.
Atlanta, GA 30333
Phone: (800) 232-4636
Internet: http://www.cdc.gov/

Cystic Fibrosis Foundation
6931 Arlington Rd.
Bethesda, MD 20814
Phone: (301) 951-4422
Phone: (800) 344-4823
Fax: (301) 951-6378
E-mail: info@cff.org
Internet: http://www.cff.org/

Epilepsy Foundation
8301 Professional Place
Landover, MD 20785
Phone: (800) 332-1000
Internet: http://www.epilepsyfoundation.org/

Huntington's Disease Society of America
505 Eighth Ave., Ste. 902
New York, NY 10018
Phone: (212) 242-1968
Fax: (212) 239-3430
E-mail: hdsainfo@hdsa.org
Internet: http://www.hdsa.org/

March of Dimes Birth Defects Foundation
1275 Mamaroneck Ave.
White Plains, NY 10605
Phone: (914) 997-4488
Internet: http://www.modimes.org/

Muscular Dystrophy Association–USA
National Headquarters
3300 E. Sunrise Dr.
Tucson, AZ 85718
Phone: (800) 572-1717

E-mail: mda@mdausa.org
Internet: http://www.mdausa.org/

National Center for Complementary and Alternative Medicine
9000 Rockville Pike
Bethesda, MD 20892
Phone: (301) 519-3153
Phone: (888) 644-6226
Fax: (866) 464-3616
E-mail: info@nccam.nih.gov
Internet: http://www.nccam.nih.gov/

National Diabetes Information Clearinghouse
1 Information Way
Bethesda, MD 20892-3560
Phone: (800) 860-8747
Fax: (703) 738-4929
E-mail: ndic@info.niddk.nih.gov
Internet: http://diabetes.niddk.nih.gov/

National Digestive Diseases Information Clearinghouse
2 Information Way
Bethesda, MD 20892-3570
Phone: (800) 891-5389
Fax: (703) 738-4929
E-mail: nddic@info.niddk.nih.gov
Internet: http://digestive.niddk.nih.gov/about/

National Down Syndrome Society
666 Broadway, 8th Fl.
New York, NY 10012
Phone: (800) 221-4602
E-mail: info@ndss.org
Internet: http://www.ndss.org/

National Eating Disorders Association
603 Stewart St., Ste. 803
Seattle, WA 98101
Phone: (206) 382-3587
Phone: (800) 931-2237
Fax: (206) 829-8501
E-mail: info@NationalEatingDisorders.org
Internet: http://www.nationaleatingdisorders.org/

National Fibromyalgia Association
2121 S. Towne Centre Place, Ste. 300
Anaheim, CA 92806
Phone: (714) 921-0150
Internet: http://www.fmaware.org/

National Heart, Lung, and Blood Institute Health Information Center
PO Box 30105
Bethesda, MD 20824-0105
Phone: (301) 592-8573
Fax: (240) 629-3246
E-mail: nhlbiinfo@nhlbi.nih.gov
Internet: http://www.nhlbi.nih.gov/

National Hemophilia Foundation
116 W. 32nd St., 11 Fl.
New York, NY 10001
Phone: (212) 328-3700
Phone: (800) 424-2634
Fax: (212) 328-3777
E-mail: handi@hemophilia.org
Internet: http://www.hemophilia.org/

National Institute of Allergy and Infectious Diseases
6610 Rockledge Dr., MSC 6612
Bethesda, MD 20892-6612
Phone: (301) 496-5717
Phone: (866) 284-4107
Fax: (301) 402-3573
Internet: http://www.niaid.nih.gov/

National Institute of Diabetes and Digestive and Kidney Diseases
Bldg. 31, Rm. 9A04, 31 Center Dr., MSC 2560
Bethesda, MD 20892-2560
Phone: (301) 496-3583
Internet: http://www.niddk.nih.gov/

National Multiple Sclerosis Society
733 Third Ave.
New York, NY 10017
Phone: (212) 986-3240
Phone: (800) 344-4867
Internet: http://www.nmss.org/

National Osteoporosis Foundation
1232 Twenty-second St. NW
Washington, DC 20037-1202
Phone: (202) 223-2226
Phone: (800) 231-4222
Internet: http://www.nof.org/

Sickle Cell Disease Association of America
231 E. Baltimore St., Ste. 800
Baltimore, MD 21202
Phone: (410) 528-1555
Phone: (800) 421-8453
Fax: (410) 528-1495
E-mail: scdaa@sicklecelldisease.org
Internet: http://www.sicklecelldisease.org/

World Health Organization
Avenue Appia 20
Geneva 27, 1211
Switzerland
Phone: (011-41-22) 791-2111
Fax: (011-41-22) 791-3111
E-mail: inf@who.int
Internet: http://www.who.int

Index

Note: **Bold** page numbers indicate main essays. *Italic* page numbers indicate figures.

A

B

C

D

E

F

G

H

M

N

O

P

R

S

T

U

V

W

X

Y

Z